CHILD HEALTH NURSING

Pain Chart

Ask client to rate pain using a line with numbers along it. Client must be a verbal child.

No Pain   Moderate Pain   Worst Pain

0   1   2   3   4   5   6   7   8   9   10

Acyanotic Heart Disease

Patent Ductus Arteriosus (PDA)   Ventricular Septal Defect (VSD)

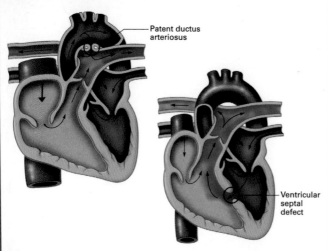

Patent ductus arteriosus

Ventricular septal defect

Left to Right Shunt: All blood that enters body circulation has been oxygenated in the lungs. There will be no cyanosis. However, some of these defects can become a right to left shunt (cyanotic heart disease) if other complications develop.

Clinical Manifestations: Acyanotic. Growth delay. Frequent respiratory infections. Murmur may be present if abnormal blood pathway exists. Exercise intolerance. CHF.

Nursing Care: Monitor G & D. Promote nutrition. Organize care to promote rest. Monitor for S & S of CHF. Promote good respiratory toilet. Protect from infection.

Cyanotic Heart Defects

Tetralogy of Fallot

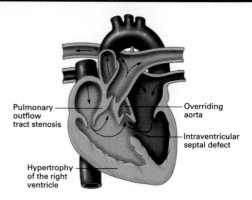

Pulmonary outflow tract stenosis

Overriding aorta

Intraventricular septal defect

Hypertrophy of the right ventricle

Right to Left Shunt: Some of the blood entering body circulation has bypassed the lungs and has not been oxygenated. Unoxygenated hemoglobin in peripheral circulation creates cyanosis. Tetralogy of Fallot is a defect consisting of four defects. The precise defects can be remembered by the acronym HIPO: **H**yperplasia of the right ventricle, **I**ntraventricular septal defect, **P**ulmonary stenosis, and **O**verriding aorta.

Clinical manifestations: Cyanosis. Elevated Hgb and Hct. Club fingers and toes. Heart murmur is usually present because of the abnormal blood pathway. Exercise intolerance and associated squatting behaviors. Growth failure and mental slowness may occur. Tet Spells (Hypercyanotic spell—worsening cyanosis, hyperpnea, limpness).

Nursing Care: Organize nursing care to allow for rest. Promote nutrition—reduce energy expenditure to achieve nutrition. Monitor for signs of CHF, respiratory infections. During Tet Spell: Place in knee chest position, provide supplemental oxygen. Morphine sulfate or propranolol may be ordered. Monitor for acidosis.

Breath Sounds

If the infant is crying, assess breath sounds, vocal resonance, and tactile fremitus when the infant takes a breath at the end of each cry. Provide a pinwheel or mobile to encourage deep breaths in toddlers.

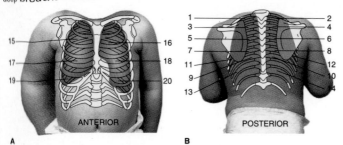

15   16
17   18
19   20

ANTERIOR

1   2
3   4
5   6
7   8
11   12
9   10
13   14

POSTERIOR

A   B

Heart Sounds

Auscultate heart sounds for quality (distinct vs muffled) and intensity (loud vs soft). Heart sounds are usually distinct and crisp in children because of their thin chest wall. Muffling or indistinct sounds may indicate heart failure.

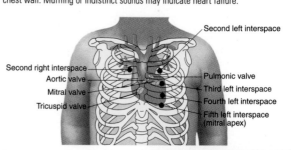

Second left interspace

Second right interspace
Aortic valve
Mitral valve
Tricuspid valve

Pulmonic valve
Third left interspace
Fourth left interspace
Fifth left interspace (mitral apex)

PEARSON

Pediatric Dosage Calculations

Calculating Medication Dosages

Calculate the dose, using the child's weight (written as mg/kg) or total body surface area (written as mg/m^2).

Recommended dose $\times$ Weight = Dose for client

$\dfrac{\text{Dose desired}}{\text{Dose on hand}} \times$ Quantity in mL = Volume to be administered

Pediatric Maintenance Fluid Requirements

Recommendation is to give fluids to the infant or child through an infusion pump; this device allows for a more accurate setting of flow rates than gravity does.

Weight (kg)	Fluid Requirements
0–10	100 mL/kg/24 hr
10–20	1000 mL + 50 mL/kg/24 hr for each kg between 11 and 20
20–70	1500 mL + 20 mL/kg/24 hr for each kg between 21 and 70
Over 70	2500 mL/24 hr (adult requirement)

Guidlines for Infusion of IV Fluids

Tubing Type	Drop Factor
Microdrip	60 drops (gtt)/mL
Macrodrip	10, 15, 20 drops (gtt)/mL, determined by brand of tubing

Calculating IV Rates

Formula

Total volume $\times$ Drop factor/Infusion time in minutes = Drops/minute

Vital Signs by Age

Age	Heart Rate Range & (Avg) in bpm*		Respiratory Rate Range in rpm**		Median Blood Pressure (mm Hg)***	
Newborn (NB)–1 mo	NB	100–170 (120)		30–80	NB	73/55
	1 mo	90–130 (110)			1 mo	86/52
6 months–1 year		80–130 (110)	6 mo	24–36	6 mo	90/53
			1 yr	20–40	1 yr	90/56
2 years		70–120 (100)		20–40		90/56
3–5 years		70–120 (100)		20–30		92/55
6–9 years		70–110 (90)		16–22	6 yrs	96/57
					9 yrs	100/61
10–15 years		60–100 (85)		16–20	10 yrs	100/61
					12 yrs	107/64
					15 yrs	114/65
18 years		60–100 (85)		12–20		121/70

*Beats per minute
**Respirations per minute; higher when awake; slower during sleep
***Blood pressure varies by gender as well as age

Growth and Development

	0–2 mo	2–4 mo	4–6 mo	6–9 mo	9–12 mo
Weight & Height	6–8 pounds (b) 20 inches (b)	Gains 5–7 oz weekly first 6 months	Doubles birthweight (6) Grows 1 in. monthly first 6 months		Triples birthweight (12) Height increases 50% (12)
Head & Fontanels	Head circumference > chest circumference(b) HC 33–35 cm (b)	Posterior fontanel closes (3)			Anterior fontanel closes (12–18)
Gross Motor		Gains head control (4)	Rolls from back to front (6)	Sits without support (8) Stands holding on (10)	Crawls (10) Walks with one hand held (12)
Fine Motor	Hand primarily closed (1)		Two-handed voluntary grasp (5)	Holds bottle (6) Transfers hand to hand (10)	Pincer grasp (12)
Sensory	Hearing & Touch (b) Turns & locates sounds (2)		Taste Preferences (6)		Follows moving objects (12); Visual acuity 20/50 or better (12)
Social	Smiles at human face (2); Solitary play	Erikson: Trust vs Mistrust (0–12)		Responds to own name (7)	Vocalizes four words (12)

	Toddler 1–3 yrs	Preschool 3–6 yrs	School-age 6–12 yrs	Adolescent 13–18 yrs
Weight & Height	Weight growth slows. Height at 2 yrs is 50% adult height	Gains 4–5 pounds/year Height increases 2–3 in./year	Gains 5 pounds/year Height increases 1–2 in./year	Weight: girls gain 15–55 pounds; boys 15–65 pounds Height: girls 3 in./yr until 16; boys 4 in./yr until later
Head & Teeth	90% adult brain size (2)	20 deciduous teeth	Loses first deciduous teeth (6) All permanent teeth except final molars (12)	Acne appears on face Final molars appear at end of period
Gross and Fine Motor	Walks without help (15m) Jumps in place (18m) Runs (2) Uses cup well (15m) Holds crayon with fingers (2–3); Copies circle (3)	Hops on one foot (4) Rides tricycle (3)	Good eye-hand coordination Acquires reading and writing skills	
Sensory	Binocular vision (15m)		Vision 20/20 (7)	
Social	Follows directions (2) Uses short sentences (2) 300 words (2); Parallel play Erikson: Autonomy vs Shame & Doubt	2100 words (5) Associative play Develops a conscience Erikson: Initiative vs Guilt	Cooperative play Enjoys team play Develops new interests Erikson: Industry vs Inferiority	Preoccupied with physical appearance Peer group very important Erikson: Identify vs role confusion

Normal Laboratory Values

Acid–Base Measurements (R)

pH: 7.38–7.42 from 14 minutes of age and older
PaO_2: 65–76 mm Hg (8.66–10.13 kPa)
$PaCO_2$: 36–38 mm Hg (4.8–5.07 kPa)
Base excess: 12–12 mEq/L, except in newborns (range 20–24)

Cholesterol, Total (S, P)

Values in mg/dL (mmol/L)

Age	Males	Females
6–7 years	115–197 (2.97–5.09)	126–199 (3.25–5.14)
8–9 years	112–119 (2.89–5.14)	124–208 (3.20–5.37)
10–11 years	108–220 (2.79–5.68)	115–208 (2.97–5.37)
12–13 years	117–202 (3.02–5.21)	114–207 (2.94–5.34)
14–15 years	103–207 (2.66–5.34)	102–208 (2.68–5.37)
16–17 years	107–198 (2.76–5.11)	106–213 (2.73–5.50)

Creatinine (S, P)

Values in mg/dL (µmol/L)

Age	Males	Females
Newborns (1–3 days)[a]	0.2–1.0 (17.7–88.4)	0.2–1.0 (17.7–88.4)
1 year	0.2–0.6 (17.7–53.0)	0.2–0.5 (17.7–44.2)
2–3 years	0.2–0.7 (17.7–61.9)	0.3–0.6 (26.5–53.0)
4–7 years	0.5–0.8 (17.7–70.7)	0.2–0.7 (17.7–61.9)
8–10 years	0.3–0.9 (26.5–79.6)	0.3–0.8 (26.5–70.7)
11–12 years	0.3–1.0 (26.5–88.4)	0.3–0.9 (26.5–79.6)
13–17 years	0.3–1.2 (26.5–106.1)	0.3–1.1 (26.5–97.2)
18–20 years	0.5–1.3 (44.2–115.0)	0.3–1.1 (26.5–97.2)

[a]Values may be higher in premature newborns.

Electrolytes

Normal: <40 mmol/L for both sodium and chloride
Clients with cystic fibrosis: >60 mmol/L for both sodium and chloride

Glucose (S, P)

Premature infants: 20–80 mg/dL (1.11–4.44 mmol/L)
Full-term infants: 30–100 mg/dL (1.67–5.56 mmol/L)
Children and adults (fasting): 60–105 mg/dL (3.33–5.88 mmol/L)

Hematocrit (B)

Values in %

Age	Males	Females
Newborns	43.4–56.1	37.4–55.9
6 months–2 years	30.9–37.0	36.2–37.2
2–6 years	31.7–37.7	32.0–37.1
6–12 years	32.7–39.3	33.0–39.6
12–18 years	34.8–43.9	34.0–40.7
>18 years	33.4–46.2	33.0–41.0

Lead (B)

<10mcg/dL (<0.48 µmol/L): Within normal range
10–19 mcg/dL (0.48–0.92 µmol/L): Prevention needed
>20 mcg/dL (>0.97 µmol/L): Evaluation, possible treatment, and environmental control
>70 mcg/dL (>3.38 µmol/L): Immediate treatment and environmental control

Partial Thromboplastin Time (P)

Children: 42–54 sec.

Prothrombin Time (P)

Children: 11–15 sec.

Potassium (S, P)

Premature infants: 4.5–7.2 mmol/L   Children: 3.5–5.8 mmol/L
Full-term infants: 3.7–5.2 mmol/L   Adults: 3.5–5.5 mmol/L

Sodium (S, P)

Newborns: 133–146 mmol/L   Children and adults: 135–148 mmol/L

Urea Nitrogen (S, P)

1–2 years: 5–15 mg/dL (1.8–5.4 mmol/L)   Thereafter: 10–20 mg/dL (3.5–7.1 mmol/L)

White Blood Cell Count (B)

Values $\times 10^3$ /mcL

Age	Males	Females
Newborns	6.8–13.3	8.0–14.3
6 months–2 years	6.2–14.5	6.4–15.0
2–6 years	5.3–11.5	5.3–11.5
6–12 years	4.5–10.5	4.7–10.3
12–18 years	4.5–10.0	4.8–10.1
>18 years	4.4–10.2	4.9–10.0

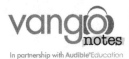
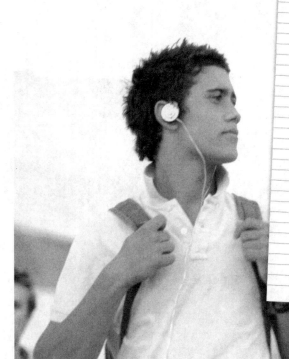

Pearson Nursing Reviews & Rationales

Child Health Nursing

Third Edition

SERIES EDITOR

MaryAnn Hogan, MSN, RN

Clinical Assistant Professor
School of Nursing
University of Massachusetts–Amherst
Amherst, Massachusetts

CONSULTING EDITORS

Judy White, RNC, MA, MSN

Nursing Faculty
Southern Union State Community College
Opelika, Alabama

Nancy H. Wagner, DNP, RN

Associate Professor
Youngstown State University
Youngstown, Ohio

Tiffany L. Johnson, MSN, RN

Professional Development Consultant
Clinical Learning
WellStar Health System
Atlanta, Georgia

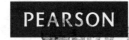

Boston   Columbus   Indianapolis   New York   San Francisco   Upper Saddle River
Amsterdam   Cape Town   Dubai   London   Madrid   Milan   Munich   Paris   Montréal   Toronto
Delhi   Mexico City   São Paulo   Sydney   Hong Kong   Seoul   Singapore   Taipei   Tokyo

Cataloging-in-Publication Data on File with the Library of Congress

Director of Readypoint™: Maura Connor
Executive Editor: Jennifer Farthing
Developmental Editor: Rachael Zipperlen
Editorial Assistant: Deirdre MacKnight
Director, Digital Product Development: Alex Marciante
Media Product Manager: Travis Moses-Westphal
Vice President, Director Sales & Marketing: David Gesell
Senior Marketing Manager: Phoenix Harvey
Marketing Coordinator: Michael Sirinides

Director of Media Production: Allyson Graesser
Media Project Manager: Rachel Collett
Managing Editor, Production: Patrick Walsh
Production Editor: GEX Publishing Services
Manufacturing Manager: Ilene Sanford
Art Director/Cover Designer: Mary Siener
Composition: GEX Publishing Services
Printer/Binder: Edwards Brothers
Cover Printer: Lehigh/Phoenix Color Hagerstown

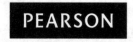

10 9 8 7 6 5 4 3 2 1

ISBN 10: 0-13-293620-8
ISBN 13: 978-0-13-293620-0

Contents

Welcome to the Pearson Nursing Reviews & Rationales Series!

This series has been specifically designed to provide a clear and concentrated review of important nursing knowledge in the following content areas:

- Anatomy & Physiology
- Nursing Fundamentals
- Nutrition & Diet Therapy
- Fluids, Electrolytes, & Acid–Base Balance
- Medical-Surgical Nursing
- Pathophysiology
- Pharmacology
- Maternal-Newborn Nursing
- Child Health Nursing
- Mental Health Nursing
- Health & Physical Assessment
- Community Health Nursing
- Leadership & Management

The books in this series are designed for use either by current nursing students as a study aid for nursing course work, for NCLEX-RN® exam preparation, or by practicing nurses seeking a comprehensive yet concise review of a nursing specialty or subject area.

This series is truly unique. One of its most special features is that it has been developed and reviewed by a large team of nurse educators from across the United States and Canada to ensure that each chapter is edited by a nurse expert in the content area under study. The series editor, MaryAnn Hogan, designed the overall series in collaboration with a core Pearson team to take full advantage of Pearson's cutting edge technology. The consulting editors for each book, also experts in that specialty area, then reviewed all chapters and test questions submitted for comprehensiveness and accuracy. Finally, MaryAnn Hogan reviewed the chapters in each book for consistency, accuracy, and applicability to the NCLEX-RN® Test Plan.

All books in the series are identical in their overall design for your convenience. As an added value, each book comes with a comprehensive support package, including access to additional questions online, complete eText, and a tear-out *NursingNotes* card for clinical reference and quick review.

Study Tips

Use of this book should help simplify your review. To make the most of your valuable study time, also follow these simple but important suggestions:

1. Use a weekly calendar to schedule study sessions.
   - Outline the timeframes for all of your activities (home, school, appointments, etc.) on a weekly calendar.
   - Find the "holes" in your calendar, which are the times when you can plan to study. Add study sessions to the calendar at times when you can expect to be mentally alert and follow your plan!
2. Create the optimal study environment.
   - Eliminate external sources of distraction, such as television, telephone, etc.
   - Eliminate internal sources of distraction, such as hunger, thirst, or dwelling on items or problems that cannot be worked on at the moment.
   - Take a break for 10 minutes or so after each hour of concentrated study both as a reward and an incentive to keep studying.
3. Use prereading strategies to increase comprehension of chapter material.
   - Skim read the headings in the chapter (because they identify chapter content).
   - Read the definitions of key terms, which will help you learn new words to comprehend chapter information.
   - Review all graphic aids (figures, tables, boxes) because they are often used to explain important points in the chapter.

4. Read the chapter thoroughly but at a reasonable speed.
   - Comprehension and retention are actually enhanced by not reading too slowly.
   - Do take the time to reread any section that is unclear to you.
5. Summarize what you have learned.
   - Use the accompanying online resource, NursingReviewsandRationales.com, to test yourself with hundreds of NCLEX-RN®-style practice questions.
   - Review again any sections that correspond to questions you answered incorrectly or incompletely.

Test-Taking Strategies

Test-taking strategies accompany the rationales for every question in the series. These strategies will assist you to select the correct answer by breaking down the question, even if you do not know the correct response. Use the following strategies to increase your success on nursing tests or examinations:

- Get sufficient sleep and have something to eat before taking a test. Avoid eating concentrated sweets, though, to prevent rapid upward and then downward surges in your blood glucose. Avoid also high-fat foods that will make you sleepy.
- Take deep breaths during the test as needed. Remember, the brain requires both oxygen and glucose as fuel.
- Read the question carefully, identifying the stem, all the options, and any critical words or phrases in either the stem or options.
  - Critical words in the stem such as "most important" indicate the need to set priorities, since more than one option is likely to contain a statement that is technically correct.
  - Remember that the presence of red flag words such as *never* or *only* in an answer option is more likely to make that option incorrect.
- Determine who is the client in the question; often this is the person with the health problem, but it may also be a significant other, relative, friend, or another nurse.
- Decide whether the stem is a true response stem or a false response stem. With a true response stem, the correct answer will be a true statement, and vice-versa.

- Determine what the question is really asking, sometimes referred to as the core issue of the question. Evaluate all answer options in relation to this issue, and not strictly to the "correctness" of the statement in each individual option.
- Eliminate options that are obviously incorrect, then go back and reread the stem. Evaluate those remaining options against the stem once more to make a final selection.
- If two answers seem similar and correct, try to decide whether one of them is more global or comprehensive. If one option includes the alternative option within it, it is likely that the more global option is the correct answer.

The NCLEX-RN® Licensing Examination

Upon graduation from a nursing program, successful completion of the NCLEX-RN® licensing examination is required to begin professional nursing practice. The NCLEX-RN® exam is a Computer Adaptive Test (CAT) that ranges in length from 75 to 265 individual (stand-alone) test items, depending on your performance during the examination. The blueprint for the exam is reviewed and revised every three years by the National Council of State Boards of Nursing using the results of a job analysis study of new graduate nurses practicing within the first six months after graduation. Each question on the exam is coded to a *Client Need Category* and an *Integrated Process*.

Client Need Categories   There are four categories of client needs, and each exam will contain a minimum and maximum percent of questions from each category. Each major category has subcategories within it. The *Client Need* categories according to the NCLEX-RN® Test Plan effective April 2010 are as follows:

- Safe Effective Care Environment
  - Management of Care (16–22%)
  - Safety and Infection Control (8–14%)
- Health Promotion and Maintenance (6–12%)
- Psychosocial Integrity (6–12%)
- Physiological Integrity
  - Basic Care and Comfort (6–12%)
  - Pharmacological and Parenteral Therapies (13–19%)
  - Reduction of Risk Potential (10–16%)
  - Physiological Adaptation (11–17%)

Integrated Processes The integrated processes identified on the NCLEX-RN® Test Plan effective April 2010, with condensed definitions, are as follows:

- Nursing Process: a scientific problem-solving approach used in nursing practice; consisting of assessment, analysis, planning, implementation, and evaluation.
- Caring: client–nurse interaction(s) characterized by mutual respect and trust and that are directed toward achieving desired client outcomes.
- Communication and Documentation: verbal and/or nonverbal interactions between nurse and others (client, family, health care team); a written or electronic recording of activities or events that occur during client care.
- Teaching and Learning: facilitating client's acquisition of knowledge, skills, and attitudes that lead to behavior change.

More detailed information about this examination may be obtained by visiting the National Council of State Boards of Nursing website at http://www.ncsbn.org and viewing the *2010 NCLEX-RN® Detailed Test Plan*.[1]

---

[1]Reference: National Council of State Boards of Nursing, Inc. *2010 NCLEX-RN® Test Plan*. Effective April, 2010. Retrieved from http://www.ncsbn.org/2010_NCLEX_RN_TestPlan.pdf.

HOW TO GET THE MOST OUT OF THIS BOOK

Each chapter has the following elements to guide you during review and study:

Chapter Objectives describe what you will be able to know or do after learning the material covered in the chapter.

Objectives

➤ Review basic principles of growth and development.
➤ Describe major physical expectations for each developmental age group.
➤ Identify developmental milestones for various age groups.
➤ Identify major stages of psychosocial and cognitive development for children at various age groups.
➤ Discuss the reactions to illness and hospitalization for children at various stages of development.
➤ Discuss the reaction to death and dying for children at various stages of development.

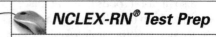

NCLEX-RN® Test Prep

Use the accompanying online resource, NursingReviewsandRationales, to test yourself with hundreds of NCLEX®-style practice questions.

Review at a Glance contains a glossary of critical terms used in the chapter, with definitions provided up-front and available at your fingertips, to help you stay focused and make the best use of your study time.

Review at a Glance

amblyopia visual condition in which brain suppresses vision in eye with weaker muscle; also known as "lazy eye"

cerumen waxy substance secreted in outer third of ear canal; also known as earwax

genogram a family map of three or more generations that records relationships, deaths, occupations, and health and illness history

lordosis anterior convex curvature of lumbar spine

objective data information obtained through physical assessment techniques and diagnostic studies

scoliosis lateral curvature of the spine

Pretest provides a 10-question quiz as a sample overview of the material covered in the chapter and helps you decide in what areas you need the most—or the least—review.

PRETEST

1 The physician orders amoxicillin (Amoxil) 500 mg IVPB q 8 hours for a pediatric client with tonsillitis. What is the appropriate nursing action?

1. Question the order because the route of administration is incorrect.
2. Give the medication as ordered.
3. Question the order because the dosage is too high.
4. Question the order because the dosing frequency is incorrect.

Practice to Pass questions are open ended, stimulate critical thinking, and reinforce mastery of the chapter information.

> ### Practice to Pass
>
> What are the risk factors contributing to the development of bronchopulmonary dysplasia (BPD)?

NCLEX Alert identifies concepts that are likely to be tested on the NCLEX-RN® examination. Be sure to learn the information highlighted wherever you see this icon.

!

Case Study, found at the end of the chapter, provides an opportunity for you to use your critical thinking and clinical reasoning skills to "put it all together." It describes a true-to-life client case situation and asks you open-ended questions about how you would provide care for that client and/or family.

Case Study

A 1-week-old client is scheduled for palliative surgery for transposition of the great vessels. You are the nurse who is supporting the parents through this illness.

1. What questions will you ask the parents prior to surgery?
2. What assessments do you make preoperatively?
3. What are the priority postoperative nursing interventions?
4. What discharge instructions will you give the parents?
5. The parents ask what emergency situations may arise and how they should respond. What do you say?

For suggested responses, see pages 352–353.

Posttest provides an additional 10-question quiz at the end of the chapter. It provides you with feedback about mastery of the chapter material following review and study. All pretest and posttest questions contain comprehensive rationales for the correct and incorrect answers, and are coded according to cognitive level of difficulty, and the NCLEX-RN® Test Plan categories of client need and integrated processes.

POSTTEST

❶ A 3-month-old infant has been admitted with a diagnosis of encephalitis. What is the priority assessment by the nurse?

1. Pupillary reaction
2. Level of consciousness
3. Ability to maintain airway
4. Response to verbal stimulation

NCLEX-RN® Test Prep: NursingReviewsandRationales.com

For those who want to prepare for the NCLEX-RN®, practicing online will help you become more familiar with the computer-based testing experience, especially for the new alternate item formats such as audio, media-enhanced, hot spot, and exhibit questions. With this new edition, use the code printed inside the front cover of the book to access Nursing Reviews & Rationales, which offers 700 practice questions using all NCLEX®-style formats. This includes the practice questions found in all chapters of the book as well as 30 additional questions per chapter. Nursing Reviews & Rationales allows you to choose two ways to prepare for the NCLEX-RN®. Both approaches personalize your practice experience according to what stage you are at in your NCLEX® preparation.

Nursing Reviews & Rationales includes the eText version of *Pearson Nursing Child Health Nursing Reviews and Rationales*, Third Edition. This eText is fully searchable and includes features like note-taking, highlighting, and more. The eText allows you to take your review with you anywhere you have an internet connection to NursingReviewsandRationales.com.

NursingNotes Card

This tear-out card provides a reference for frequently used facts and information related to the subject matter of the book. These are designed to be useful in the clinical setting, when quick and easy access to information is so important!

About the Child Health Nursing Book

Chapters in this book cover "need-to-know" information about child health nursing, including pediatric growth and development and care of the child with respiratory, cardiac, neurological, renal, gastrointestinal, musculoskeletal, and other health problems. The final chapter focuses on special situations, including autism, child abuse, poisoning, suicide, and others. The term *parent* or *parents* has been used in this book to indicate the primary caretaker(s) for the child. The author understands and appreciates that there are a variety of family configurations in which a child can grow and thrive.

Acknowledgments

This book is a monumental effort of collaboration. Without the contributions of many individuals, this edition of *Child Health Nursing: Reviews and Rationales* would not have been possible. Thank you to all the contributors and reviewers who devoted their time and talents to the third edition. The contributors are Judy White, RNC, MA, MSN, Southern Union State Community College, Opelika, Alabama; Nancy H. Wagner, DNP, RN, Youngstown State University, Youngstown, Ohio; and Tiffany L. Johnson, MSN, RN, Professional Development Consultant, Clinical Learning, WellStar Health System. The reviewers are Mikki Meadows-Oliver, PhD, RN, Yale School of Nursing, New Haven, Connecticut; and Marie H. Thomas, PhD, RN, Forsyth Technical Community College, Winston-Salem, North Carolina.

Thanks also to the contributors and reviewers who assisted with the previous editions of this book: Vera Brancato, EdD, MSN, RN, BC, Kutztown University, Kutztown, Pennsylvania, Kathleen Falkenstein, PhD, CPNP, Drexel University, Philadelphia, Pennsylvania; Judy white, RNC, MA, MSN, Southern Union State Community College, Opelika, Alabama; Jacqueline B. Arnett, RN, BSN, North Seattle Community College, Seattle, Washington; J. Mari Beth Barr, PhD, RNC, Missouri Southern State College, Joplin, Missouri;

Jennifer Jeames Coleman, MSN, RN, Samford University, Birmingham, Alabama; Donna Miles Curry, RN, PhD, Wright State University, Dayton, Ohio; Vera Dauffenbach, MSN, EdD, RN, Bellin College of Nursing, Green Bay, Wisconsin; Joseann Helmes DeWitt, MSN, RN, C, CLNC, Our Lady of the Lake College, Natchez, Mississippi; Leona M. Florek, Holyoke Community College, Holyoke, Massachusetts; Gwendolyn T. Martin, MS, RN, CNS, CPN, Texas Woman's University, Dallas, Texas; Gina M. Orta, MS, RN, Texas Woman's University, Dallas, Texas; Kathleen Peterson-Sweeney, MS, RN, CPNP, State University of New York, Brockport, New York; Kimberly A. Serroka, MSN, RN, Youngstown State University, Youngstown, Ohio; Nancy H. Wagner, MSN, RN, Youngstown State University, Youngstown, Ohio; Marilyn L. Weitzel, MSN, RN, Doctoral Candidate, University of South Alabama, Mobile, Alabama; and Judy E. White, RNC, MA, MSN, Southern Union Community College, Opelika, Alabama; Eva Caldwell, RN, EdD, Armstrong Atlantic State University, Savannah, Georgia; Dawn M. Pope, MS, RN, CS-PNP, University of Wisconsin-Oshkosh, Oshkosh, Wisconsin; Deborah A. Redd-Terrell, RN, MS, CS, CFNP, Harry S. Truman College, Flossmoor, Illinois; Gwendolyn P. Taylor, RN, MSN, Augusta Technical College, Thomson, Georgia; Rosemarie C. Westberg, RN, MSN, CPN, Northern Virginia Community College, Annandale, Virginia; Sharon A. Wilkerson, PhD, RN, Purdue University, West Lafayette, Indiana; and Beatrice Crofts Yorker, JD, RN, MS, CS, FAAN, San Francisco State University, San Francisco, California. Their work will surely assist both students and practicing nurses alike to extend their knowledge in the area of child health.

I owe a special debt of gratitude to the wonderful team at Pearson Nursing for their enthusiasm for this project, as well as their good humor, expertise, and encouragement as the series developed. Maura Connor, Director of Readypoint™, was unending in her creativity, support, encouragement, and belief in the need for this series. Jennifer Farthing, Executive Editor, Readypoint™, coordinated this revision with insight, talent, and zeal, and fostered a culture of true collaboration and team work. Rachael Zipperlen, Developmental Editor, devoted many long hours to coordinating different facets of this project. Her high standards and attention to detail contributed greatly to the final "look" of this book. Editorial Assistant, Deirdre MacKnight, helped to keep the project moving forward on a day-to-day basis, and I am grateful for her efforts as well. A very special thank you goes to the designers of the book and the production team, led by Patrick Walsh, Managing Editor, who brought the ideas and manuscript into final form.

Thank you to the team at GEX Publishing Services, led by Ashley Lewis and Kelly Morrison, Project Managers, for the detail-oriented work of creating this book. I greatly appreciate their hard work, attention to detail, and spirit of collaboration.

Finally, I would like to acknowledge and gratefully thank my children Michael Jr., Kathryn, Kristen, and William, who sacrificed precious hours of family time so this book could be revised. I would also like to thank my students, past and present, for continuing to inspire me with their quest for knowledge and passion for nursing. You are the future!

– *MaryAnn Hogan*

Growth and Development

1

Chapter Outline

Objectives

➤ Review basic principles of growth and development.
➤ Describe major physical expectations for each developmental age group.
➤ Identify developmental milestones for various age groups.
➤ Identify major stages of psychosocial and cognitive development for children at various age groups.
➤ Discuss the reactions to illness and hospitalization for children at various stages of development.
➤ Discuss the reaction to death and dying for children at various stages of development.

NCLEX-RN® Test Prep

Use the accompanying online resource, NursingReviewsandRationales, to test yourself with hundreds of NCLEX®-style practice questions.

Review at a Glance

anticipatory guidance process of understanding upcoming developmental needs and then teaching caregivers to meet those needs

cephalocaudal development process by which development proceeds from head downward through body and towards feet

chronological age age in years

critical periods times when an individual is especially responsive to certain environmental effects, sometimes called sensitive periods

development an increase in capability or function; a more complex concept that is a continuous, orderly series of conditions that lead to activities, new motives for activities; and eventual patterns of behavior

developmental age age based on functional behavior and ability to adapt to environment; does not necessarily correspond to chronological age

differentiation development from simple operations to more complex activities and functions

egocentrism an inability to put oneself in another's place; unable to see things from any other perspective other than one's own; cannot see another's point of view or any reason to do so

growth an increase in physical size

growth spurt brief periods of rapid increase in growth rate

object permanence knowledge that an object or person continues to exist when not seen, heard, or felt

proximodistal development process by which development proceeds from center of body outward to extremities

regression use of behavior that is more appropriate to an earlier stage of development, often used to cope with stress or anxiety

ritualism toddler's need to maintain sameness and reliability; provides a sense of comfort

separation anxiety distress behavior observed in young children separated from familiar caregivers

therapeutic play planned play techniques that provide an opportunity for children to deal with their fears and concerns related to illness or hospitalization

PRETEST

1 The nurse discusses dental care with the parents of a 3-year-old. The nurse explains that by the age of 3 years, their child should have _____ deciduous teeth.

Fill in your answer below:
_____ deciduous teeth

---

2 The mother of a 6-month-old infant is concerned that the infant's anterior fontanel is still open. The nurse would explain to the mother that further evaluation is needed if the anterior fontanel is still open after which age?

1. 10 months
2. 6 months
3. 18 months
4. 12 months

---

3 The nurse has discussed with a group of new mothers appropriate support of the young infant to prevent injuries from falls. The mother who needs further education is one who makes which statement?

1. "My baby is not allowed to have his walker near the stairs."
2. "I never leave my baby unattended on my bed."
3. "By the time my baby is 6 months old he will be able to sit without support."
4. "Before my child is standing, I need to place the crib mattress at its lowest level."

---

4 The 9-year-old child is at the 98th percentile for weight and at the 40th percentile for height. The school nurse determines that this child is which of the following?

1. Underweight or small in stature
2. Overweight or large in stature
3. Experiencing a prepubescent growth spurt
4. Normal for size

---

5 In discussing sexual maturation with a health class, the nurse would include the information that secondary sex characteristics begin to appear at what age in girls and boys?

1. 10 years in girls, 12 years in boys
2. 12 years in girls, 16 years in boys
3. 8 years in boys, 10 years in girls
4. 12 years in girls and boys

---

6 A recently hospitalized 2-year-old client screams and shouts that he wants a "bottle." His parents are puzzled, and state that he has been drinking from a cup for the past year. The nurse would include which information in an explanation to the parents?

1. Irritability is exhibited in all age groups.
2. Temper tantrums often represent the child's need for parental attention.
3. Various forms of punishment are necessary when such behaviors occur.
4. Regression to an earlier behavior often helps the child cope with stress and anxiety.

---

7 A friend is shopping for a toy to give to her nephew. The friend knows nothing about children and asks what would be the most appropriate toy to give an 18-month-old child. Based on growth and developmental skills, which item would the nurse recommend? Select all that apply.

1. A rocking horse
2. A music box
3. A pull toy
4. A stuffed animal
5. A cloth and cardboard book

8 The nurse is preparing an 8-year-old child for a procedure. What is the most appropriate nursing intervention considering the child's stage of growth and development?

1. Provide visual aids, such as dolls, puppets, and diagrams in the explanation.
2. Provide a written pamphlet for the child to review prior to the procedure.
3. Discourage any emotional outbursts.
4. Request that parents wait outside while the nurse provides instructions to the child.

9 The nurse explains to new parents that the American Academy of Pediatrics recommends iron-fortified formula be continued in a child's dietary intake up until what age?

1. 6 months
2. 12 months
3. 18 months
4. 24 months

10 Piaget identifies that the 2- to 7-year-old child is in a preoperational stage. The nurse observes a 2½-year-old girl taking a toy from another and recognizes the child is unable to put herself in the place of another because the toddler is displaying which of the following?

1. Centration
2. Negativism
3. Egocentrism
4. Selfishness

➤ *See pages 21–22 for Answers and Rationales.*

I. INTRODUCTION TO GROWTH AND DEVELOPMENT

A. Definition of terms

1. The terms "growth" and "development" are often used interchangeably but have specific meanings
   a. **Growth**: an increase in physical size of a whole or any of its parts
   b. **Development**: continuous, orderly series of conditions that lead to activities, new motives for activities, and eventual patterns of behavior
2. **Chronological age** is defined as age in years, which differs from **developmental age**, which refers to age based on functional behavior and ability to adapt to the environment
3. *Adjusted age* is used when describing developmental age of premature infants; the number of weeks premature is subtracted from the chronological age to determine infant's developmental age or level; use of adjusted age is usually stopped by age 2 years

B. Patterns of growth and development

1. Each child displays definite predictable patterns of growth and development
2. These patterns of growth and development are universal and basic to all human beings
3. Individual differences: although sequence is predictable, rates of growth vary, and individual variation exists in age at which developmental milestones are reached
4. Directional trends: growth and development follow a specific pattern
   a. **Cephalocaudal development** (head to tail): process by which development proceeds from head downward through body towards feet
   b. **Proximodistal development** (near to far): process by which development proceeds from center of body outward to extremities
   c. **Differentiation**: development from simple operations to more complex activities and functions

     5. Sequential trends: an orderly sequence; each child normally passes through every stage
       a. Each stage is affected by preceding stage and affects those stages that follow
       b. Critical periods: time period in which child is especially responsive to certain environmental effects; sometimes called sensitive periods
       c. Positive and negative stimuli enhance or defer achievement of a skill or function

C. Factors influencing development
     1. Genetics: a family history of diseases may be inherited by unique genes that are linked to specific disorders; chromosomes carry genes that determine physical characteristics, intellectual potential, and personality
     2. Nutrition: has greatest influence on physical growth and intellectual development; adequate nutrition provides essentials for physiologic needs, which promote health and prevent illness
     3. Prenatal and environmental factors: include nutrition from mother; exposures in utero to alcohol, smoking, infections, and drugs; environmental exposures, such as radiation and chemicals; all influence growth and development of developing child
     4. Family and community: a stimulating environment from family helps a child reach his or her potential; family structure and community support services influence environment in the process of growth and development of a child
     5. Cultural factors: customs, traditions, and attitudes of cultural groups influence child's growth and development regarding physical health, social interaction, and assumed roles

D. Developmental stages
     1. Prenatal period
       a. Germinal: conception to 2 weeks
       b. Embryonic: 2 weeks to 8 weeks
       c. Fetal: 8 weeks to 40 weeks (birth)
     2. Infancy period
       a. Neonatal: birth to 28 days
       b. Infancy: 1 to 12 months
     3. Early childhood period
       a. Toddler: 1 to 3 years
       b. Preschooler: 3 to 6 years
     4. Middle childhood period: the "school-age" period from 6 to 12 years
     5. Later childhood period: 13 to 18 years
       a. Prepubertal: 10 to 13 years
       b. Adolescence: 13 to 18 years

E. Importance of anticipatory guidance
     1. Anticipatory guidance is a process of understanding upcoming developmental needs and then teaching caregivers to meet those needs
     2. Information about what parents are to expect in each developmental stage includes the following:
       a. Health habits
       b. Prevention of illness and injury
       c. Prevention of poisonings
       d. Nutrition
       e. Dental care
       f. Sexuality
     3. Health promotion guidance also helps to develop strategies to enhance social development, family and community relationships, school and vocational achievement

II. BIOLOGIC GROWTH AND DEVELOPMENT

A. Neonatal period (birth to 1 month)
1. General appearance: newborn's head is one-quarter of body length; child is top heavy with short lower extremities
2. Weight: 6 to 8 lbs.; gains 5 to 7 oz (142 to 198 grams) weekly for first 6 months
3. Height: 20 in. (50 cm); grows 1 in. (2.5 cm) monthly for first 6 months
4. Head circumference: 33 to 35 cm (13 to 14 in.); head circumference is greater than chest circumference

B. Growth during infancy (1 to 12 months)
1. Weight: doubles birth weight in 5 to 6 months; triples birth weight in 1 year
2. Height: increases 50% by 1 year
3. Head growth is rapid; brain increases in weight 2.5 times by 1 year
   a. Head circumference exceeds chest circumference
   b. Posterior fontanel closes at 2 to 3 months
   c. Anterior fontanel closes by 12 to 18 months
4. Reflexes present at birth
   a. Moro: startle reflex elicited by loud noise or sudden change in position; disappears by age 6 months
   b. Tonic neck: elicited when infant lies supine and head is turned to one side; infant will assume a "fencing position"; disappears by age 6 months
   c. Gag, cough, blink, pupillary: protective reflexes
   d. Grasp: infant's hands and feet will grasp when hand or foot is stimulated; disappears by age 3 months
   e. Rooting: elicited when side of mouth is touched, causing infant to turn to that side; disappears by 4 months
   f. Babinski: fanning of toes when sole of foot is stroked upward; disappears between 1 and 2 years of age, usually after infant begins to walk
5. Reflexes that appear during infancy
   a. Parachute: involves extension of arms when suspended in prone position and lowered suddenly
   b. Landau: when infant is suspended horizontally, head is raised
   c. Labyrinth righting: provides orientation of head in space
   d. Body righting: when hips are turned to the side, the body follows
6. Gross motor development: developmental maturation in posture, head balance, sitting, creeping, standing, and walking
   a. Gains head control by 4 months
   b. Rolls from back to side by 4 months
   c. Rolls from abdomen to back by 5 months
   d. Rolls from back to abdomen by 6 months
   e. Sits alone without support by 8 months
   f. Stands holding furniture by 9 months
   g. Crawls with abdomen on floor (may go backward initially) by 10 months
   h. Creeps with abdomen off floor by 11 months
   i. Cruises (walking upright while holding furniture) by 10–12 months
   j. Can sit down from upright position by 10–12 months
   k. Walks well with one hand held by 12 months
7. Fine motor development: use of hands and fingers to grasp objects
   a. Hand predominantly closed at 1 month
   b. Desires to grasp at 3 months
   c. Two-handed, voluntary grasp at 5 months
   d. Holds bottle, grasps feet at 6 months

     e. Transfers from hand to hand by 7 months

     f. Pincer grasp established by 10 months

     g. Refined pincer grasp (e.g., picks up raisin) with thumb and finger by 12 months; see Box 1-1 for suggested recommendations regarding when to introduce various foods in infancy

8. Sensory development

     a. Hearing and touch well developed at birth

     b. Sight not fully developed until 6 years; differentiates light and dark at birth; prefers human face; smiles at 2 months

     c. Usually searches and turns head to locate sounds by 2 months

     d. Has taste preferences by 6 months

     e. Responds to own name by 7 months

     f. Able to follow moving objects; visual acuity 20/50 or better; amblyopia may develop by 12 months

     g. Can vocalize four words by 1 year

Box 1-1	**Recommendation**	**Rationale**
Introduction of Solid Foods in Infancy	Introduce rice cereal at 4–6 months.	Rice cereal is easy to digest, has low allergenic potential, and contains iron.
	Introduce fruits or vegetables at 6–8 months.	Fruits and vegetables provide needed vitamins.
	Introduce meats at 8–10 months.	Meats are harder to digest, have high protein load, and should not be fed until close to 1 year of age.
	Use single-food prepared baby foods rather than combination meals.	Combination meals usually contain more sugar, salt, and fillers.
	Introduce one new food at a time, waiting at least three days to introduce another. Delay eggs, strawberries, wheat, corn, fish and nut products until close to age 2–3 years.	If a food allergy or intolerance develops, it will be easy to identify. The foods listed are most commonly associated with food allergy.
	Avoid carrots, beets, and spinach before 4 months of age. Have well water evaluated for nitrates (recommended level <10 mg/L).	Nitrates in these foods and in water near agricultural runoff can be converted to nitrite by young infants, causing methemoglobinemia.
	Infants can be fed mashed portions of table foods such as carrots, rice, and potatoes.	This is a less expensive alternative to jars of commercially prepared baby food; it allows parents of various cultural groups to feed ethnic foods to infants.
	Avoid adding sugar, salt, spices when mixing own baby foods.	Infants need not become accustomed to these flavors; they may get too much sodium from salt or develop gastric distress from some spices.
	Avoid honey until at least 1 year of age.	Infants cannot detoxify *Clostridium botulinum* spores sometimes present in honey and can develop botulism.

9. When an infant is born prematurely, it is important to consider an infant's adjusted age rather than chronological age when looking at milestones
10. Nutrition
    a. Human breast milk is most complete and easily digested
    b. Commercially prepared iron-fortified formulas used for bottle-feeding closely resemble nutritional content of human milk; recommended for first 12 months

    c. Solids are introduced no sooner than age 6 months to avoid exposure to allergens
    d. Iron-fortified rice cereal is introduced first because of its low allergenic potential
    e. Introduction of fruits, vegetables, and meats follow (refer again to Box 1-1 for sequencing to reduce risk of food allergy or aid in its detection)
    f. Eruption of deciduous or "baby" teeth occurs by age 5 to 6 months; central incisors erupt first; increase in drooling and saliva occurs; slight elevated temperature may be associated with teething
    g. Gradual weaning from breast to bottle to cup usually occurs during second 6 months of infancy
    h. Juices are currently recommended to be delayed until age 1 year and then limited to no more than 4 to 6 oz per day
    i. Junior foods or chopped table foods are introduced by age 12 months
    j. No more than 28–30 oz of formula per 24 hours should be given to infants to avoid iron-deficiency anemia
    k. Infant nutritional requirement: at age 1–6 months, there is a need for 108 kcal/kg/day and for protein 9.1 gram/day; at age 6–12 months, there is a need for 98 kcal/kg/day and protein 11 grams/day
11. Safety
    a. Car safety seats
        1) Infants *must* be restrained in an approved rear-facing car safety seat in the middle of the back seat of the car until they are 20 lbs. and 1 year of age (if 20 lbs. before 1 year must still be rear-facing)
        2) Latest American Academy of Pediatrics (AAP) recommendation is to keep toddler rear-facing until age 2 years or reaching highest weight or height allowed by car seat manufacturer; thereafter, toddlers should use rear-facing car seat with a harness up to highest weight/height allowed by manufacturer, followed by a booster seat
        3) See AAP website for guidelines and a listing of suggested car safety seats (www.aap.org)
    b. Cribs: keep side rails of crib up; new federal guidelines virtually eliminate drop-down crib sides; distance between crib slats should be no more than $2^3/_8$ inches apart
    c. Never leave infant unattended on table, bed, or bathtub
    d. Check temperature of bath water, formula, foods
    e. Avoid giving bottles at naps or bedtime (may cause dental caries)
    f. Teach injury prevention
        1) Aspiration of foreign objects (buttons, toys, peanuts, hot dogs)
        2) Suffocation (plastic bags, strangulation)
        3) Falls
        4) Poisonings
        5) Burns (electric cords, wall outlets, radiators, pots and pans on stoves)
12. Play (solitary)
    a. Provide black/white contrasts for premature and newborn infants
    b. Hang mobile 8 to 10 inches from infant's face
    c. Provide sensory stimuli (bath water) and tactile stimuli (feel of various shapes of objects), large toys, balls (see Box 1-2)

Box 1-2	**Birth to 2 months**

Box 1-2

Favorite Toys and Activities in Infancy

Birth to 2 months
- Mobiles, black-and-white patterns, mirrors
- Music boxes, singing, tape players, soft voices
- Rocking and cuddling
- Moving legs and arms while listening to singing and talking
- Varying stimuli—different rooms, sounds, visual images

3 to 6 months
- Rattles
- Stuffed animals
- Soft toys with contrasting colors
- Noise-making objects that are easily grasped

6 to 9 months
- Teething toys
- Social interaction with adults and other children
- Soft balls

9 to12 months
- Large blocks
- Toys that pop apart and back together
- Nesting cups and other objects that fit into one another or stack
- Surprise toys such as jack-in-the-box
- Games such as peek-a-boo
- Push and pull toys

Source: Bindler, Ruth C.; Ball, Jane W.; Cowen, Kay J., *Clinical handbook for child health nursing: Partnering with children and families,* 2nd Ed., ©2010. Reprinted and Electronically reproduced by permission of Pearson Education, Inc. Upper Saddle River, NJ.

    d. Expose to environmental sounds: rattles, musical toys
    e. Use variety of primary-colored objects during infancy
    f. Place unbreakable mirror in crib for infants to focus on their face
    g. Provide toys that let infants practice skills to grasp and manipulate objects
    h. Vocalization provides pleasure in relationships with people (smiling, cooing, laughing)

13. Recommended immunization schedule (Figure 1-1)
    a. Hepatitis B: 1st (after birth), 2nd (1 to 4 months), 3rd (6 to 18 months)
    b. Rotavirus: 1st (2 months), 2nd (4 months), 3rd (6 months)
    c. Diphtheria-tetanus-acellular pertussis (DTaP): 1st (2 months), 2nd (4 months), 3rd (6 months), 4th (15 to 18 months), 5th (4 to 6 years)
    d. *Haemophilus influenzae* type B (Hib): 1st (2 months), 2nd (4 months), 3rd (6 months), 4th (12 to 18 months)
    e. Inactivated poliovirus vaccine (IPV): 1st (2 months), 2nd (4 months), 3rd (6 to 18 months), 4th (4 to 6 years)
    f. Pneumococcal vaccine (PCV): 1st (2 months), 2nd (4 months), 3rd (6 months), 4th (12 to 15 months); PCV13 administered to the older child
    g. Measles-mumps-rubella (MMR): 1st (12 to 15 months), 2nd (4 to 6 years)
    h. Varicella: (12 to 15 months), 2nd (4 to 6 years)
    i. Influenza: annually beginning at age 6 months and older; for the first dose of flu vaccine, a child 6 months–8 years should receive two doses, separated by at least 4 weeks
    j. Hepatitis A: 1st (12–23 months), 2nd (at least 6 months later) in selected areas

Figure 1-1 A and B

Recommended Childhood and Adolescent Immunization Schedule in the United States

Recommended Immunization Schedule for Persons Aged 0 Through 6 Years—United States • 2011
For those who fall behind or start late, see the catch-up schedule

Vaccine ▼ Age ►	Birth	1 month	2 months	4 months	6 months	12 months	15 months	18 months	19–23 months	2–3 years	4–6 years	
Hepatitis B[1]	HepB	HepB				HepB						
Rotavirus[2]			RV	RV	RV[2]							Range of recommended ages for all children
Diphtheria, Tetanus, Pertussis[3]			DTaP	DTaP	DTaP	see footnote[3]	DTaP				DTaP	
Haemophilus influenzae type b[4]			Hib	Hib	Hib[4]	Hib						
Pneumococcal[5]			PCV	PCV	PCV	PCV				PPSV		
Inactivated Poliovirus[6]			IPV	IPV		IPV					IPV	
Influenza[7]						Influenza (Yearly)						Range of recommended ages for certain high-risk groups
Measles, Mumps, Rubella[8]						MMR		see footnote[8]			MMR	
Varicella[9]						Varicella		see footnote[9]			Varicella	
Hepatitis A[10]						HepA (2 doses)				HepA Series		
Meningococcal[11]										MCV4		

This schedule includes recommendations in effect as of December 21, 2010. Any dose not administered at the recommended age should be administered at a subsequent visit, when indicated and feasible. The use of a combination vaccine generally is preferred over separate injections of its equivalent component vaccines. Considerations should include provider assessment, patient preference, and the potential for adverse events. Providers should consult the relevant Advisory Committee on Immunization Practices statement for detailed recommendations: http://www.cdc.gov/vaccines/pubs/acip-list.htm. Clinically significant adverse events that follow immunization should be reported to the Vaccine Adverse Event Reporting System (VAERS) at http://www.vaers.hhs.gov or by telephone, 800-822-7967. Use of trade names and commercial sources is for identification only and does not imply endorsement by the U.S. Department of Health and Human Services.

1. **Hepatitis B vaccine (HepB).** (Minimum age: birth)
   At birth:
   • Administer monovalent HepB to all newborns before hospital discharge.
   • If mother is hepatitis B surface antigen (HBsAg)-positive, administer HepB and 0.5 mL of hepatitis B immune globulin (HBIG) within 12 hours of birth.
   • If mother's HBsAg status is unknown, administer HepB within 12 hours of birth. Determine mother's HBsAg status as soon as possible and, if HBsAg-positive, administer HBIG (no later than age 1 week).
   Doses following the birth dose:
   • The second dose should be administered at age 1 or 2 months. Monovalent HepB should be used for doses administered before age 6 weeks.
   • Infants born to HBsAg-positive mothers should be tested for HBsAg and antibody to HBsAg 1 to 2 months after completion of at least 3 doses of the HepB series, at age 9 through 18 months (generally at the next well-child visit).
   • Administration of 4 doses of HepB to infants is permissible when a combination vaccine containing HepB is administered after the birth dose.
   • Infants who did not receive a birth dose should receive 3 doses of HepB on a schedule of 0, 1, and 6 months.
   • The final (3rd or 4th) dose in the HepB series should be administered no earlier than age 24 weeks.

2. **Rotavirus vaccine (RV).** (Minimum age: 6 weeks)
   • Administer the first dose at age 6 through 14 weeks (maximum age: 14 weeks 6 days). Vaccination should not be initiated for infants aged 15 weeks 0 days or older.
   • The maximum age for the final dose in the series is 8 months 0 days
   • If Rotarix is administered at ages 2 and 4 months, a dose at 6 months is not indicated.

3. **Diphtheria and tetanus toxoids and acellular pertussis vaccine (DTaP).** (Minimum age: 6 weeks)
   • The fourth dose may be administered as early as age 12 months, provided at least 6 months have elapsed since the third dose.

4. **Haemophilus influenzae type b conjugate vaccine (Hib).** (Minimum age: 6 weeks)
   • If PRP-OMP (PedvaxHIB or Comvax [HepB-Hib]) is administered at ages 2 and 4 months, a dose at age 6 months is not indicated.
   • Hiberix should not be used for doses at ages 2, 4, or 6 months for the primary series but can be used as the final dose in children aged 12 months through 4 years.

5. **Pneumococcal vaccine.** (Minimum age: 6 weeks for pneumococcal conjugate vaccine [PCV]; 2 years for pneumococcal polysaccharide vaccine [PPSV])
   • PCV is recommended for all children aged younger than 5 years. Administer 1 dose of PCV to all healthy children aged 24 through 59 months who are not completely vaccinated for their age.
   • A PCV series begun with 7-valent PCV (PCV7) should be completed with 13-valent PCV (PCV13).
   • A single supplemental dose of PCV13 is recommended for all children aged 14 through 59 months who have received an age-appropriate series of PCV7.
   • A single supplemental dose of PCV13 is recommended for all children aged 60 through 71 months with underlying medical conditions who have received an age-appropriate series of PCV7.

   • The supplemental dose of PCV13 should be administered at least 8 weeks after the previous dose of PCV7. See *MMWR* 2010:59(No. RR-11).
   • Administer PPSV at least 8 weeks after last dose of PCV to children aged 2 years or older with certain underlying medical conditions, including a cochlear implant.

6. **Inactivated poliovirus vaccine (IPV).** (Minimum age: 6 weeks)
   • If 4 or more doses are administered prior to age 4 years an additional dose should be administered at age 4 through 6 years.
   • The final dose in the series should be administered on or after the fourth birthday and at least 6 months following the previous dose.

7. **Influenza vaccine (seasonal).** (Minimum age: 6 months for trivalent inactivated influenza vaccine [TIV]; 2 years for live, attenuated influenza vaccine [LAIV])
   • For healthy children aged 2 years and older (i.e., those who do not have underlying medical conditions that predispose them to influenza complications), either LAIV or TIV may be used, except LAIV should not be given to children aged 2 through 4 years who have had wheezing in the past 12 months.
   • Administer 2 doses (separated by at least 4 weeks) to children aged 6 months through 8 years who are receiving seasonal influenza vaccine for the first time or who were vaccinated for the first time during the previous influenza season but only received 1 dose.
   • Children aged 6 months through 8 years who received no doses of monovalent 2009 H1N1 vaccine should receive 2 doses of 2010–2011 seasonal influenza vaccine. See *MMWR* 2010;59(No. RR-8):33–34.

8. **Measles, mumps, and rubella vaccine (MMR).** (Minimum age: 12 months)
   • The second dose may be administered before age 4 years, provided at least 4 weeks have elapsed since the first dose.

9. **Varicella vaccine.** (Minimum age: 12 months)
   • The second dose may be administered before age 4 years, provided at least 3 months have elapsed since the first dose.
   • For children aged 12 months through 12 years the recommended minimum interval between doses is 3 months. However, if the second dose was administered at least 4 weeks after the first dose, it can be accepted as valid.

10. **Hepatitis A vaccine (HepA).** (Minimum age: 12 months)
    • Administer 2 doses at least 6 months apart.
    • HepA is recommended for children aged older than 23 months who live in areas where vaccination programs target older children, who are at increased risk for infection, or for whom immunity against hepatitis A is desired.

11. **Meningococcal conjugate vaccine, quadrivalent (MCV4).** (Minimum age: 2 years)
    • Administer 2 doses of MCV4 at least 8 weeks apart to children aged 2 through 10 years with persistent complement component deficiency and anatomic or functional asplenia, and 1 dose every 5 years thereafter.
    • Persons with human immunodeficiency virus (HIV) infection who are vaccinated with MCV4 should receive 2 doses at least 8 weeks apart.
    • Administer 1 dose of MCV4 to children aged 2 through 10 years who travel to countries with highly endemic or epidemic disease and during outbreaks caused by a vaccine serogroup.
    • Administer MCV4 to children at continued risk for meningococcal disease who were previously vaccinated with MCV4 or meningococcal polysaccharide vaccine after 3 years if the first dose was administered at age 2 through 6 years.

The Recommended Immunization Schedules for Persons Aged 0 Through 18 Years are approved by the Advisory Committee on Immunization Practices (http://www.cdc.gov/vaccines/recs/acip), the American Academy of Pediatrics (http://www.aap.org), and the American Academy of Family Physicians (http://www.aafp.org).
Department of Health and Human Services • Centers for Disease Control and Prevention

(continued)

Figure 1-1 A and B   *(continued)*

Recommended Immunization Schedule for Persons Aged 7 Through 18 Years—United States • 2011
For those who fall behind or start late, see the schedule below and the catch-up schedule

Vaccine ▼ Age ▶	7–10 years	11–12 years	13–18 years
Tetanus, Diphtheria, Pertussis[1]		Tdap	Tdap
Human Papillomavirus[2]	see footnote [2]	HPV (3 doses)(females)	HPV Series
Meningococcal[3]	MCV4	MCV4	MCV4
Influenza[4]	Influenza (Yearly)		
Pneumococcal[5]	Pneumococcal		
Hepatitis A[6]	HepA Series		
Hepatitis B[7]	Hep B Series		
Inactivated Poliovirus[8]	IPV Series		
Measles, Mumps, Rubella[9]	MMR Series		
Varicella[10]	Varicella Series		

Range of recommended ages for all children

Range of recommended ages for catch-up immunization

Range of recommended ages for certain high-risk groups

This schedule includes recommendations in effect as of December 21, 2010. Any dose not administered at the recommended age should be administered at a subsequent visit, when indicated and feasible. The use of a combination vaccine generally is preferred over separate injections of its equivalent component vaccines. Considerations should include provider assessment, patient preference, and the potential for adverse events. Providers should consult the relevant Advisory Committee on Immunization Practices statement for detailed recommendations: **http://www.cdc.gov/vaccines/pubs/acip-list.htm**. Clinically significant adverse events that follow immunization should be reported to the Vaccine Adverse Event Reporting System (VAERS) at **http://www.vaers.hhs.gov** or by telephone, **800-822-7967**.

1. **Tetanus and diphtheria toxoids and acellular pertussis vaccine (Tdap).**
   (Minimum age: 10 years for Boostrix and 11 years for Adacel)
   - Persons aged 11 through 18 years who have not received Tdap should receive a dose followed by Td booster doses every 10 years thereafter.
   - Persons aged 7 through 10 years who are not fully immunized against pertussis (including those never vaccinated or with unknown pertussis vaccination status) should receive a single dose of Tdap. Refer to the catch-up schedule if additional doses of tetanus and diphtheria toxoid–containing vaccine are needed.
   - Tdap can be administered regardless of the interval since the last tetanus and diphtheria toxoid–containing vaccine.
2. **Human papillomavirus vaccine (HPV).** (Minimum age: 9 years)
   - Quadrivalent HPV vaccine (HPV4) or bivalent HPV vaccine (HPV2) is recommended for the prevention of cervical precancers and cancers in females.
   - HPV4 is recommended for prevention of cervical precancers, cancers, and genital warts in females.
   - HPV4 may be administered in a 3-dose series to males aged 9 through 18 years to reduce their likelihood of genital warts.
   - Administer the second dose 1 to 2 months after the first dose and the third dose 6 months after the first dose (at least 24 weeks after the first dose).
3. **Meningococcal conjugate vaccine, quadrivalent (MCV4).** (Minimum age: 2 years)
   - Administer MCV4 at age 11 through 12 years with a booster dose at age 16 years.
   - Administer 1 dose at age 13 through 18 years if not previously vaccinated.
   - Persons who received their first dose at age 13 through 15 years should receive a booster dose at age 16 through 18 years.
   - Administer 1 dose to previously unvaccinated college freshmen living in a dormitory.
   - Administer 2 doses at least 8 weeks apart to children aged 2 through 10 years with persistent complement component deficiency and anatomic or functional asplenia, and 1 dose every 5 years thereafter.
   - Persons with HIV infection who are vaccinated with MCV4 should receive 2 doses at least 8 weeks apart.
   - Administer 1 dose of MCV4 to children aged 2 through 10 years who travel to countries with highly endemic or epidemic disease and during outbreaks caused by a vaccine serogroup.
   - Administer MCV4 to children at continued risk for meningococcal disease who were previously vaccinated with MCV4 or meningococcal polysaccharide vaccine after 3 years (if first dose administered at age 2 through 6 years) or after 5 years (if first dose administered at age 7 years or older).
4. **Influenza vaccine (seasonal).**
   - For healthy nonpregnant persons aged 7 through 18 years (i.e., those who do not have underlying medical conditions that predispose them to influenza complications), either LAIV or TIV may be used.
   - Administer 2 doses (separated by at least 4 weeks) to children aged 6 months through 8 years who are receiving seasonal influenza vaccine for the first

time or who were vaccinated for the first time during the previous influenza season but only received 1 dose.
   - Children 6 months through 8 years of age who received no doses of monovalent 2009 H1N1 vaccine should receive 2 doses of 2010-2011 seasonal influenza vaccine. See *MMWR* 2010;59(No. RR-8):33–34.
5. **Pneumococcal vaccines.**
   - A single dose of 13-valent pneumococcal conjugate vaccine (PCV13) may be administered to children aged 6 through 18 years who have functional or anatomic asplenia, HIV infection or other immunocompromising condition, cochlear implant or CSF leak. See *MMWR* 2010;59(No. RR-11).
   - The dose of PCV13 should be administered at least 8 weeks after the previous dose of PCV7.
   - Administer pneumococcal polysaccharide vaccine at least 8 weeks after the last dose of PCV to children aged 2 years or older with certain underlying medical conditions, including a cochlear implant. A single revaccination should be administered after 5 years to children with functional or anatomic asplenia or an immunocompromising condition.
6. **Hepatitis A vaccine (HepA).**
   - Administer 2 doses at least 6 months apart.
   - HepA is recommended for children aged older than 23 months who live in areas where vaccination programs target older children, or who are at increased risk for infection, or for whom immunity against hepatitis A is desired.
7. **Hepatitis B vaccine (HepB).**
   - Administer the 3-dose series to those not previously vaccinated. For those with incomplete vaccination, follow the catch-up schedule.
   - A 2-dose series (separated by at least 4 months) of adult formulation Recombivax HB is licensed for children aged 11 through 15 years.
8. **Inactivated poliovirus vaccine (IPV).**
   - The final dose in the series should be administered on or after the fourth birthday and at least 6 months following the previous dose.
   - If both OPV and IPV were administered as part of a series, a total of 4 doses should be administered, regardless of the child's current age.
9. **Measles, mumps, and rubella vaccine (MMR).**
   - The minimum interval between the 2 doses of MMR is 4 weeks.
10. **Varicella vaccine.**
   - For persons aged 7 through 18 years without evidence of immunity (see *MMWR* 2007;56[No. RR-4]), administer 2 doses if not previously vaccinated or the second dose if only 1 dose has been administered.
   - For persons aged 7 through 12 years, the recommended minimum interval between doses is 3 months. However, if the second dose was administered at least 4 weeks after the first dose, it can be accepted as valid.
   - For persons aged 13 years and older, the minimum interval between doses is 4 weeks.

The Recommended Immunization Schedules for Persons Aged 0 Through 18 Years are approved by the Advisory Committee on Immunization Practices (**http://www.cdc.gov/vaccines/recs/acip**), the American Academy of Pediatrics (**http://www.aap.org**), and the American Academy of Family Physicians (**http://www.aafp.org**).
Department of Health and Human Services • Centers for Disease Control and Prevention

Source: Recommended Childhood Immunization Schedule—United States. January–December, 2011. http://www.cdc.gov/vaccines/recs/schedules/child-schedule.htm (February 2, 2011) and Courtesy of www.cdc.gov.
(Figure 1-1 A) http://www.cdc.gov/vaccines/recs/schedules/downloads/child/0-6yrs-schedule-bw.pdf
(Figure 1-1 B) http://www.cdc.gov/vaccines/recs/schedules/downloads/child/7-18yrs-schedule-bw.pdf

Practice to Pass

What would you explain as normal motor development for a 10-month-old infant?

C. Growth during the toddler years (1 to 3 years)

1. Weight: growth rate slows considerably; weight is 4 times the birth rate by 2½ years
2. Height: at 2 years height is 50% of future adult height
3. Head circumference: 19½ to 20 in. (49 to 50 cm) by 2 years; increases only 3 cm in second year; achieves 90% of adult-sized brain by 2 years
4. Anterior fontanel closes by 18 months
5. Gross motor development: still clumsy at this age
   a. Walks without help (usually by 15 months)
   b. Jumps in place by 18 months
   c. Goes up stairs (with 2 feet on each step) by 24 months
   d. Runs fairly well (wide stance) by 24 months
6. Fine motor development
   a. Uses cup well by 15 months
   b. Builds a tower of two cubes or blocks by 15 months
   c. Holds crayon with fingers by 24 to 30 months
   d. Good hand–finger coordination by 30 months
   e. Copies a circle by 3 years
7. Sensory development
   a. Binocular vision well developed by 15 months
   b. Knows own name by 12 months; refers to self
   c. Follows simple directions by 2 years
   d. Identifies geometric forms by 18 months
   e. Uses short sentences by 18 months to 2 years
   f. Remembers and repeats 3 numbers by 3 years
   g. Able to speak 300 words by 2 years
8. **Object permanence** is knowledge that an object or person continues to exist when not seen, heard, or felt
9. Ritualistic behavior is exhibited during toddler period; **ritualism** is toddler's need to maintain sameness and reliability; provides sense of comfort
10. Nutrition
    a. Growth slows at age 12 to 18 months; thus appetite and need for intake decrease
    b. Toddlers are picky, ritualistic eaters
     c. Limit milk to less than 32 oz/day to prevent iron-deficiency anemia
    d. Avoid large pieces of food such as hot dogs, grapes, cherries, peanuts
    e. Able to feed self completely by 3 years
    f. Deciduous teeth (approx. 20) are present by 2½ to 3 years
    g. Teach good dental practices (brushing, fluoride); do not allow to take a bottle to bed
    h. Toddler nutritional requirement: at 1–3 years, there is a need for 102 kcal/kg/day and protein 11 grams/day
11. Safety
    a. Continue to use car seat properly; see guidelines as outlined previously in chapter
    b. Supervise indoor play and outdoor activities
    c. Teach injury prevention
       1) Childproof home environment: stairways, cupboards, medicine cabinet, outlets
       2) Suffocation: plastic bags, pacifier, toys, unused refrigerators
       3) Burns: ovens, heaters, sunburns, check water and food temperature
       4) Falls: stairs, windows, balconies, walkers
       5) Aspiration/poisonings: medications, store garage items out of reach; it is no longer recommended to have ipecac in home as antidote for poisoning

  12. Play (parallel)
   a. Begins as imaginative and make-believe play; may imitate adult in play
   b. Provide blocks, wheel toys, push toys, puzzles, crayons to develop motor and coordination abilities
   c. Toddlers enjoy repetitive stories and short songs with rhythm
  13. Recommended immunizations (refer back to Figure 1-1)

D. Growth during preschool years (3 to 6 years)
  1. Weight: growth is slow and steady; gains 4 to 5 lbs./year
  2. Height: increases 2 to 3 in./year
  3. Motor development
   a. Skips and hops on one foot by 4 years
   b. Rides tricycle by 3 years
   c. Throws and catches ball well by 5 years
   d. Balances on alternate feet by 5 years
   e. Knows 2100 words by 5 years
   f. Increased strength and refinement of fine and gross motor abilities
  4. Nutrition
   a. Similar to toddlers' eating patterns
   b. Demonstrates food preferences: likes and dislikes
   c. Influenced by others' eating habits
   d. Preschool nutritional requirement: 90 kcal/kg/day and protein 13 grams/day
   e. Reinforce good dental hygiene: regular exams, brushing, fluoride, less concentrated sugar
  5. Safety
   a. All children should be in a safety or booster seat until 8 years or 80 lb (height of 4 ft, 9 in.)
   b. Able to learn safety habits
   c. Teach injury prevention
    1) Traffic safety
    2) Strangers
    3) Fire prevention/safety
    4) Water safety; drowning
  6. Play (associative)
   a. Enjoys imitative and dramatic play
   b. Imitates same-sex role in play
   c. Provide toys to develop motor and coordination skills (tricycle, clay, paints, swings, sliding board)
   d. Parental supervision of television
   e. Enjoys "sing-along" songs with rhythm
  7. Recommended immunizations (refer back to Figure 1-1)
   a. Review necessary immunizations prior to entering kindergarten
   b. Boosters
    1) 5th DTaP (4 to 6 years)
    2) 4th IPV (4 to 6 years)
    3) 2nd MMR (4 to 6 years)
    4) 2nd Varicella (4 to 6 years)

E. Growth during school-age years (6 to 12 years)
  1. Weight: steady, slow growth; gains approximately 5 lbs./year
  2. Height: increases 1 to 2 in./year; boys and girls differ little at first, but by end of this period girls will gain more weight and height compared to boys
  3. Motor/sensory development
   a. Bone growth faster than muscle and ligament development

Practice to Pass

The mother of a 2 ½-year-old tells you that her child is into everything. What safety precautions will you discuss with her today?

    b. Susceptible to greenstick fractures

    c. Movements become more limber, graceful, and coordinated

    d. Have greater stamina and energy

    e. Vision 20/20 by 6 to 7 years; myopia may appear by 8 years

  4. Nutrition

    a. Risk of obesity in this age group

    b. Identify those falling above 95th percentile and below 5th percentile in weight and height on plotted growth charts

    c. School-age nutritional requirement: 85 kcal/kg/day; protein 19–35 grams/day

    d. Tendency to eat "junk" foods, empty calories

    e. Secondary sex characteristics begin at 10 years in girls; 12 years in boys

    f. Loses first deciduous teeth at age 6; by age 12 has all permanent teeth, except final molars

  5. Safety

    a. Incidence of accidents/injuries less likely

    b. Teach proper use of sports equipment

    c. Discourage risk-taking behaviors (smoking, alcohol, drugs, sex)

    d. Introduce sex education

    e. Teach injury prevention

      1) Bicycle safety, including use of safety helmet by law

      2) Firearms

      3) Smoking education

      4) Hobbies/handicrafts

  6. Play (cooperative)

    a. Comprehends rules and rituals of games

    b. Enjoys team play; helps learn values and develop sense of accomplishment

    c. Enjoys athletic activities such as swimming, soccer, hiking, bicycling, basketball, baseball, football

    d. Provide construction toys: puzzles, erector sets, Legos

    e. Good eye/hand coordination: interested in video and computer games (needs monitoring and time limits with this activity)

    f. Enjoys music, adventure stories, competitive activities

  7. Recommended immunizations (refer back to Figure 1-1)

    a. Recheck records to identify any missed immunizations

    b. Tetanus, diphtheria, and pertussis (Tdap) recommended every 10 years as replacement to Td; some may receive Td

    c. If child has not received 2nd MMR, administer prior to 7th grade (11 to 12 years)

    d. If child has never received varicella immunization, administer at 11 to 12 years; will need two doses

F. Growth during adolescence (13 to 18 years)

  1. Weight: rapid period of growth causes anxiety; girls gain 15 to 55 lbs. (7 to 25 kg); boys gain 15 to 65 lbs. (7 to 29 kg)

  2. Height: attain final 20% of mature height; girls: height increases approximately 3 in./year, slows at menarche, stops at 16 years; boys: increases 4 in./year, growth spurt approximately at 13 years, slows in late teens

  3. Puberty

    a. Related to hormonal changes

    b. Apocrine glands become active, may develop body odor

    c. Appearance of acne on face, back, trunk

    d. Development of secondary sex characteristics: girls experience breast development, menarche (average age 12½ years), pubic hair; boys experience enlargement

---

Practice to Pass

A 6-year-old child will enter kindergarten this fall. List all immunizations that he or she is required to have received.

of testes (13 years), increase in scrotum and penis size, nocturnal emission, pubic hair, vocal changes, possibly gynecomastia

4. Nutrition
   a. **Growth spurt**: brief period of rapid increase in growth
   b. "Hollow leg stage": appetite increases
   c. Nutrition requirements: 60 to 80 kcal/kg/day—1500 to 3000 kcal/day (11 to 14 years); 2100 to 3900 kcal/day (15 to 18 years); protein requirement ranges from 34–52 grams/day
   d. At risk for fad diets; food choices influenced by peers
   e. Require increased calcium for skeletal growth
   f. Continue emphasis on prevention of caries and good dental hygiene
   g. Final molars erupt at end of adolescent period; orthodontia common dental need

5. Safety
   a. Accidents are leading cause of death: motor vehicle accidents (MVA), sports, firearms, suicide
   b. May be interested in body art including tattooing, branding; may be at risk for cutting
   c. Support needed for LGBT (lesbian, gay, bisexual, and transgender) groups; adolescents may also question their sexuality and experience stress over "coming out"
   d. Provide drug and alcohol education
   e. Provide sex education
   f. Discourage risk-taking activities
   g. Adolescents may display lack of impulse control, reckless behaviors, and a sense of invulnerability
   h. Teach health promotion: breast self-exams (BSE), testicular self-exams (TSE)
   i. Teach injury prevention
      1) Proper use of sports equipment (protective gear)
      2) Diving, drowning
      3) Provide driver's education
      4) Use of seat belts
      5) Violence and weapon prevention
      6) Crisis intervention (stress, depression, eating disorders, attempted suicide)
      7) Provide information about the risks of body piercing, tattooing, and cutting
   j. Reinforce rules when necessary

6. Play/activities
   a. Enjoys sports, school activities, peer group activities (movies, dances, eating out, music, videos, computers)
   b. Interest in heterosexual relationships common

7. Recommended immunizations (see Figure 1-1 again)
   a. Review records for any missed immunizations
   b. Tetanus, diphtheria and pertussis (Tdap) recommended every 10 years as a replacement to Td; some may receive Td; hepatitis A in selected areas
   c. Varicella 2 immunizations 1 month apart if older than age 13 at first immunization
   d. Human Papillomavirus (HPV 3) immunizations given with 2nd dose at 1–2 months after first dose and 3rd dose at 6 months after first dose; administered to girls aged 11–26 with some receiving vaccine at 9 years; vaccine available to males
   e. Meningococcal conjugate vaccine (MCV4) recommended at 11–12 years of age followed by a booster at age 16; administered at 2–3 years of age to high-risk groups

III. GROWTH AND DEVELOPMENT THEORIES

A. Stages of Piaget's theory of cognitive development

1. Sensorimotor (birth to 2 years)

   a. An infant learns about world through senses and motor activity

   b. Progresses from reflex activity through simple repetitive behaviors to imitative behaviors

   c. Develops a sense of "cause and effect"

   d. Language enables child to better understand world

   e. Curiosity, experimentation, and exploration result in the learning process

   f. Object permanence is fully developed

2. Preoperational (2 to 7 years)

   a. Forms symbolic thought

   b. Exhibits **egocentrism**—unable to put oneself in the place of another

   c. Unable to understand conservation (e.g., clay shapes, glasses of liquid)

   d. Increasing ability to use language

   e. Play becomes more socialized

   f. Can concentrate on only one characteristic of an object at a time (centration)

3. Concrete operational (7 to 11 years)

   a. Thoughts become increasingly logical and coherent

   b. Able to shift attention from one perceptual attribute to another (decentration)

   c. Concrete thinkers: view things as "black or white," right or wrong, no in between or "gray areas"

   d. Able to classify and sort facts, do problem solving

   e. Acquires conservation skills

4. Formal operations (11 years to death)

   a. Able to logically manipulate abstract and unobservable concepts

   b. Adaptable and flexible

   c. Able to deal with contradictions

   d. Uses scientific approach to problem solve

   e. Able to conceive the distant future

B. Stages of Erickson's theory of psychosocial development

1. Trust vs. mistrust (birth to 1 year)

   a. Task of first year of life is to establish trust in people providing care

   b. Mistrust develops if basic needs are inconsistently or inadequately met

2. Autonomy vs. shame and doubt (1 to 3 years)

   a. Increased ability to control self and environment

   b. Practices and attains new physical skills, developing autonomy

   c. Symbolizes independence by controlling body secretions, saying "no" when asked to do something, and directing motor activity

   d. If successful, develops self-confidence and willpower; if criticized or unsuccessful, develops a sense of shame and doubt about his or her abilities

3. Initiative vs. guilt (3 to 6 years)

   a. Explores the physical world with all the senses, initiates new activities, and considers new ideas

   b. Demonstrates initiative by being able to formulate and carry out a plan of action

   c. Develops a conscience

   d. If successful, develops direction and purpose; if criticized, leads to feelings of guilt and a lack of purpose

4. Industry vs. inferiority (6 to 12 years)

   a. Middle years of childhood; displays development of new interests and involvement in activities

---

Practice to Pass

The nurse observes a 2-year-old child having a tantrum. What should the response to the parents be?

      b. Learns to follow rules

      c. Acquires reading, writing, math, and social skills

      d. If successful, develops confidence and enjoys learning about new things; if compared to others, may develop feeling of inadequacy; inferiority may develop if too much is expected

    5. Identity vs. role confusion (12 to 18 years)

      a. Rapid and marked physical changes

      b. Preoccupation with physical appearance

      c. Examines and redefines self, family, peer group, and community

      d. Experiments with different roles

      e. Peer group very important

      f. If successful, develops confidence in self-identity and optimism; if unable to establish meaningful definition of self, develops role confusion

IV. CHILD'S REACTION TO ILLNESS AND HOSPITALIZATION

A. Infants and toddlers

    1. Parent–child relationship is disturbed

    2. Unpredictable routine of hospital promotes feelings of distrust

    3. Infants and toddlers experience **separation anxiety**, which is distress behavior that is observed in young children, between the ages of 6 and 30 months, when separated from familiar caregivers; separation anxiety peaks around age 15 months

      a. Stages of separation anxiety

        1) Protest: child appears sad, agitated, angry, inconsolable, watches desperately for parents to return

        2) Despair: child appears sad, hopeless, withdrawn; acts ambivalent when parents return

        3) Detachment: child appears happy, interested in environment, becomes attached to staff members; may ignore parents

      b. Nursing interventions related to separation anxiety

        1) Goal is to preserve child's trust

        2) Reassure child that parents will return

        3) Provide "rooming in" to encourage parent–child attachment

        4) Have parents leave a personal article, picture, or favorite toy with child

        5) Maintain usual routine and rituals whenever possible

        6) Allow choices, whenever possible, to return control to parent and child

    4. Responses to pain

      a. Infants will have increases in blood pressure and heart rate and decrease in arterial oxygen saturation

      b. Harsh, tense, or loud crying

      c. Facial grimacing, flinching, thrashing of extremities

      d. Toddlers will verbally indicate discomfort ("no," "ouch," "hurts")

      e. Generalized restlessness, uncooperative, clings to family member

    5. **Regression**: use of behavior that is more appropriate to an earlier stage of development, often used to cope with stress or anxiety

      a. Result is lack of control, toddler may become frustrated, returns to bottle, temper tantrums, incontinence

      b. Help parents to understand changes in behavior; avoid punishment

B. Preschoolers

    1. Major fears

      a. Mutilation: has general lack of understanding of body integrity

      b. Intrusive procedures: will misinterpret words, has active imagination

    2. Very egocentric and present oriented

3. Perceives illness as punishment; associates own actions with disease; may believe hospitalization is punishment for bad behavior
4. Some degree of separation anxiety still exists; may become uncooperative, develop nightmares, become withdrawn or aggressive
5. Nursing interventions
   a. Encourage parents to participate in child care
   b. Allow child to express feelings
   c. Give simple explanations; avoid medical terminology
   d. Provide **therapeutic play** (planned play techniques that provide an opportunity for children to deal with fears and concerns related to illness or hospitalization)
   e. Allow child to manipulate and play with equipment
   f. Maintain trusting relationship with parents and child; allow time for questions
   g. Praise child, focus on desired behavior, and give rewards (such as stickers)
6. May show signs of regression, like the toddler (loss of bowel and bladder control)
7. Response to pain
   a. All children have a major fear of needles; preschoolers will deny pain to avoid an injection
   b. Restlessness, irritability, cries, kicks with experiences of pain
   c. Able to describe the location and intensity of pain

C. **School-age children**
1. Major fears
   a. Pain and bodily injury
   b. Loss of control
   c. Fears often related to school, peers, and family
2. Ask relevant questions, want to know reasons for procedures and tests
3. Have a more realistic understanding of their disease
4. Become distressed over separation from family and peers
5. Nursing interventions
   a. Communicate openly and honestly; explain rules
   b. Clarify any misconceptions
   c. Encourage child's participation in care to maintain sense of control and independence
   d. Provide visiting for siblings and peers
   e. Use age-appropriate therapeutic play to provide an opportunity for children to deal with their fears and concerns related to illness or hospitalization
   f. Art therapy to assist child to express feelings
   g. Provide explanations; use visual aids such as diagrams, models, and body outlines
   h. Praise the child; focus on the desired behavior
6. Response to pain
   a. Able to describe pain, concerned with disability and death
   b. Girls express pain more than boys
   c. Demonstrate overt behaviors: biting, kicking, crying, and bargaining
   d. Cues to pain: facial expression, silence, false sense of being "okay"

D. **Adolescents**
1. Major fears
   a. Loss of independence
   b. Loss of identity
   c. Body image disturbance
   d. Rejection by others
2. Separation from peers is a source of anxiety
3. Physical appearance has major importance to how adolescents perceive themselves

    4. Behavior exhibited by loss of control: anger, withdrawal, uncooperativeness, power struggles

    5. Reluctant to ask questions; questions competency of others, will verify answers from more than one individual to determine if others are being truthful

    6. Often believe they are invincible, nothing can hurt them, resulting in risk-taking and noncompliant behaviors

    7. Nursing interventions
      a. Involve adolescent in plan of care
      b. Support relationships with family and peers
      c. Provide consistent and truthful explanations; can use abstract terms
      d. Accept emotional outbursts
      e. Promote communication between adolescents and their parents

    8. Response to pain
      a. Associates pain with being different from peers
      b. May exhibit projected confidence, conceited attitude, withdraws, rejects others
      c. Increase muscle tension and body control
      d. Understands cause and effect; able to describe pain

E. Nursing diagnoses for hospitalized child

    1. Imbalanced Nutrition: Less Than Body Requirements related to unfamiliar foods, separation from caregiver, strange environment, or disease process

    2. Ineffective Coping related to anxiety of hospitalization and procedures

    3. Diversional Activity Deficit related to separation from normal activities and peers

    4. Interrupted Family Processes related to hospitalization

    5. Self-Care Deficit related to physical disability, change in environment, and regression

    6. Disturbed Sleep Pattern related to unfamiliar environment, separation from caregiver, or discomfort

    7. Pain related to disease process or specific injury

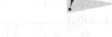

Practice to Pass

The nurse is to start an IV infusion on a 5-year-old child. What interventions can be used to decrease anxiety of this intrusive procedure?

V. CHILD'S REACTION TO DEATH AND DYING

A. Infants and toddlers

    1. Both lack an understanding of the concept of death

    2. Infants react to loss of caregiver with behaviors such as crying, sleeping more, and eating less

    3. Aware someone is missing, may experience separation anxiety

    4. Toddlers may develop fearfulness, become more attached to remaining parent, cease walking and talking

B. Preschoolers

    1. View death as temporary and reversible

    2. Magical thinking and egocentricity lead to belief that dead person will come back

    3. View death as a punishment; believe bad thoughts and actions cause death

    4. First exposure to death is frequently death of a pet

    5. Common behaviors: nightmares, bowel and bladder problems, crying, anger, out-of-control behaviors

    6. Preschoolers will ask a lot of questions, may display fascination with death

C. School-age children

    1. View death as irreversible, but not necessarily inevitable

    2. By age 10, understand death is universal and will happen to them

    3. May believe death serves as a punishment for wrongdoing

    4. May deny sadness and attempt to act like an adult

    5. Common behaviors: difficulty with concentration in school, psychosomatic complaints, acting-out behaviors

D. Adolescents
1. View death as irreversible, universal, and inevitable
2. Seen as a personal but distant event
3. Develop a better understanding between illness and death
4. Sense of invincibility conflicts fear of death
5. Common behaviors: feelings of loneliness, sadness, fear, depression; acting out behaviors may include risk taking, delinquency, suicide attempts, promiscuity

E. Nursing diagnoses for child experiencing death and dying
1. Anticipatory Grieving related to impending death of a child/parent
2. Anxiety related to diagnosis and/or impending death
3. Ineffective Coping related to death of a child/parent
4. Disturbed Sleep Pattern related to grieving, anxiety, sadness, feelings of depression

Practice to Pass

The nurse talks with a 15-year-old student about the sudden death of a grandparent. What are the expected reactions of adolescents to death and dying?

Case Study

A 6-month-old female infant is brought into the pediatric clinic for a well-baby visit. You, as the pediatric nurse, will be assigned to care for this family.

1. Identify the primary growth and development expectations for a 6-month-old.
2. What type common behavior is expected of this 6-month-old towards the nurse?
3. What immunization(s) are recommended at this age to maintain health and wellness?
4. Identify what types of toys would be appropriate for play for this 6-month-old child.
5. What information would you give these parents regarding anticipatory guidance?

For suggested responses, see page 351.

POSTTEST

1 A mother asks the pediatric nurse what she should begin to feed her 6-month-old infant. What should the nurse include in a response?

1. Egg whites are the least allergenic food to be introduced into the baby's diet.
2. Rice cereal is the first solid introduced that is least allergenic of the cereals.
3. Formula is the only source of nutrition given for the first year.
4. Fruits and vegetables are good sources of iron.

2 A 1-year-old male child is scheduled for a routine exam at the pediatric clinic. The child's birth weight was 8 lbs. If the child has followed normal growth patterns, he should weigh _____ pounds at 1 year of age.

Fill in your answer below:
_____ pounds

3 The nurse who is providing injury prevention anticipatory guidance to parents of a 3-year-old child should include which items of information? Select all that apply.

1. The use of child-resistant containers and cupboard safety closures
2. The routine use of syrup of ipecac for accidental poisonings
3. Drug and alcohol education
4. The proper use of sports equipment
5. Keeping the poison control center's number close to the phone

4 After providing a lecture on puberty for 5th- and 6th-grade girls, the school nurse asks the group to place the secondary sexual characteristics in their order of appearance. The nurse evaluates the students learned the information if they responded with which order to the characteristics below? Place the characteristics below in order or appearance.

1. The appearance of pubic hair
2. The occurrence of first menarche
3. The appearance of breast buds
4. The slowing of growth

5 The mother discusses with the nurse that her toddler asks every night for a bedtime story. The mother asks why the child does this. The nurse would explain that this behavior demonstrates which of the following?

1. Ritualism
2. Object permanence
3. Dependency
4. Conservation

6 Whenever the parents of a 10-month-old leave their hospitalized child for short periods, the child begins to cry and scream. The nurse explains that the child is exhibiting which of the following?

1. A need to remain with his parents at all times
2. An episode of separation anxiety
3. A time of discomfort
4. A state of being extremely spoiled

7 A teenage male refuses to wear the clothes his mother bought for him. He states he wants to look like the other kids at school and wear the types of clothes they wear. The nurse explains this behavior is an example of teenage rebellion related to internal conflicts of which of the following?

1. Autonomy vs. shame and doubt
2. Trust vs. mistrust
3. Identity vs. role confusion
4. Initiative vs. inferiority

8 An 18-month-old arrives at the pediatric clinic for an examination and scheduled immunizations. The nurse identifies that which immunizations are recommended for a child of this age? Select all that apply.

1. Hepatitis B
2. Diphtheria, tetanus, and pertussis (DTaP)
3. Pneumococcal vaccine (PCV)
4. Measles, mumps, rubella (MMR)
5. Rotovirus (RV)

9 The mother of a 5-year-old expresses concern about her child who believes that "Grandma is still alive" three months after the grandmother's death. What explanation could the nurse offer the mother?

1. Magical thinking often accounts for a preschooler who believes that dead people will come back.
2. There is a need for psychological counseling for this child and family.
3. This is a form of regression exhibited by the preschooler.
4. The child is in denial regarding Grandma's death.

10 Hospitalization of a child has resulted in disturbance of the dynamics of family life. Which nursing diagnosis would be most appropriate for the nurse to formulate?

1. Diversional Activity Deficit related to separations from siblings and peers
2. Disturbed Sleep Pattern related to unfamiliar surroundings
3. Ineffective Family Processes related to hospitalization
4. Ineffective Individual Coping related to procedures

➤ *See pages 22–24 for Answers and Rationales.*

POSTTEST

ANSWERS & RATIONALES

Pretest

1 **Answer: 20** **Rationale:** Children have 20 deciduous teeth that erupt between 6 months and 24 months of age. The deciduous teeth are lost beginning at age 6 years through age 12, and they are replaced by permanent teeth. **Cognitive Level:** Applying **Client Need:** Health Promotion and Maintenance **Integrated Process:** Teaching and Learning **Content Area:** Foundational Sciences **Strategy:** Critical words are *3-year-old* and *dental care*. Knowledge of normal growth and development of the correct number of teeth helps to choose the correct answer. **Reference:** Ball, J., Bindler, R., & Cowen, K. (2010). *Child health nursing: Partnering with children & families* (2nd ed.). Upper Saddle River, NJ: Pearson/Prentice Hall, p. 216.

2 **Answer: 3** **Rationale:** Fontanels are inspected and palpated for size, tenseness, and pulsation. The anterior fontanel should be soft, flat, and pulsatile with the child in the sitting position. The anterior fontanel should be completely closed by age 12 to 18 months. If the fontanel is found to be open after 18 months, the child is referred for further evaluation. **Cognitive Level:** Applying **Client Need:** Health Promotion and Maintenance **Integrated Process:** Teaching and Learning **Content Area:** Foundational Sciences **Strategy:** Critical words are *6-month-old* and *concern that anterior fontanel is still open*. Use knowledge of normal closure of anterior fontanel to choose the correct answer. **Reference:** Ball, J., Bindler, R., & Cowen, K. (2010). *Child health nursing: Partnering with children & families* (2nd ed.). Upper Saddle River, NJ: Pearson/ Prentice Hall, p. 205.

3 **Answer: 3** **Rationale:** Infants sit without support at 8 months of age. Baby walkers can topple over and should not be near the stairs. Infants may be able to roll over at 4 months and should be placed in a crib, playpen, or restricted environment to avoid falling. By placing the crib mattress at the lowest level, the standing child will not fall out of bed. **Cognitive Level:** Analyzing **Client Need:** Health Promotion and Maintenance **Integrated Process:** Teaching and Learning **Content Area:** Foundational Sciences **Strategy:** Critical words are *young infant* and *needs further education*. This indicates that the correct answer is an incorrect statement. Use knowledge of infant safety measures to choose correctly. **Reference:** Ball, J., Bindler, R., & Cowen, K. (2010). *Child health nursing: Partnering with children & families* (2nd ed.). Upper Saddle River, NJ: Pearson/Prentice Hall, p. 152.

4 **Answer: 2** **Rationale:** The NCHS growth charts use the 5th and 95th percentiles as criteria for determining those children who fall outside the normal limits for growth. Children whose height and weight are above the 95th percentile are considered overweight or large for stature. Prepubescent growth spurts are between 10 to 12 years for girls and 12 to 14 years for boys. This is not a normal proportion for height and weight for this 9-year-old. **Cognitive Level:** Analyzing **Client Need:** Health Promotion and Maintenance **Integrated Process:** Nursing Process: Diagnosis **Content Area:** Foundational Sciences **Strategy:** The critical words are *9-year-old child* and *98th percentile for weight* and *40th percentile for height*. Knowledge of the growth charts and normal growth is needed to answer the question correctly. **Reference:** Ball, J., Bindler, R., & Cowen, K. (2010). *Child health nursing: Partnering with children & families* (2nd ed.). Upper Saddle River, NJ: Pearson/Prentice Hall, p. 155?.

5 **Answer: 1** **Rationale:** Secondary sex characteristics begin at 10 to 12 years for girls and 12 to 14 years for boys. The growth in girls is accompanied by an increase in breast size, development of pubic hair, and lastly menstruation. In boys, the growth spurt includes growth in size of the penis and testes, and pubic hair development. **Cognitive Level:** Applying **Client Need:** Health Promotion and Maintenance **Integrated Process:** Teaching and Learning **Content Area:** Foundational Sciences **Strategy:** Critical words are *secondary sex characteristics* and *begin*. Knowledge of normal development of secondary sex characteristics is needed to answer this question. **Reference:** Ball, J., Bindler, R., & Cowen, K. (2010). *Child health nursing: Partnering with children & families* (2nd ed.). Upper Saddle River, NJ: Pearson/Prentice Hall, p. 164.

6 **Answer: 4** **Rationale:** Requesting a bottle after drinking from a cup for a number of months reflects regression, often seen in toddlers as they cope with hospitalization or other stressful times. The child is communicating stress by regressing to a previous behavior. The child is not having a temper tantrum. Hospitalized children should not be punished for behaviors resulting from stress and illness. **Cognitive Level:** Analyzing **Client Need:** Psychosocial Integrity **Integrated Process:** Communication and Documentation **Content Area:** Foundational Sciences **Strategy:** Critical phrases are *2-year-old screams that he wants a bottle* and *has been drinking from a cup*. Knowledge of regression as a temporary coping mechanism in reaction to hospitalization is needed to answer this question. **Reference:** Ball, J., Bindler, R., & Cowen, K. (2010). *Child health nursing: Partnering with children & families* (2nd ed.). Upper Saddle River, NJ: Pearson/Prentice Hall, p. 131.

7 **Answer: 1, 3, 5** **Rationale:** Music boxes and stuffed toys are appropriate for an infant. The 18-month-old child will enjoy toys that encourage or allow movement, such as the rocking horse and push or pull toys. Quiet activities can include toddler books, usually made of cloth or cardboard. **Cognitive Level:** Applying **Client Need:** Health Promotion and Maintenance **Integrated Process:** Teaching and Learning **Content Area:** Foundational Sciences **Strategy:** The core issue of the question is the age of the child, which is 18 months. Picture the child using the toy to determine the appropriate age for the toy. **Reference:** Ball, J., Bindler, R., & Cowen, K. (2010). *Child health nursing: Partnering with children & families* (2nd ed.). Upper Saddle River, NJ: Pearson/Prentice Hall, p. 160.

8 **Answer: 1** **Rationale:** Visual aids such as doll, puppets, and outlines of the body can be used to illustrate the cause and treatment of the child's illness. Use of such equipment provides information for the school-age child to understand and cope with feelings about the procedure. Written pamphlets should be given to the parents to review prior to the procedure. Children should be allowed to cry or verbalize their feelings without guilt as long as they hold still. Parents should be given a choice to accompany their child during the procedure. **Cognitive Level:** Applying **Client Need:** Psychosocial Integrity **Integrated Process:** Nursing Process: Implementation **Content Area:** Foundational Sciences **Strategy:** Critical phrases are *preparing an 8-year-old child for a procedure* and *intervention*. Knowledge of coping mechanisms appropriate for the age of the child to deal with illness is needed. **Reference:** Ball, J., Bindler, R., & Cowen, K. (2010). *Child health nursing: Partnering with children & families* (2nd ed.). Upper Saddle River, NJ: Pearson/Prentice Hall, pp. 492–493.

9 **Answer: 2** **Rationale:** The American Academy of Pediatrics (AAP) recommends that all formulas be fortified with iron and continued for the first 12 months. Most formulas also have docosahexaenoic acid (DHA) and arachidonic acid (ARA) added to them, which are fatty acids, important for the development of a baby's brain and eyes. Whole milk should not be introduced to infants until after 1 year of age. Pasteurized cow's milk is deficient in iron, zinc, and vitamin C, and has a high renal solute load. Solid foods are introduced between 4 and 6 months of age. **Cognitive Level:** Applying **Client Need:** Health Promotion and Maintenance **Integrated Process:** Teaching and Learning **Content Area:** Foundational Sciences **Strategy:** Critical words are *iron-fortified formula* and *continued until what age*. Knowledge of formula feeding and infant nutrition is needed. **Reference:** Ball, J., Bindler, R., & Cowen, K. (2010). *Child health nursing: Partnering with children & families* (2nd ed.). Upper Saddle River, NJ: Pearson/Prentice Hall, p. 275.

10 **Answer: 3** **Rationale:** Egocentrism occurs when the child cannot see things from another one's view. Centration is focusing only on one aspect of a situation. Negativism occurs especially during the toddler period when the child exhibits independence by saying "no." Selfishness occurs when the child only cares about their own feelings but does not pertain to inability to see things from another's perspective. **Cognitive Level:** Analyzing **Client Need:** Health Promotion and Maintenance **Integrated Process:** Nursing Process: Diagnosis **Content Area:** Foundational

Sciences **Strategy:** Critical words are *preoperational stage* and *2½- year-old girl taking a toy from another*. Knowledge of Piaget's stages of development is necessary to answer the question correctly. **Reference:** Ball, J., Bindler, R., & Cowen, K. (2010). *Child health nursing: Partnering with children & families* (2nd ed.). Upper Saddle River, NJ: Pearson/Prentice Hall, p. 135.

Posttest

1 **Answer: 2** **Rationale:** Introduction of solid food is recommended at age 4 to 6 months, when the gastrointestinal system has matured sufficiently to handle complex nutrients. The suck reflex and tongue-thrust reflex diminish at 4 months of age. Rice cereal is the first solid food because it is a rich source of iron, easily digested, and rarely induces allergic reactions. Fruits and vegetables, which are good sources of vitamins and fiber, are introduced after cereal, one at a time to determine allergic reactions. Egg whites are highly allergenic. **Cognitive Level:** Applying **Client Need:** Health Promotion and Maintenance **Integrated Process:** Nursing Process: Implementation **Content Area:** Foundational Sciences **Strategy:** Critical words are *begin to feed* and *6-month-old*. Knowledge of introduction of solid food is necessary to choose the correct answer. **Reference:** Potts, N., & Mandleco, B. (2012). *Pediatric nursing: Caring for children and their families* (3rd ed.). Clifton Park, NY: Delmar, p. 244.

2 **Answer: 2, 4** **Rationale:** The first year of life is one of rapid growth. The birth weight usually doubles by 6 months and triples by the end of the first year. **Cognitive Level:** Analyzing **Client Need:** Health Promotion and Maintenance **Integrated Process:** Nursing Process: Assessment **Content Area:** Foundational Sciences **Strategy:** This question requires knowledge of infant growth patterns and then mathematically calculating three times the birth weight. **Reference:** Ball, J., Bindler, R., & Cowen, K. (2010). *Child health nursing: Partnering with children & families* (2nd ed.). Upper Saddle River, NJ: Pearson/Prentice Hall, p. 277.

3 **Answer: 1, 5** **Rationale:** Using child-resistant containers and cupboard safety closures help keep toddlers and preschoolers from coming in contact with poisonous substances. Educating the family about the importance of the poison control center is essential in anticipatory guidance for the well-being of the child. Syrup of ipecac is no longer recommended used for inducement of emesis after home poisonings, especially after ingestion of corrosives. Drug and alcohol education is appropriate for the school-age child or adolescent. Instructions on the appropriate use of sports equipment are helpful for the older child. **Cognitive Level:** Applying **Client Need:** Reduction of Risk Potential **Integrated Process:** Nursing Process: Implementation **Content Area:** Foundational Sciences **Strategy:** Critical words are *anticipatory guidance* and *3-year-old*. Consider the activities of a 3-year-old to determine which anticipatory guidance should be given. Knowledge of normal growth and development and injury prevention is necessary to answer the question correctly. **Reference:** Potts, N., & Mandleco, B. (2012). *Pediatric nursing: Caring for children and their families* (3rd ed.). Clifton Park, NY: Delmar, pp. 323–325. Healthy Children. (2011). AAP recommendations on car seats. Retrieved from "http://www.healthychildren.org/English/news/pages/AAP-Updates-Recommendations-on-Car-Seats.aspx"

4 **Answer: 3, 1, 2, 4** **Rationale:** The development of secondary sex characteristics begins around 9 to 11 years of age with the appearance of breast buds. The appearance of pubic hair occurs second after the appearance of breast buds. Menarche follows approximately one year later as third in the order of occurrence. Lastly, following menarche, there is an abrupt deceleration of linear growth. **Cognitive Level:** Applying **Client Need:** Health Promotion and Maintenance **Integrated Process:** Nursing Process: Implementation **Content Area:** Foundational Sciences **Strategy:** Critical words are *girls* and *ordering the signs of puberty*. Knowledge of the development of secondary sex characteristics and puberty is needed to answer the question correctly. **Reference:** Potts, N., & Mandleco, B. (2012). *Pediatric nursing: Caring for children and their families* (3rd ed.). Clifton Park, NY: Delmar, p. 358.

5 **Answer: 1** **Rationale:** Ritualism allows the toddler to have a sense of control and to feel more secure and confident. Often the child asks for the same story to be read. Object permanence is a developmental task of during the infant period when the infant realizes that objects or humans continue to exist even if they are not visible. Dependency occurs when the infant depends totally on the caregiver for all needs. Conservation is a concept during the school-age years when the child understands that properties of objects do not change even if moved to another location. **Cognitive Level:** Analyzing **Client Need:** Health Promotion and Maintenance **Integrated Process:** Nursing Process: Implementation **Content Area:** Foundational Sciences **Strategy:** Critical words are *toddler*, *every night*, and *bedtime story*. Consider each of the terms and definitions to determine which relates to frequent repetition. **Reference:** Potts, N., & Mandleco, B. (2012). *Pediatric nursing: Caring for children and their families* (3rd ed.). Clifton Park, NY: Delmar, pp. 292–293.

6 **Answer: 2** **Rationale:** Separation anxiety occurs between the ages of 6 months to 30 months. The child demonstrates crying and screaming when the parent or significant person leaves them alone or with a stranger. It is unrealistic for an infant to need to be in the presence of a parent at all times. The situation depicts a child who is upset about the parent leaving the hospital room, not discomfort. The situation does not exemplify spoiling. **Cognitive Level:** Analyzing **Client Need:** Psychosocial Integrity **Integrated Process:** Teaching and Learning **Content Area:** Foundational Sciences **Strategy:** Core concepts are the age of the child and recent hospitalization.

Knowledge of coping mechanisms of infants and separation anxiety reaction are needed to answer the question correctly. **Reference:** Ball, J., Bindler, R., & Cowen, K. (2010). *Child health nursing: Partnering with children & families* (2nd ed.). Upper Saddle River, NJ: Pearson/Prentice Hall, p. 490.

7 **Answer: 3** **Rationale:** Erikson's theory of psychosocial development states that the child is faced with conflicts that need to be resolved during various stages of personality development. Identity vs. role confusion (12 to 19 years) is a period when adolescents search for answers regarding their future. During this time, the child rejects the identity presented by his parents and attempts to create his own identity. Identity is often based on peers. Autonomy vs. shame and doubt occurs during the toddler period of development. Trust vs. mistrust occurs during the infant period of development. Initiative vs. inferiority occurs during the preschool period. **Cognitive Level:** Applying **Client Need:** Health Promotion and Maintenance **Integrated Process:** Teaching and Learning **Content Area:** Foundational Sciences **Strategy:** Critical words are *teenage* and *wants to look like the other kids*. Knowledge of Erikson's stages of psychosocial development is needed to answer this question correctly. **Reference:** Ball, J., Bindler, R., & Cowen, K. (2010). *Child health nursing: Partnering with children & families* (2nd ed.). Upper Saddle River, NJ: Pearson/Prentice Hall, pp. 133–134.

8 **Answer: 1, 2** **Rationale:** The third dose of hepatitis B may be administered at 6–18 months of age. The fourth DtaP may be administered at 15–18 months of age. The PCV and RV series should be completed before 18 months. The first MMR vaccine should be administered between 12–15 months, with the booster dose given at 4–6 years. **Cognitive Level:** Applying **Client Need:** Health Promotion and Maintenance **Integrated Process:** Nursing Process: Planning **Content Area:** Child Health **Strategy:** Critical words are *18-month-old* and *recommended immunizations*. Knowledge of the Routine Immunization Recommendations is needed to answer this question correctly. **Reference:** Ball, J., Bindler, R., & Cowen, K. (2010). *Child health nursing: Partnering with children & families* (2nd ed.). Upper Saddle River, NJ: Pearson/Prentice Hall, p. 622.

9 **Answer: 1** **Rationale:** Preschoolers often think that death is reversible. They also exhibit magical thinking, believing that something occurs because of their egocentricity or that they "thought it." The reversibility of death is a common thought process of the preschooler. No psychological counseling is needed at this time. The situation does not exemplify regression. Reversibility, not denial, is a common thought in the preschooler's thought process. **Cognitive Level:** Analyzing **Client Need:** Psychosocial Integrity **Integrated Process:** Nursing Process: Implemen-tation **Content Area:** Foundational Sciences **Strategy:** Critical words are *5-year-old*, *still* *alive*, and *after the grandmother's death*. Knowledge of Piaget's characteristics of thought for preschoolers is necessary to answer the question correctly. **Reference:** Ball, J., Bindler, R., & Cowen, K. (2010). *Child health nursing: Partnering with children & families* (2nd ed.). Upper Saddle River, NJ: Pearson/Prentice Hall, p. 715.

10 **Answer: 3** **Rationale:** Ineffective Family Processes can occur when there is a disturbance of everyday or usual family life. Short-stay or long-term hospitalization disturbs family dynamics related to emotions, jobs, school attendance, etc. Diversional Activity Deficit relates to the child not having a lack of usual activity. Disturbed Sleep Pattern may occur but it does not relate to the disturbance of family dynamics. Ineffective Individual Coping depicts anxiety or fear occurring before a procedure or surgery. **Cognitive Level:** Analyzing **Client Need:** Psychosocial Integrity **Integrated Process:** Nursing Process: Diagnosis **Content Area:** Child Health **Strategy:** Concepts of hospitalization and family dynamics are needed to answer this question correctly. **Reference:** Ball, J., Bindler, R., & Cowen, K. (2010). *Child health nursing: Partnering with children & families* (2nd ed.). Upper Saddle River, NJ: Pearson/Prentice Hall, p. 493.

References

Ball, J., Bindler, R., & Cowen, K. (2010). *Child health nursing: Partnering with children & families* (2nd ed.). Upper Saddle River, NJ: Pearson Education.

Hockenberry, M., & Wilson, D. (2011). *Wong's nursing care of infants and children* (9th ed.). St. Louis, MO: Elsevier.

Jarvis, C. (2012). *Physical examination and health assessment* (6th ed.). St. Louis, MO: Elsevier.

London, M., Ladewig, P., Ball, J., Bindler, R., and Cowen, K. (2011). *Maternal & child nursing care* (3rd ed.). Upper Saddle River, NJ: Pearson Education.

Perry, S., Hockenberry, M., Lowdermilk, D. & Wilson, D. (2010). *Maternal-child nursing care* (4th ed.). St. Louis, MO: Elsevier.

Pillitteri, A. (2010). *Maternal & child health nursing: Care of the childbearing & childrearing family* (6th ed.). Philadelphia: Lippincott Williams & Wilkins.

Nursing Process, Physical Assessment, and Common Laboratory Tests

2

Chapter Outline

Nursing Process
Nursing History

Physical Assessment of the Child
Common Laboratory Tests

Denver Developmental
Screening Test II (Denver II)

Objectives

➤ Discuss the areas of medical history to be included in the assessment of a child.
➤ Describe the physical assessment of a child.
➤ Identify the four areas evaluated by the Denver Developmental Screening Test (Denver II).

NCLEX-RN® Test Prep

Use the accompanying online resource, NursingReviewsandRationales, to test yourself with hundreds of NCLEX®-style practice questions.

Review at a Glance

amblyopia visual condition in which brain suppresses vision in eye with weaker muscle; also known as "lazy eye"

cerumen waxy substance secreted in outer third of ear canal; also known as earwax

facies expression and appearance of face

fremitus vibrations of voice transmitted through chest wall of a person speaking; can be palpated with hands on chest or back or auscultated with a stethoscope

genogram a family map of three or more generations that records relationships, deaths, occupations, and health and illness history

lordosis anterior convex curvature of lumbar spine

Mongolian spots bluish-colored area usually located in sacral region of newborn Asian, Native American, and African-American infants; usually disappears in childhood

objective data information obtained through physical assessment techniques and diagnostic studies

scoliosis lateral curvature of the spine

strabismus lack of eye muscle coordination caused by one muscle being weaker than the other

subjective data information obtained from child and family using interview techniques

PRETEST

1 A 7-month-old infant has all of the following abilities. Place the skills in the order of appearance from earliest to most recently acquired skills.

1. Smiling at self in a mirror
2. Transferring a rattle from one hand to the other
3. Rolling from back to abdomen
4. Pulling feet to mouth

2 The school health nurse is scheduled to do routine vision testing with a group of students. The nurse would assess each child's visual acuity using which of the following tests?

1. The Snellen eye chart
2. An ophthalmoscopic exam
3. The cover-uncover test
4. The Weber test

3 Children are usually brought to the clinic for health care by a parent. Beginning at what age is it appropriate for the nurse to question the child about presenting symptoms?

1. 3 years
2. 5 years
3. 7 years
4. 9 years

4 When recording the health history of a child, what information that is uniquely pertinent to children is important for the nurse to obtain?

1. Past hospitalizations
2. Coping strategies
3. Immunization status
4. Past accidents

5 While taking the family history of a child, the mother states that her brother had been diagnosed with diabetes mellitus. Mark the affected individual on the genogram. Draw an "X" in the correct area on the image shown.

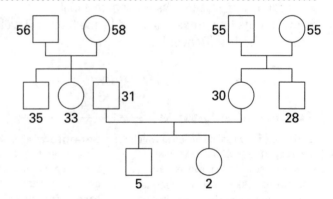

6 When plotting a child's height and weight on a growth grid, the nurse understands that which range generally represents the normal percentile range for children?

1. 10th to 90th percentile
2. 25th to 75th percentile
3. 50th to 100th percentile
4. 15th to 95th percentile

7 When assessing a child who reports abdominal pain, what is the most appropriate nursing action?

1. Palpate the most painful area first
2. Palpate for rebound tenderness
3. Avoid painful areas until the end of the assessment
4. Use deep palpation for abdominal tenderness

8 When sharing the purpose of the Denver Developmental Screening Test (Denver II) with parents of an 18-month-old, what should the nurse explain to the parents?

1. The Denver II is a test that will predict future intellectual ability.
2. The Denver II is a screening test used to detect children who may be slow in development.
3. The Denver II is used for early detection of speech disorders.
4. The Denver II measures psychological, cognitive, and social development.

9 What order should the nurse utilize when performing a physical assessment on a sleeping 8-month-old baby? Place the assessments in proper sequence.

1. Measure the occipital-frontal head circumference
2. Auscultate the heart and lungs
3. Check the eyes for the red reflex
4. Inspect the genitalia

10 When preparing to assess a preschool child, the nurse should do which of the following? Select all that apply.

1. Give detailed explanations to alleviate the child's anxiety
2. Give reassurance and feedback to the child during the assessment
3. Suggest that the child act like "the big kids" when he or she is assessed.
4. Say that the shirt is the only clothing that must be removed
5. Ask if the child prefers to sit on the parent's lap during the assessment.

➤ *See pages 48–49 for Answers and Rationales.*

I. NURSING PROCESS

A. Assessment
1. **Subjective data**: information obtained from child and family using interview techniques
2. **Objective data**: information obtained through physical assessment techniques and diagnostic studies
3. Provides a basis for identifying problems and serves as a baseline against which to compare further assessments
4. Data should be recorded systematically

B. Nursing diagnosis
1. Statement of actual or potential health problems that can be resolved, diminished, or changed by nursing interventions
2. Standardized labels assigned to specific nursing diagnoses by North American Nursing Diagnosis Association (NANDA)
3. Has three parts: problem statement, etiology, and signs and symptoms

C. Planning
1. Setting client outcomes that allow nurses to develop courses of action that assist client to achieve improved or optimal functioning
2. Includes determination of priorities
3. Requires setting long- and short-term goals
4. Includes selecting interventions that assist client to achieve goals
5. Becomes part of client's record

D. Implementation
1. Phase in which nurse works with client, family, and health care team to perform interventions designated in care plan

    2. Independent functions: carrying out interventions prescribed by nurse on care plan that have been initiated without direction or supervision of another health care professional; based on assessment of client's needs

    3. Dependent functions: carrying out orders prescribed by health care providers

    4. Interdependent functions: actions performed jointly by nurses and other health care team members (sometimes called collaborative functions)

E. Evaluation

    1. Examines client's progress toward long- and short-term goals

    2. Identifies factors that contribute to ability to achieve or not achieve goals

    3. Allows for modification or continuance of care plan

II. NURSING HISTORY

A. Major source of subjective data from family and child

B. Provides opportunity to observe parent–child interactions

C. Communication strategies

    1. Provide privacy and comfort

    2. Use therapeutic techniques, such as open-ended questions, clarification, and summarizing as appropriate

    3. Employ active listening

    4. Observe nonverbal behavior for consistency with words and tone of voice

    5. Show empathy

D. Demographic and biographical information

    1. Child's name, nickname, parents' names

    2. Addresses of child and parents

    3. Telephone numbers and emergency contacts

    4. Ages of child, siblings, parents

    5. Ethnic identification and religion

E. Reason for seeking care

    1. Sometimes called "chief complaint"

    2. May be wellness- or illness-oriented

    3. Record in words of the informant, parent, or child

F. History of present illness

    1. Onset and location

        a. Date and time

        b. Sudden or gradual

        c. Generalized or anatomically precise location

        d. Sequence of events

    2. Quality or character

        a. Description of symptoms

        b. Worsening, improving, or staying the same

    3. Quantity or severity

        a. Relates to amounts (ex: vomit) or a rating scale (ex: pain)

        b. How symptoms interfere with daily activities

    4. Duration or timing

    5. Aggravating or alleviating factors (that make it worse or better)

    6. Perceptions of parent and/or child

    7. Associated factors

G. Past medical history

    1. Birth history

        a. Length of pregnancy

        b. Mother's health

Practice to Pass

How should the nurse provide a comfortable environment for taking a health history of a young child?

    c. Access to prenatal care

    d. Medications taken during pregnancy

    e. Alcohol, tobacco, or street-drug use

    f. Duration of labor

    g. Type of delivery

    h. Apgar scores, if known

    i. Birth weight, length, head circumference

    j. Postnatal health problems

    k. Feeding

        1) Formula, including type

        2) Breastfeeding, including length of time

2. Past illnesses

3. Hospitalizations, injuries, accidents, or surgeries

4. Allergies

    a. Medication

    b. Food

    c. Environmental

5. Immunizations including boosters

6. Habits and behaviors

    a. Sleep

    b. Discipline

    c. Socialization

    d. Exercise or activity

    e. Behavior issues

    f. Wellness behaviors

    g. Use of alcohol, drugs, nicotine, or caffeine

    h. Sexuality issues

7. Medications taken regularly

    a. Prescription

    b. Over-the-counter

    c. Home or folk remedies

8. Developmental data

    a. Age at which child achieved specific developmental milestones, including first held head erect, first rolled over, first sat unsupported, first steps, first used words appropriately, bowel and bladder control

    b. Current developmental performance measured by a screening tool such as Denver II, if known

    c. Academic performance, if in school

9. Nutritional data

    a. Early infancy (birth to 6 months)

    b. Later infancy (6 to 12 months)

    c. Toddler

    d. Preschool

    e. School-age

    f. Adolescence

    g. Timing and frequency of meals and snacks

    h. Ethnic or cultural considerations in food choices

    i. Use a 24-hour diet recall or food frequency record to assess adequacy of diet

10. Family history

    a. Primarily for purpose of discovering potential or actual existence of hereditary or familial diseases in child or parents

b. Includes a **genogram** (pictorial representation of family "tree") that includes hereditary diseases, ages and causes of death, and chronic conditions (see Figure 2-1); males noted by squares and females by circles; create genogram with three generations

c. Family structure

1) Family composition: immediate and extended members of family

2) Previous marriages, divorces, separations, or deaths of spouses

3) Home and community environment: type of dwelling, sleeping arrangements, safety features, relationships with neighbors

4) Occupations and education of family members, including work schedules

5) Cultural and religious traditions, including language spoken at home

d. Family function

1) Family interactions and roles: amount of intimacy and closeness among family members, ways family members relate to one another

2) Power, decision making, and problem solving: maintenance and clarity of boundaries between parents and children, understanding of who makes rules in family and what happens when they are broken

3) Communication: clarity and directness of communication among family members, patterns of relating to one another, agreement between verbal and non-verbal communication

4) Expression of feelings and individuality: ability to freely express feelings of anger, joy, sadness, etc., and freedom to grow as an individual

11. Review of physical systems

a. Includes a specific review of each body system

b. Begin with a broad question about the child's overall health

c. Integument

1) Pruritus

2) Rashes, including location

3) Acne

4) Bruising

5) Hair growth or loss

6) Disorders or deformities of nails

d. Head

1) Headaches

2) Dizziness or injuries

Practice to Pass

What are some questions the nurse should ask to assess cultural and religious traditions in a child's family?

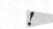

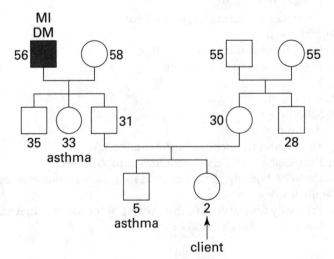

Figure 2-1

Sample genogram. Shaded area shows paternal grandfather had a myocardial infarction (MI) and has diabetes mellitus (DM). Brother and paternal aunt have asthma.

    e. Eyes

        1) Visual problems: bumping into things, squinting, blurred vision, holding books close or sitting close to television or computer

        2) Rubbing eyes

        3) Eye infections

        4) Glasses or contact lenses

    f. Ears

        1) Earaches: frequency and treatment

        2) Evidence of hearing loss, needing to repeat requests, loud voice

        3) Previous hearing testing

    g. Nose

        1) History of nosebleeds

        2) Constant or frequent runny or stuffy nose

        3) Problems with sense of smell

    h. Mouth

        1) Mouth breathing

        2) Dental visits, child's dentist

        3) Tooth-care habits: brushing, flossing

        4) Toothaches

    i. Throat

        1) Sore throats

        2) Difficulty swallowing or choking

        3) Hoarseness or voice problems

    j. Neck

        1) Stiffness or problems moving

        2) Difficulty in holding head erect

    k. Chest

        1) Breast enlargement or development

        2) Breast self-examination for adolescents

    l. Respiratory

        1) Frequency of colds

        2) Coughing or wheezing

        3) Difficulty breathing

        4) Sputum production

        5) History of pneumonia or tuberculosis (TB)

        6) Date of last TB test

    m. Cardiovascular

        1) Cyanosis or fatigue on exertion

        2) History of heart murmurs, anemia, or rheumatic fever

        3) Blood type, if known

    n. Gastrointestinal

        1) Nausea or vomiting

        2) Jaundice

        3) Change in bowel habits, diarrhea, or constipation

    o. Genitourinary

        1) Pain on urination

        2) Unpleasant odor to urine

        3) Enuresis

        4) Testicular self-examination, for adolescents

    p. Gynecological

        1) Date or age of menarche

        2) Date of last menstrual period

        3) Pain on menstruation

           4) Vaginal discharge

           5) Last Pap smear, if sexually active

           6) Contraception use, if sexually active

        q. Musculoskeletal

           1) Weakness

           2) Clumsiness or lack of coordination

           3) Back or joint pain

           4) Muscle pain or cramps

           5) Abnormal gait or posturing or spasticity

           6) History of fractures or sprains

           7) Usual activity level

        r. Neurological

           1) History of seizures

           2) Speech problems

           3) Nightmares or fears

           4) Dizziness or tremors

           5) Learning disabilities or problems with attention at home or school

    12. Review of psychosocial systems

        a. Family composition

           1) Family members in home and their relationship to child

           2) Marital status of parents

           3) Parents' educational level

           4) Persons participating in care of child

           5) Recent changes or crises in family

        b. Financial resources

           1) Family members' employment status or occupation

           2) Health insurance coverage

        c. Home environment

           1) Safe play area

           2) Well or community water supply

           3) Availability of heat, electricity, etc.

           4) Transportation arrangements

           5) Neighborhood safety issues

        d. Child care arrangements

           1) Day-care resources needed/available

           2) School attended

         e. Daily living habits

           1) Peer relationships

           2) Sleep, rest, activity patterns

           3) Social activities

           4) Self-esteem and body image

        f. Child's temperament

III. PHYSICAL ASSESSMENT OF THE CHILD

A. General considerations

    1. Developmental level of child is most important consideration for a successful assessment (see Table 2-1)

    2. Each health care visit becomes a learning experience for child and parents; it becomes an opportunity for positive relationships

    3. Use terms understandable to and appropriate for child and parents

    4. Allow child to become familiar with examiner prior to beginning examination

Table 2-1	Age-Specific Approaches to Physical Assessment
Age	**Approach**
Infant	Child lying flat or held in parent's arms
	Use distraction with older infant
	Assess heart, pulse, lungs, respirations, and fontanels while quiet, then head-to-toe
	Eyes, ears, and mouth near end
	Check reflexes as body parts are examined
	Moro reflex last
Toddler	Minimal contact initially
	Allow to inspect equipment
	Assess heart and lungs while quiet, then head-to-toe
	Eyes, ears, and mouth last
Preschool	Allow to handle equipment
	Head-to-toe if cooperative
	Same as toddler if uncooperative
School-age	Respect privacy
	Explain procedures
	Head-to-toe
	Genitalia last
Adolescent	Explain findings
	Proceed as for school-age child

    5. Save distressful or intrusive parts of examination for last
    6. Encourage active participation of child or parents when possible
    7. Prepare child and parents for new or painful procedures
    8. Examine child in a comfortable and secure position
    9. Perform assessment in an organized sequence
    10. Reassure child throughout examination
    11. Praise cooperation

B. Methods of restraint
    1. May be necessary with infants, toddlers, or uncooperative children
    2. When examining eyes, ears, nose, or throat, examiner may need to have a parent or other adult hold child supine with arms extended alongside head
    3. "Hug" method has child sit on parent's lap with legs to one side and one arm tucked under parent's arm while parent holds other arm securely; child's legs may need to be held between parent's legs to prevent kicking
    4. Ask another adult if parent is distressed and cannot help

C. Growth measurements
    1. Plot results on growth charts; length/height to age, weight to age, length to weight, head circumference
    2. Overall pattern of growth is more important than any single measurement
    3. Use 10th and 90th percentiles to determine which children are outside typical limits
    4. Length/height
        a. Recumbent length (birth to 36 months) with child supine and legs extended
        b. Use crown to heel measurement (see Figure 2-2a)
        c. Children older than 2 years may stand shoeless as straight as possible at stadiometer

Figure 2-2

A. Measuring infant length. Have an assistant hold the infant's head in the midline while you gently push down on the knees until the legs are straight. Position the heels of the feet on the footboard and record the length to the nearest 0.5 cm or 1/4 inch. B. Measuring head circumference. Wrap the tape around the head at the supraorbital prominence, above the ears, and around the occipital prominence, the point of largest circumference of the head.

Source: Bindler, Ruth C.; Ball, Jane W.; Cowen, Kay J., *Clinical handbook for child health nursing: Partnering with children and families,* 2nd Ed., ©2010. Reprinted and Electronically reproduced by permission of Pearson Education, Inc. Upper Saddle River, NJ.

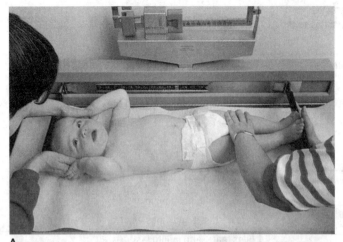

A

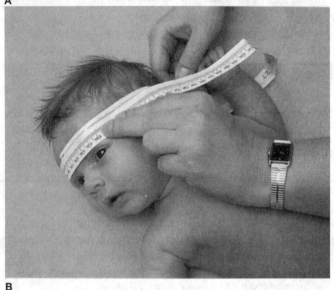

B

5. Weight
   a. Use appropriately sized beam scale
   b. Weigh naked infant lying or sitting
   c. Weigh older children on upright scale dressed only in underpants or light gown
   d. Calculate body mass index (BMI) for children over age 3
6. Head circumference

   a. Measure at every physical assessment for infants and toddlers under age 2 years
   b. Is best indication of brain growth
   c. Place measuring tape over most prominent part of occiput and just above supra-orbital ridges (see Figure 2-2b)

   d. Always measure head circumference of child suspected of having a neurological problem or developmental delay
   e. Use paper or nonstretching tape
   f. Repeat measurement to confirm findings
   g. Percentiles should be comparable to child's height and weight
   h. Head circumference exceeds chest circumference until between 1 and 2 years of age

7. Chest circumference
   a. Is usually done at birth and early infancy
   b. Place measuring tape at level of nipple with child supine
   c. Take measurement midway between inspiration and expiration
   d. Head and chest circumference should be approximately equal between 1 and 2 years of age
   e. During childhood, chest circumference exceeds head circumference by two to three inches

D. Vital signs (see Table 2-2)
   1. Temperature
      a. Rectal, axillary, skin, tympanic or temporal when assessing infants
      b. Oral route may be used in children over 5 years of age
      c. Use rectal only when necessary because of discomfort and intrusiveness; should never be used in children who have a low white blood cell count or who are immunosuppressed
      d. May be altered by exercise, crying, stress, or environmental conditions
      e. Record method used, along with results
      f. When using electronic thermometers, follow manufacturer's directions carefully regarding instrument placement in mouth or ear
   2. Pulse
      a. Try to measure with child at rest, sleeping, or lying quietly
      b. Apical pulse for children younger than 2 years
      c. Count for one full minute
      d. Radial pulse in children over 2 years of age
      e. Palpate brachial artery in arm and femoral or popliteal arteries in legs to evaluate pulses
      f. Rate may be altered by anxiety, activity, pain, crying, medications, or disease
      g. Record rate, rhythm, quality, and amplitude
   3. Respirations
      a. Try to measure while child is at rest, sleeping, or lying quietly
      b. Measure rate in infants and young children to age 6 or 7 by observing abdominal movements
      c. Measure rate in older children by observing rise and fall of chest
      d. Record rate, rhythm, and quality
      e. May be altered by anxiety, activity, medications, fever, or disease

Table 2-2 Normal Vital Signs for Infants and Children

Age	Average Pulse	Average Respirations	Average Blood Pressure
Newborn	120	35	73/50
1 year	120	30	90/56
2 years	110	25	91/55
4 years	100	25	92/55
6 years	100	22	96/57
10 years	90	20	100/61
14 years			
Female	85	16	114/65
Male	80	16	114/65
18 years			
Female	75	16	121/70
Male	70	16	121/70

Practice to Pass

What are several strategies the nurse should use to ensure an adequate physical assessment of a toddler?

4. Blood pressure
   a. Measure annually in children over 3 years of age
   b. Select cuff width that covers 75% of length of upper arm
   c. Cuff should encircle arm circumference without overlapping
   d. Use Doppler or electronic device for infants
   e. Child should be quiet for three to five minutes prior to measurement; result may be altered by anxiety, activity, crying, medications, or disease

E. **General appearance**
   1. Cumulative, subjective impression of a child's physical appearance, nutrition status, behavior, hygiene, personality, posture and body movement, interactions with parents and nurse, speech and development
   2. Observe **facies** (facial expression and appearance of child) for clues about illness, pain, fear, etc.

F. **Skin, hair, and nails**
   1. Inspect and palpate
   2. Skin: note color, texture, temperature, moisture, turgor, edema, rashes, or lesions
      a. Congenital dermae melanocytosis or **Mongolian spots**: bluish-colored areas common on buttocks or lower back of dark-skinned infants; they disappear with age
      b. Storkbites, café au lait spots, or nevus flammeus (port-wine stains) are common birthmarks
      c. Bruises in various stages of healing or unusual locations or circular burn areas may indicate child abuse
      d. Acne vulgaris may be present in adolescents
   3. Hair: observe for color, distribution, characteristics, quality, infestations, and texture
   4. Nails: note color, texture, shape, and condition; clubbing frequently indicates cardiopulmonary disease

G. **Head, neck, and cervical lymph nodes**
   1. Inspect and palpate head, neck, and lymph nodes
   2. Head: note shape and symmetry
      a. Anterior fontanel: closes by 12 to 18 months
      b. Posterior fontanel: closes by 2 to 3 months
      c. Infant should be able to hold head erect by 4 months of age
      d. Newborn skull may show molding from birth process or flattening from repeated lying in same position
      e. Note symmetry by having older child make faces
   3. Neck and lymph nodes: note size, mobility, swelling, temperature, and tenderness
      a. Thyroid is difficult to palpate in infants because of thick neck
      b. Palpate submaxillary, sublingual, and parotid glands
      c. Observe trachea for midline placement
      d. Determine mobility of neck

H. **Mouth, throat, nose, and sinuses**
   1. Inspect mouth, nose, and throat, and palpate sinuses
   2. Mouth and throat
      a. Examine last in young children; it is intrusive and may provoke fear
      b. Note tooth eruption, condition of gums, lips, teeth, palates, tonsils, tongue, and buccal mucosa
      c. Deciduous teeth erupt by about 6 months of age; all 20 appear by about age 2½ years
      d. Teeth begin to fall out at about 6 years when permanent teeth erupt; this progresses until all 32 teeth erupt by late adolescence

       e. Tonsils may normally appear enlarged, as tonsillar tissue reaches adult size during childhood

       f. Signs of abuse could include presence of a sexually transmitted infection in mouth or throat

  3. Nose and sinuses

       a. Push up tip of nose and shine light into each nostril

       b. Note structure, patency of nares, discharge, tenderness, and any color or swelling of turbinates

       c. Percuss and palpate sinuses of children over age 3; sinuses of infants and young children not palpable

I. Eyes

  1. Inspect external eye

       a. Note position, slant, epicanthal folds, eyelid placement, swelling, discharge, color of sclera and conjunctiva, redness, eyebrows, and lashes

       b. Epicanthal folds are normal in Asian children, suggestive of Down syndrome in others

       c. Outer canthus should be in line with upper portion of pinna

  2. Visual acuity tests (see Table 2-3)

       a. Snellen Letter Chart for school-age children

       b. Snellen Symbol Chart (E Chart) for preschool-age

       c. Faye Symbol Chart (pictures) for preschool-age

       d. Visual acuity difficult to assess in infants; tested by observing infant's ability to fixate and follow objects

       e. Should be able to differentiate colors by 5 years

  3. Extraocular muscle tests

       a. Cover-uncover test: cover one eye and have child look at object; observe uncovered eye for movement; remove cover and observe that eye for movement

       b. Eye movement during cover-uncover test may indicate **strabismus** (lack of eye muscle coordination), which can lead to **amblyopia** (blindness caused by weak eye muscle)

       c. Hirschberg test: shine light on cornea while child looks straight ahead; light should reflect symmetrically in center of both pupils

       d. Unequal reflection may indicate strabismus

  4. Ophthalmoscopic examination

       a. Same procedure as for adults

       b. Save until last; may require restraint or distraction

       c. Red reflex should be present

       d. Expected finding: pupils equal, round, and reactive to light and accommodation (PERRLA)

       e. Permanent eye color by 9 months

J. Ears

  1. Inspect and palpate external ear for placement, discharge, and lesions

Table 2-3 Visual Acuity by Age

Age	Visual Acuity
Birth	20/300
4–6 months	20/200
12 months	20/100
2 years	20/50–20/40
4–6 years	20/30–20/20
7 years	20/20

    2. Inspect internal ear with otoscope
- **a.** Save until last; this usually requires restraint in infants and young children
- **b.** With infants, pull pinna down and back because canal is short and straight
- **c.** With older child, pull pinna up and back like adult
- **d.** Observe for **cerumen** (ear wax), foreign bodies, or discharge
- **e.** Tympanic membrane should be pearly gray to light pink with landmarks visible
- **f.** Tympanic membranes redden during crying
- **g.** Assess mobility of tympanic membrane with pneumatic otoscope
- **h.** Tympanic membrane should move with pressure

    3. Hearing acuity
- **a.** Tested in infants by noting reaction to loud noise
- **b.** Newborns exhibit moro (startle) reflex and blink eyes
- **c.** Older children may be tested with whispered voice
- **d.** Audiometry testing of all children should be done prior to entering school

K. Thorax and lungs

    1. Inspect shape of thorax and respiratory effort
- **a.** Evaluate respirations for rate, depth (deep or shallow), quality (effortless, difficult, or labored), and rhythm (regular or irregular)
- **b.** Evaluate breath sounds for noise, grunting, snoring, etc.

    2. Palpate back or chest for respiratory movement and **fremitus** (conduction of voice sounds through respiratory tract)

    3. Percuss lungs
- **a.** Hyperresonance is normal in infants and young children because of thinness of chest wall
- **b.** Begin with anterior lung from apex to base with child lying or sitting

    4. Auscultate lungs
- **a.** Encourage deep breathing in children by having them blow a pinwheel, cotton ball, or other readily available object
- **b.** Breath sounds may seem louder or harsher because of thin chest wall
- **c.** Use both open bell and closed diaphragm of stethoscope

    5. Inspect and palpate breasts
- **a.** Newborns may have enlarged or engorged breasts due to influence of maternal hormones
- **b.** Breast exam and teaching of breast self-exam for adolescents

L. Heart

    1. Inspect and palpate precordium for heaves and apical impulse

    2. Perform early in exam because quiet environment and child are essential
- **a.** Apical pulse at 4th intercostal space (ICS) until age 7 years
- **b.** Apical pulse at 5th ICS after age 7 years
- **c.** Apical pulse just medial to left midclavicular line (MCL) until age 7 years
- **d.** Apical pulse at left MCL by age 7 years

    3. Auscultate heart sounds
- **a.** Note rate, which should be regular and same as radial pulse
- **b.** Sinus arrhythmia (rate speeds up with inspiration and slows with expiration) is common in children
- **c.** Evaluate rhythm, which should be even and regular
- **d.** Evaluate quality for clarity as opposed to muffled
- **e.** Note intensity, which should not be heavy or pounding
- **f.** Evaluate for presence of murmurs
- **g.** Sounds are louder and higher pitched and of shorter duration in infants and children

M. Abdomen

1. To promote relaxation and cooperation, have child place one hand beneath examiner's, use age-appropriate distraction, or use conversation focused on topic of interest to child; inspect shape
   a. Abdomen is prominent when standing and supine in infants and children until age 4 years
   b. After age 4 years, abdomen is somewhat prominent when standing but flat when supine
   c. Scaphoid abdomen indicates malnutrition or dehydration
   d. Umbilicus should be pink without redness or discharge
   e. Umbilical hernias fairly common, especially in African-American children
2. Auscultate bowel sounds the same as for adults
3. Palpate for masses or tenderness
   a. Liver palpable 1 to 2 cm (0.4 to 0.8 in.) below right costal margin in young children
   b. Spleen, kidneys, and bladder palpated same as for adults
   c. Begin with light palpation and progress to deeper
   d. Palpate tender or painful areas last
   e. Palpate for inguinal or femoral hernias

N. Genitalia

1. Always wear gloves during examination
2. Assess development of secondary sexual characteristics with Tanner's Sexual Maturity Rating scale
3. Male
   a. Inspect penis and urinary meatus
   b. Foreskin should be retractable by 3 months, if uncircumcised
   c. Redness, discharge, or lacerations of external genitalia or perineum in young children may indicate abuse
   d. Inspect and palpate scrotum and testes to determine if both are descended
   e. In young children, testicle may withdraw into inguinal canal because of cremasteric reflex
   f. Block cremasteric reflex in infants by beginning palpation at inguinal ring and moving down to scrotum
   g. Check for inguinal hernias by having child blow or bear down
4. Female
   a. Inspect external genitalia for evidence of discharge, redness or enlarged vaginal opening, which may indicate abuse in young children
   b. Internal examination and Pap test within 3 years of onset of vaginal intercourse or no later than 21 years of age (ACOG: American College of Obstetricians and Gynecologists)

O. Anus and rectum

1. Inspect for patency in infants
2. Skin should be smooth and free of lesions or tearing
3. Internal exam not done unless symptoms suggest a problem

P. Musculoskeletal

1. Inspect neck, extremities, hips, and spine for symmetry, increased or decreased mobility, and anatomical defects
   a. Extremities should be warm, mobile, with pulses strong and equal bilaterally
   b. Newborn's feet may be turned in but can be manipulated to normal position without resistance
   c. True deformities do not return to normal position with manipulation

          1) *Metatarsus varus*: forefoot turned in

          2) *Talipes varus*: adduction of forefoot and inversion of entire foot

          3) *Talipes equinovarus*: clubfoot, adduction of forefoot, inversion of entire foot, and pointing downward of entire foot

          4) Medial tibial torsion: entire foot turned in while knee remains straight

          5) Medial femoral torsion: entire leg turned in along with foot

  2. Assess for congenital hip dislocation

    a. Assessed until about 1 year

    b. Use Ortolani's maneuver

      1) With infant supine, flex knees while holding thumbs on mid-thighs and fingers over greater trochanters

      2) Abduct legs, moving knees outward and down toward table

    c. Use Barlow's maneuver

      1) With infant supine, flex knees while holding thumbs on mid-thighs and fingers over greater trochanters

      2) Adduct legs until thumbs touch

    d. Gluteal folds should be equal, hips abduct easily, and legs should be same length

  3. Assess spine and posture

    a. Newborn spine is flexible and rounded

    b. Cervical curve develops by 3 to 4 months

    c. Lumbar curve develops by 12 to 18 months

    d. Normal toddler has **lordosis** (exaggerated curvature of lumbar spine)

    e. Check for **scoliosis** (lateral curvature of spine) in school-age children and adolescents by looking at spine as child is bent over with knees straight

  4. Assess gait, joints, and muscles

    a. Observe unobtrusively during history

    b. Toddlers have wide-based gait and are usually bowlegged (genu varum)

    c. Children 2 to 7 are often mildly knock-kneed (genu valgum)

    d. Scissoring gait in which thighs cross over each other with each step is common in cerebral palsy

    e. Joints should have full range of motion, and muscles should be equally strong bilaterally

Q. Neurologic

  1. Integrate into overall assessment as much as possible

  2. Assess child over 2 years the same as adult

  3. Newborn and infant assessment

    a. Observe symmetry of spontaneous movements, appearance, positioning, posture, and responsiveness to parents and environment

    b. Assess level of consciousness, behavior, adaptation, and speech

    c. Use Glasgow Coma Scale to quantify level of consciousness (LOC); use Preverbal Glasgow Coma Scale for infants and young children, and Glasgow Coma Scale for older child and adult

  4. Autonomic infant reflexes

    a. Rooting reflex

      1) Touch infant's lip or cheek, and infant should turn head toward stimulation and open mouth

      2) Should disappear by 3 to 4 months

    b. Sucking reflex

      1) Infant should suck vigorously when gloved finger inserted into infant's mouth

      2) Disappears by 10 to 12 months

    c. Palmar grasp reflex

      1) Pressing fingers against palmar surface of infant's hand produces grasp strong enough to pull infant to sitting position

      2) Disappears by 3 to 4 months

    d. Plantar grasp reflex

      1) Touching ball of foot causes toes to curl downward tightly

      2) Disappears by 8 to 10 months

    e. Tonic neck reflex

      1) With infant supine, turn head to one side; arm and leg on side to which head is turned will extend and opposite extremities will flex

      2) Appears at about 2 months and disappears by 4 to 6 months

    f. Moro reflex

      1) Also called startle reflex

      2) When a loud noise is created, the infant flexes and abducts legs, laterally extends arms, forms a "C" with thumb and forefinger, and fans other fingers

      3) Immediately followed by anterior flexion and adduction of arms

      4) Disappears by 3 months

    g. Babinski reflex

      1) While holding infant's foot, stroke up lateral edge across ball of foot

      2) Positive reflex is fanning of toes

      3) Some infants have normal adult response of flexion of toes

      4) Either response should be symmetrical bilaterally

      5) Disappears within 2 years

    h. Stepping reflex

      1) Holding infant upright with support under arms, let feet touch a surface and infant appears to take steps in a walking motion

      2) Disappears by 2 months

  5. Presence of reflexes beyond expected times indicates CNS problem

  6. Cranial nerves and deep tendon reflexes are same as for adults

  7. Hand preference develops during preschool years

  8. Observe for "soft" neurologic signs

    a. Gray area between normal and abnormal, those things which may change with maturation

    b. Short attention span, easy distractibility

    c. Impulsiveness

    d. Poor coordination

    e. Language and articulation problems

    f. Problems with learning, especially reading, writing, and arithmetic

IV. COMMON LABORATORY TESTS

  A. Routine blood chemistry tests

    1. Red blood count (RBC) or erythrocytes

      a. Normal range for children 3.2 to 5.2 million/mm^3

      b. Elevated in severe diarrhea or dehydration

      c. Decreased in anemias, leukemia, and after hemorrhage

    2. Hematocrit (Hct)

      a. Normal range for children 30 to 54%

      b. Elevated in dehydration

      c. Decreased in anemias or after blood loss

      d. Routine screening of toddlers and young, school-age children desirable

  3. Hemoglobin (Hgb)
      a. Normal range for children 10.3 to 18 grams/dL
      b. Increased in polycythemia or chronic obstructive pulmonary disease
      c. Decreased in anemias, after blood loss, or excessive fluid intake
      d. Routine screening of toddlers and young, school-age children desirable
  4. Platelet (thrombocyte) count
      a. Normal range for children 150,000 to 465,000/mm^3
      b. Increased in infections, acute blood loss, and splenectomy
      c. Decreased in cancer, renal or liver disease, and aplastic anemia
  5. White blood count (WBC) or leukocytes
      a. Normal range in children 5000 to 13,000/mm^3
      b. Increased in acute infections, burns, leukemia, and sickle cell anemia
      c. Decreased in cancer, aplastic anemia, and viral infections

B. Serum electrolytes
  1. Potassium (K$^+$)
      a. Normal range in children 3.5 to 5.5 mEq/L
      b. Increased (hyperkalemia) in renal failure, severe burns or tissue trauma, or metabolic acidosis
      c. Decreased (hypokalemia) in vomiting, diarrhea, dehydration, gastric suctioning, or metabolic alkalosis
  2. Sodium (Na$^+$)
      a. Normal range in children 135 to 145 mEq/L
      b. Increased in dehydration, severe vomiting, and diarrhea
      c. Decreased in gastric suctioning, burns, or tissue injury
  3. Chloride (Cl$^-$)
      a. Normal range in children 95 to 105 mEq/L
      b. Increased in dehydration, high serum Na$^+$ level, metabolic acidosis
      c. Decreased in vomiting, diarrhea, acute infections, burns, or metabolic alkalosis
  4. Magnesium (Mg^{++})
      a. Normal range in children 1.6 to 2.6 mEq/L
      b. Increased in severe dehydration, renal failure, early diabetes mellitus, and leukemia
      c. Decreased in protein malnutrition, hypokalemia, or chronic diarrhea
  5. Calcium (Ca^{++})
      a. Normal range in children 4.4 to 5.8 mEq/L
      b. Increased in multiple fractures or hyperparathyroidism
      c. Decreased in lack of calcium or vitamin D intake, burns, or diarrhea

C. Lead
  1. Accumulates in the body with exposure and can lead to significant health problems; more common in children under age 6 years
  2. Desirable levels are below 9 mcg/dL; levels between 10 to 25 mcg/dL suggest need for more frequent monitoring; depending on source used, pharmacologic chelation therapy may be indicated for levels above 25 mcg/dL or above 45 mcg/dL
  3. Increased in exposure to high levels of lead through heater fumes, lead-based paint, unglazed pottery, or batteries
  4. Desirable to screen toddlers and children who are considered at high risk because of possible environmental exposure

D. Glucose
  1. Normal range in children 60 to 105 mg/dL
  2. Increased in diabetes mellitus, burns, severe infections
  3. Deceased in hypoglycemia or malnutrition

E. Cholesterol
  1. Normal range in children 130 to 170 mg/dL
  2. Increased in hypercholesterolemia or uncontrolled diabetes mellitus

3. Decreased in starvation or hyperthyroidism
4. Screen children and adolescents if positive family history of high cholesterol

F. **Triglycerides**
1. Normal range in children <40 mg/dL at birth to 75–80 by age 18 years
2. Increased in high-carbohydrate diet, hyperlipoproteinemia, or uncontrolled diabetes mellitus
3. Decreased in protein malnutrition
4. Screen children and adolescents if positive family history of elevated triglycerides

Practice to Pass

How will the nurse decide which laboratory screening tests would be appropriate for a 7-year-old child?

V. DENVER DEVELOPMENTAL SCREENING TEST II (DENVER II)

A. **Purpose**
1. Detection of potential developmental problems in young children
2. Used to confirm suspicion of developmental delay
3. Can be used to monitor children at risk for developmental delays

B. **Description (see Figure 2-3)**
1. Designed to be used on well-children between birth and 6 years
2. The test assesses performance on age-appropriate tasks
3. Should not be used in place of diagnostic evaluation or physical assessment
4. Assesses four areas of functioning
   a. Personal–social: getting along with people and caring for personal needs
   b. Fine motor–adaptive: hand–eye coordination, manipulation of small objects, and problem solving
   c. Language: hearing, understanding, and using language
   d. Gross motor: sitting, walking, jumping, and large muscle movement
5. "Test behavior" items completed at conclusion of test to rate child's behavior
6. Becomes basis for nursing care plan to provide activities that promote development in weak areas

C. **Test administration**
1. Age calculation is very important and must be done according to guidelines
2. Age may be adjusted for prematurity between birth and 2 years only
3. Items that require "report" from parent should be scored first
4. Easy tasks are administered first with praise given regardless of pass or fail on that item
5. Materials from test kit (blocks, etc.) should be used next
   a. Only material used for specific testing item should be visible to child
   b. Keep all other materials out of sight until needed
6. For infants, all items that need to be administered with baby lying down should be done at same time
7. In each testing area, begin with items to left of child's age line and move right
8. Generally, administer items to right of any passes until three failures are recorded
9. Scoring
   a. P (Pass): successful performance of an item, or caregiver reports that child does item
   b. F (Fail): unsuccessful performance of an item, or caregiver reports that child does not do item
   c. NO (No opportunity): only used for "report" items; child does not have opportunity to do item
   d. R (Refused): child refuses to attempt item
   e. C (Caution): when child fails or refuses an item on which age line falls between 75th and 90th percentile
   f. D (Delayed): when child fails or refuses item that 90% of standardized sample passed

Practice to Pass

How should the nurse explain the Denver II to an anxious parent?

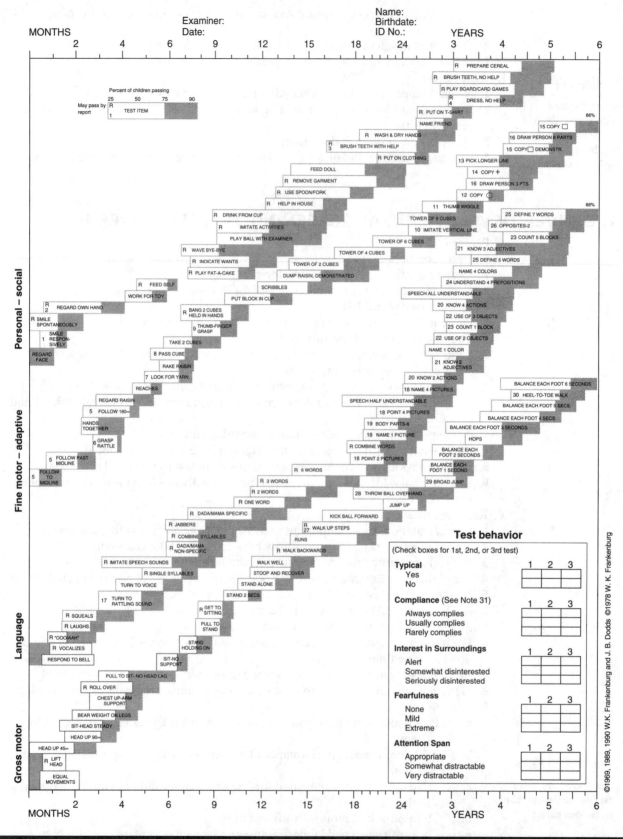

Figure 2-3

Denver Developmental Screening Test II (Denver II)

Source: ©1969, 1989, 1990 W.K. Frankenburg and J.B. Dodds ©1978 W.K. Frankenburg ©2009 Wilhelmine R. Frankenburg — Contact DDM, Inc. 1-800-419-4729 or Sales@denverii.com.

DIRECTIONS FOR ADMINISTRATION

1. Try to get child to smile by smiling, talking, or waving. Do not touch him/her.
2. Child must stare at hand several seconds.
3. Parent may help guide toothbrush and put toothpaste on brush.
4. Child does not have to be able to tie shoes or button/zip in the back.
5. Move yarn slowly in an arc from one side to the other, about 8" above child's face.
6. Pass if child grasps rattle when it is touched to the backs or tips of fingers.
7. Pass if child tries to see where yarn went. Yarn should be dropped quickly from sight from tester's hand without arm movement.
8. Child must transfer cube from hand to hand without help of body, mouth, or table.
9. Pass if child picks up raisin with any part of thumb and finger.
10. Line can vary only 30 degrees or less from tester's line.
11. Make a fist with thumb pointing upward and wiggle only the thumb. Pass if child imitates and does not move any fingers other than the thumb.

| 12. Pass any enclosed form. Fail continuous round motions. | 13. Which line is longer? (Not bigger.) Turn paper upside down and repeat. (pass 3 of 3 or 5 of 6). | 14. Pass any lines crossing near midpoint. | 15. Have child copy first. If failed, demonstrate. |

When giving items 12, 14, and 15, do not name the forms. Do not demonstrate 12 and 14.

16. When scoring, each pair (2 arms, 2 legs, etc.) counts as one part.
17. Place one cube in cup and shake gently near child's ear, but out of sight. Repeat for other ear.
18. Point to picture and have child name it. (No credit is given for sounds only.)
    If less than 4 pictures are named correctly, have child point to picture as each is named by tester.

   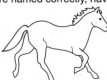   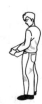

19. Using doll, tell child: Show me the nose, eyes, ears, mouth, hands, feet, tummy, hair. Pass 6 of 8.
20. Using pictures, ask child: Which one flies?... says meow?... talks?... barks?... gallops? Pass 2 of 5, 4 of 5.
21. Ask child: What do you do when you are cold?... tired?... hungry? Pass 2 of 3, 3 of 3.
22. Ask child: What do you do with a cup? What is a chair used for? What is a pencil used for?
    Action words must be included in answers.
23. Pass if child correctly places <u>and</u> says how many blocks are on paper. (1, 5).
24. Tell child: Put block **on** table; **under** table; **in front of** me, **behind** me. Pass 4 of 4.
    (Do not help child by pointing, moving head or eyes.)
25. Ask child: What is a ball?... lake?... desk?... house?... banana?... curtain?... fence?... ceiling? Pass if defined in terms of use, shape, what it is made of, or general category (such as banana is fruit, not just yellow). Pass 5 of 8, 7 of 8.
26. Ask child: If a horse is big, a mouse is_____? If fire is hot, ice is_____? If sun shines during the day, the moon shines during the _____? Pass 2 of 3.
27. Child may use wall or rail only, not person. May not crawl.
28. Child must throw ball overhand 3 feet to within arm's reach of tester.
29. Child must perform standing broad jump over width of test sheet (8 1/2 inches).
30. Tell child to walk forward, ⚬⚬⚬⚬⚬ → heel within 1 inch of toe. Tester may demonstrate.
    Child must walk 4 consecutive steps.
31. In the second year, half of normal children are non-compliant.

OBSERVATIONS:

D. Test interpretation
1. Normal: no delays, maximum of one caution
2. Suspect: two or more cautions, or one or more delays
3. Untestable: refusal on one or more items to left of child's age
4. Referral only after retest is also suspect or untestable and other assessments (physical or history) indicate a need

Case Study

The nurse is preparing to do a health history and physical assessment on a 5-year-old child whose family is new to the area.

1. Why does the nurse want to establish quickly the reason for the visit?

2. How can the nurse make the mother and child feel comfortable?

3. What strategies should the nurse employ to gain the trust and cooperation of the child?

4. What measures will the nurse use to establish the child's nutritional status?

5. What laboratory tests might the nurse want to consider ordering for this child?

For suggested responses, see page 351.

POSTTEST

① When using the otoscope to examine the ears of a 2-year-old child, the nurse should pull the pinna in which direction? Select an arrow. Draw an "X" in the correct area on the image shown.

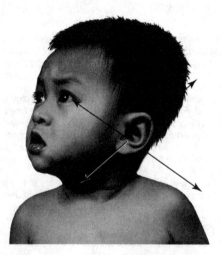

② To assess the length of an 18-month-old child who is brought to the clinic for routine examination, the nurse should do which of the following?

1. Measure arm span to estimate adult height.
2. Use a tape measure.
3. Use a horizontal measuring board.
4. Have the child stand at the stadiometer.

POSTTEST

3 At what age would the pediatric nurse change the sequence of the examination of a child from that of chest and thorax first to head-to-toe?

1. Infant
2. Toddler
3. Preschool child
4. School-age child

4 A mother of a pediatric client who is considering going to nursing school asks the pediatric nurse how the nurse plans the child's care. The nurse's best response would be that the nursing framework used is which of the following?

1. A process that evaluates the etiology of a disease
2. A conceptual scheme that relies exclusively on nursing judgment about the child's health
3. The nursing process, which aids in identifying and solving both actual and potential health problems
4. An efficient basis for communicating client data among nurses

5 The pediatric nurse should plan to include the cover-uncover test screening for strabismus and amblyopia into the physical assessment of children at which developmental level?

1. All children under 18 years old
2. Infants
3. Preschool children
4. School-age children

6 The nurse who is examining an infant would document a positive Babinski reflex after noting which of the following?

1. Curling downward of the toes
2. Dorsiflexion of the toes
3. Fanning of the toes
4. Withdrawing the foot from the stimulus

7 The nurse is performing a Denver Developmental Screening Test on a child. The child's mother asks what the nurse will be checking. What would the nurse's response include? Select all that apply.

1. Physical maturity
2. The social interaction of the child
3. Language skills
4. Fine motor skills
5. Gross motor skills

8 The pediatric nurse would perform abdominal percussion to assess which of the following? Select all that apply.

1. Generalized tenderness
2. Local inflammation
3. Density of tissues and organs
4. Size and placement of liver
5. Borders and size of abdominal organs

9 When assessing a 4-year-old child with a persistent cough, the nurse would assess respirations by observing which muscle group?

1. Thoracic
2. Abdominal
3. Accessory
4. Intercostal

10 The nurse is assessing a newborn while the mother watches. While assessing the fontanel, the nurse explains that the posterior fontanel will close by the time the infant reaches the age of _____ months. Record an answer that is a whole number.

Fill in your answer below:
_____ months

➤ *See pages 49–51 for Answers and Rationales.*

POSTTEST

ANSWERS & RATIONALES

Pretest

1 **Answer: 4, 1, 3, 2** **Rationale:** An infant of 7 months just begins to transfer objects from one hand to the other. Pulling feet to mouth begins at about 4 months, smiling at self begins at about 5 months, and rolling over begins at about 6 months of age. **Cognitive Level:** Analyzing **Client Need:** Health Promotion and Maintenance **Integrated Process:** Nursing Process: Assessment **Content Area:** Foundational Sciences **Strategy:** Key concept is normal growth and development and order of skill development. **Reference:** Ball, J., Bindler, R., & Cowen, K. (2010). *Child health nursing: Partnering with children & families,* (2nd ed.). Upper Saddle River, NJ: Pearson/Prentice Hall, p. 152.

2 **Answer: 1** **Rationale:** The Snellen eye chart measures visual acuity by assessing from a set distance how well a child can see. An ophthalmoscope looks at the internal parts of the eye, the cover-uncover test measures eye muscle coordination, and the Weber test measures hearing. **Cognitive Level:** Applying **Client Need:** Health Promotion and Maintenance **Integrated Process:** Nursing Process: Assessment **Content Area:** Child Health **Strategy:** Critical words are *vision testing* and *acuity.* Use knowledge of health screening for visual acuity to answer the question correctly. **Reference:** Ball, J., Bindler, R., & Cowen, K. (2010). *Child health nursing: Partnering with children & families,* (2nd ed.). Upper Saddle River, NJ: Pearson/ Prentice Hall, p. 208.

3 **Answer: 3** **Rationale:** By age 7, most children are able to clearly, and in chronological order, describe symptoms. Their vocabulary is extensive enough to have words to describe what they are feeling, time of onset, and changes from the norm. **Cognitive Level:** Analyzing **Client Need:** Health Promotion and Maintenance **Integrated Process:** Communication and Documentation **Content Area:** Foundational Sciences **Strategy:** Critical words are *beginning at what age* and *question the child about presenting symptoms.* Knowledge of the core concepts of growth and development and communication skills of children will help to answer this question. **Reference:** Potts, N. & Mandleco, B. (2012). *Pediatric nursing: Caring for children and their families,* (3rd ed.). Clifton Park, NY: Delmar, pp. 536–538.

4 **Answer: 3** **Rationale:** It is important for the nurse to know the immunization record and status for any child. If a child is not up to date with immunizations it is up to the nurse to plan with the family a schedule to get necessary immunizations. Hospitalizations, coping mechanisms, and accidents are important for the nurse, but immunizations are uniquely important for pediatric clients. **Cognitive Level:** Analyzing **Client Need:** Health Promotion and Maintenance **Integrated Process:** Communication and Documentation **Content Area:** Child Health **Strategy:** Critical

words are *recording the health history* and *uniquely pertinent to children.* Core knowledge of the importance of up-to-date immunizations for children is necessary to answer the question. **Reference:** Ball, J., Bindler, R., & Cowen, K. (2010). *Child health nursing: Partnering with children & families,* (2nd ed.). Upper Saddle River, NJ: Pearson/Prentice Hall, pp. 192, 628.

5 **Answer:**

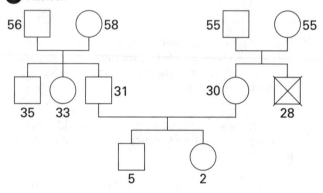

Rationale: Females are indicated by circles and males by squares. The child is indicated so the individual will be one generation up on the mother's side. The mother is indicated as number 30. Therefore, the uncle of the child is number 28. **Cognitive Level:** Applying **Client Need:** Health Promotion and Maintenance **Integrated Process:** Nursing Process: Assessment **Content Area:** Child Health **Strategy:** Start with the client and go up one generation. **Reference:** Ball, J., Bindler, R., & Cowen, K. (2010). *Child health nursing: Partnering with children & families,* (2nd ed.). Upper Saddle River, NJ: Pearson/ Prentice Hall, p. 193.

6 **Answer: 1** **Rationale:** The normal range for most children falls somewhere between the 10th and 90th percentile. The other ranges do not accommodate as many variations in height and weight that are considered normal. **Cognitive Level:** Applying **Client Need:** Health Promotion and Maintenance **Integrated Process:** Nursing Process: Assessment **Content Area:** Foundational Sciences **Strategy:** Critical words are *growth grid* and *normal percentile range for children.* Knowledge of the appropriate growth measurements is necessary to answer the question correctly. **Reference:** Ball, J., Bindler, R., & Cowen, K. (2010). *Child health nursing: Partnering with children & families,* (2nd ed.). Upper Saddle River, NJ: Pearson/ Prentice Hall, p. 286.

7 **Answer: 3** **Rationale:** Save the painful area for last to avoid abdominal guarding and to gain the child's trust. Always tell the child before touching a tender area. Light palpation, not deep palpation, would be used when assessing a painful or tender area. **Cognitive Level:** Analyzing

Client Need: Physiological Adaptation **Integrated Process:** Nursing Process: Assessment **Content Area:** Child Health **Strategy:** Critical phrases are *when assessing a child* and *complains of abdominal pain*. Knowledge of conducting a physical assessment of the child is needed to answer the question correctly. **Reference:** Potts, N. & Mandleco, B. (2012). *Pediatric nursing: Caring for children and their families*, (3rd ed.). Clifton Park, NY: Delmar, p. 459.

8 **Answer: 2** **Rationale:** The Denver II is used to screen children for possible developmental delays in the areas of gross-motor skills, language, fine-motor skills, and personal-social development. The Denver II does not measure intelligence, cognitive difficulties, or speech difficulties. **Cognitive Level:** Applying **Client Need:** Health Promotion and Maintenance **Integrated Process:** Teaching and Learning **Content Area:** Foundational Sciences **Strategy:** Critical words are *Denver II* and *the purpose*. Knowledge of developmental tests and their purpose is necessary to answer the question. **Reference:** Potts, N. & Mandleco, B. (2012). *Pediatric nursing: Caring for children and their families*, (3rd ed.). Clifton Park, NY: Delmar, p. 1264.

9 **Answer: 2, 1, 4, 3** **Rationale:** Examination should proceed in an orderly fashion from head to foot. Measuring head circumference should be done after auscultating heart and lungs. Auscultation is always easiest in a sleeping or quiet baby and should be done first. Checking the eyes is considered invasive and should be saved for the end of the examination. Inspecting the genitalia would be done third, working in general from head to toe. **Cognitive Level:** Applying **Client Need:** Health Promotion and Maintenance **Integrated Process:** Nursing Process: Assessment **Content Area:** Child Health **Strategy:** This question asks for ordering the procedure. The core concept is cooperation from the baby. **Reference:** Ball, J., Bindler, R., & Cowen, K. (2010). *Child health nursing: Partnering with children & families*, (2nd ed.). Upper Saddle River, NJ: Pearson/Prentice Hall, pp. 196–240.

10 **Answer: 2, 5** **Rationale:** Preschool children need to have reassurance that all is going well during the assessment. The preschool child may sit in the parent's lap for certain parts of the assessment. A short, concise explanation should be given to the preschool child. They are direct and concrete. The preschool child should not be expected to act like "the big kids," especially during a stressful time. The preschool child should remove all clothing except underwear to adequately inspect the entire body. **Cognitive Level:** Applying **Client Need:** Health Promotion and Maintenance **Integrated Process:** Nursing Process: Implementation **Content Area:** Foundational Sciences **Strategy:** Critical words are *to examine a preschool child*. Use knowledge of physical assessment of the preschooler. **Reference:** Ball, J., Bindler, R., & Cowen, K. (2010). *Child health nursing: Partnering with children & families*, (2nd ed.). Upper Saddle River, NJ: Pearson/Prentice Hall, p. 197.

Posttest

1 **Answer:**

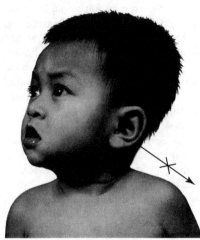

Rationale: The ear canal in infants and young children is shorter, wider, and more horizontally positioned than in older children. To adequately examine the tympanic membrane in young children, the pinna must be pulled back and down. **Cognitive Level:** Applying **Client Need:** Health Promotion and Maintenance **Integrated Process:** Nursing Process: Assessment **Content Area:** Child Health **Strategy:** Critical words are *using the otoscope* and *to examine a 2-year-old*. Knowledge of the normal anatomy and physiology of the ear canal is necessary to answer the question correctly. **Reference:** Ball, J., Bindler, R., & Cowen, K. (2010). *Child health nursing: Partnering with children & families*, (2nd ed.). Upper Saddle River, NJ: Pearson/Prentice Hall, p. 211.

2 **Answer: 3** **Rationale:** The horizontal measuring board allows for accurate length of an 18-month-old. It is helpful to lightly hold the legs in a straight position to attain accuracy. Arm span measurement does not accurately predict adult height. Using a tape measure does not provide accurate length since the 18-month-old client usually moves during the procedure. An 18-month-old is too young to stand at the stadiometer. Preschoolers will cooperate and complete the task. **Cognitive Level:** Applying **Client Need:** Health Promotion and Maintenance **Integrated Process:** Nursing Process: Assessment **Content Area:** Foundational Sciences **Strategy:** Critical words a re *length* and *18-month-old*. Use knowledge of assessment of children of different ages to determine the correct answer. The age of the child will determine the correct measurement style. **Reference:** Ball, J., Bindler, R., & Cowen, K. (2010). *Child health nursing: Partnering with children & families*, (2nd ed.). Upper Saddle River, NJ: Pearson/Prentice Hall, p. 198.

3 **Answer: 4** **Rationale:** The school-age years are the first time a child is able to reliably cooperate with the examiner and not squirm, talk, or otherwise interrupt the exam. It is beneficial to listen to breath sounds at the beginning of the examination while the infant is quiet. The toddler will most likely be more cooperative at the beginning of the examination before he or she is feeling bothered. Some preschool children will agree to the head-to-toe examination, but most talk and interrupt as the examination progresses. The preschooler usually prefers parents' closeness during the examination. **Cognitive Level:** Analyzing **Client Need:** Health Promotion and Maintenance **Integrated Process:** Nursing Process: Assessment **Content Area:** Foundational Sciences **Strategy:** Critical words are *sequence of the examination* and *head-to-toe*. Knowledge of the assessment of the child at different ages and developmental stages is needed to answer the question correctly. The core concept is the ability of the child to cooperate during an examination. **Reference:** Ball, J., Bindler, R., & Cowen, K. (2010). *Child health nursing: Partnering with children & families*, (2nd ed.). Upper Saddle River, NJ: Pearson/Prentice Hall, p. 197.

4 **Answer: 3** **Rationale:** The nursing process includes nursing assessment and development of a NANDA diagnoses related to the problem and client outcomes. Nursing frameworks do not evaluate the etiology of disease. Nurses plan care that utilizes assessment data about the client. Communicating client data among nurses is an institutional plan, not a nursing framework for positive client outcomes. **Cognitive Level:** Applying **Client Need:** Management of Care **Integrated Process:** Nursing Process: Planning **Content Area:** Child Health **Strategy:** Critical words are *asks how the nurse plans the child's care*. Knowledge of the nursing process is necessary to answer the question correctly. **Reference:** Ball, J., Bindler, R., & Cowen, K. (2010). *Child health nursing: Partnering with children & families*, (2nd ed.). Upper Saddle River, NJ: Pearson/Prentice Hall, p. 9.

5 **Answer: 3** **Rationale:** Strabismus is detected with the cover-uncover test that can first be reliably administered to children over the age of 2. Strabismus may be detected testing the corneal light reflex after 6 months of age. It is important to detect the problem early to prevent amblyopia. By school-age, vision loss would have occurred. **Cognitive Level:** Analyzing **Client Need:** Health Promotion and Maintenance **Integrated Process:** Nursing Process: Assessment **Content Area:** Child Health **Strategy:** Critical words are *screening* and *strabismus and amblyopia*. Knowledge of the assessment of the child at different ages and developmental stages is necessary to answer the question correctly. **Reference:** Ball, J., Bindler, R., & Cowen, K. (2010). *Child health nursing: Partnering with children & families*, (2nd ed.). Upper Saddle River, NJ: Pearson/Prentice Hall, p. 207.

6 **Answer: 3** **Rationale:** A positive Babinski in infants is a fanning of the toes when a stimulus is applied to the foot along the lateral edge and across the ball. The response is normal and disappears by about age 2. **Cognitive Level:** Applying **Client Need:** Health Promotion

and Maintenance **Integrated Process:** Nursing Process: Assessment **Content Area:** Child Health **Strategy:** The core concept being tested is normal reflexes in infants. Use nursing knowledge of growth and development to answer the question. **Reference:** Ball, J., Bindler, R., & Cowen, K. (2010). *Child health nursing: Partnering with children & families*, (2nd ed.). Upper Saddle River, NJ: Pearson/Prentice Hall, p. 244.

7 **Answer: 2, 3, 4, 5** **Rationale:** The Denver Developmental Screening Test II evaluates four areas: Personal/Social, Fine motor/adaptive, Language, and Gross motor. The Denver II does not include assessment of physical maturity. **Cognitive Level:** Applying **Client Need:** Health Promotion and Maintenance **Integrated Process:** Nursing Process: Assessment **Content Area:** Foundational Sciences **Strategy:** Specific knowledge about the components of the Denver II screening exam is needed to answer the question. Use concepts related to knowledge of child development and screening tests to answer the question. **Reference:** Ball, J., Bindler, R., & Cowen, K. (2010). *Child health nursing: Partnering with children & families*, (2nd ed.). Upper Saddle River, NJ: Pearson/Prentice Hall, pp. 330–331.

8 **Answer: 3, 5** **Rationale:** Indirect percussion can be used to evaluate borders and sizes of abdominal organs and masses. Percussion produces sounds of varying loudness and pitch, and these sound help to identify the density of organs and tissues. The nurse assesses the liver with palpation and percussion, but not for placement. Inflammation is assessed with inspection, and tenderness is assessed with palpation. **Cognitive Level:** Analyzing **Client Need:** Health Promotion and Maintenance **Integrated Process:** Nursing Process: Assessment **Content Area:** Child Health **Strategy:** The core issue of the question is the ability to differentiate between palpation, auscultation, and percussion assessments. Use knowledge of physical assessment skills to determine the correct answer. **Reference:** Ball, J., Bindler, R., & Cowen, K. (2010). *Child health nursing: Partnering with children & families*, (2nd ed.). Upper Saddle River, NJ: Pearson/Prentice Hall, p. 195.

9 **Answer: 2** **Rationale:** Infants and young children use the diaphragm and abdominal muscles for respiration, so the nurse would watch the rise and fall of the abdomen to count respirations. Use of accessory or intercostal muscles may be observed in respiratory distress. **Cognitive Level:** Applying **Client Need:** Health Promotion and Maintenance **Integrated Process:** Nursing Process: Assessment **Content Area:** Child Health **Strategy:** The core concept being tested is the normal respiratory function of a child of this age. Critical words are *4-year-old with a persistent cough* and *muscle group*. Use knowledge of physical assessment and respiratory assessment to make a selection. **Reference:** Ball, J., Bindler, R., & Cowen, K. (2010). *Child health nursing: Partnering with children & families*, (2nd ed.). Upper Saddle River, NJ: Pearson/Prentice Hall, p. 221.

10 **Answer: 3** **Rationale:** The posterior fontanel closes by 3 months of age. The anterior fontanel closes by 18 months. **Cognitive Level:** Applying **Client Need:** Health Promotion and Maintenance **Integrated Process:** Teaching and Learning **Content Area:** Foundational Sciences **Strategy:** The core concept is normal growth and development of the head. Specific knowledge is needed to answer the question. **Reference:** Ball, J., Bindler, R., & Cowen, K. (2010). *Child health nursing: Partnering with children & families,* (2nd ed.). Upper Saddle River, NJ: Pearson/Prentice Hall, p. 205.

References

Ball, J., Bindler, R. & Cowen, K. (2010). *Child health nursing: Partnering with children and families* (2nd ed.). Upper Saddle River, NJ: Pearson Education.

Berman, A. & Snyder, S. (2012). *Kozier & Erb's Fundamentals of nursing: Concepts, process, and practice* (9th ed.). Upper Saddle River, NJ: Pearson Education, Inc.

Hockenberry, M. & Wilson, D. (2009). *Wong's essentials of pediatric nursing* (8th ed.). St. Louis, MO: Elsevier.

Hockenberry, M. & Wilson, D. (2011). *Wong's nursing care of infants and children* (9th ed.). St. Louis, MO: Elsevier.

Jarvis, C. (2012). *Physical examination and health assessment* (6th ed.). St. Louis, MO: Elsevier.

Kee, J. (2010). *Laboratory and diagnostic tests* (8th ed.). Upper Saddle River, NJ: Pearson Education, Inc.

London, M., Ladewig, P., Ball, J., Bindler, R., & Cowen, K. (2011). *Maternal & child nursing care* (3rd ed.). Upper Saddle River, NJ: Pearson Education.

ANSWERS & RATIONALES

3

Eye, Ear, Nose, and Throat Problems

Chapter Outline

Disorders of the Eye

Disorders of the Ear

Disorders of the Throat

Disorders of the Nose

 NCLEX-RN® Test Prep

Use the accompanying online resource, NursingReviewsandRationales, to test yourself with hundreds of NCLEX®-style practice questions.

Objectives

➤ Identify data essential to the assessment of alterations in health of the sensory organs in a child.
➤ Discuss the clinical manifestations and pathophysiology of alterations in health of the sensory organs in a child.
➤ Discuss therapeutic management of a child with alterations in health of the sensory organs.
➤ Describe nursing management of a child with alterations in health of the sensory organs.

Review at a Glance

amblyopia "lazy eye" results when one eye does not receive sufficient stimulation; can cause eventual loss of vision in affected eye

conjunctivitis inflammation of conjunctiva

corneal light reflex (Hirschberg test) a screening test for strabismus and symmetrical alignment of eyes

cover-uncover test a screening test for "lazy eye"

epistaxis nosebleed

otitis media inflammation of middle ear

pharyngitis inflammation of pharynx

sensory impairment a general term that indicates sensory disability that may range in severity from mild to

profound; includes hearing and visual impairment

strabismus misalignment of eyes; abnormal turning of eye inward or outward

tonsillitis inflammation of tonsils, resulting in tonsillar enlargement, frequently occurs with pharyngitis

PRETEST

1 The physician orders amoxicillin (Amoxil) 500 mg IVPB q 8 hours for a pediatric client with tonsillitis. What is the appropriate nursing action?

1. Question the order because the route of administration is incorrect.
2. Give the medication as ordered.
3. Question the order because the dosage is too high.
4. Question the order because the dosing frequency is incorrect.

2 The nurse administers cefprozil (Cefzil) as ordered to a 22-month-old client with bacterial pharyngitis. The nurse notes patches of white on the child's oral mucosa that cannot be removed. Which condition does the nurse suspect?

1. Allergic reaction to the medication manifested by stomatitis
2. A herpes simplex virus infection
3. Oral thrush caused by *Candida albicans*
4. Presence of mumps infection

3 A pediatric client has been diagnosed with otitis media. The nurse should place highest priority on teaching the parent which of the following?

1. How to administer ear drops
2. Importance of completing full course of antibiotic therapy
3. About myringotomy and tympanostomy tube insertion
4. About eliminating environmental allergens

4 What should the nurse include when developing the care plan for a child who is postoperative for a tonsillectomy? Select all that apply.

1. Apply warm, moist compresses to the neck area.
2. Observe for excessive swallowing.
3. Maintain the child in a supine position.
4. Offer warm liquids with a straw for the child to sip.
5. Report any trickle of bright red blood.

5 The nurse is caring for a child with a common cold (nasopharyngitis). The primary goal of nursing care is directed toward which of the following?

1. Preventing injury
2. Promoting nutrition
3. Relieving symptoms
4. Administering antibiotics

6 The nurse obtains a health history on a preschool pediatric client. Which of the following signs should alert the nurse to possible hearing impairment in the child?

1. Distractibility and short attention span
2. Disinterest in reading storybooks
3. Turning up the volume on the family television set
4. Temper tantrums

7 The nurse is caring for a 1-month-old client who is blind secondary to retinopathy of prematurity. The nurse is teaching the parents about activities to promote their infant's development. Which of the following statements by the nurse is correct?

1. "Infants with visual impairment respond to tactile stimuli rather than auditory stimuli."
2. "Talking, holding, and singing to your baby are appropriate activities at this age."
3. "You should expect your baby to smile in response to your voice by 4 months of age."
4. "Position the baby side-lying in the crib at all times, and avoid loud noises, which could startle the infant."

8 The nurse is assessing a child with conjunctivitis (pink eye). Which of the following signs would the nurse most likely assess?

1. Serous drainage from the affected eye
2. Severe eye pain
3. Periorbital edema
4. Crusting of eyelids and eyelashes

9 The nurse teaches a child with conjunctivitis measures to prevent the spread of infection. The nurse concludes that further teaching is needed when the child states which of the following?

1. "I will wash my hands frequently."
2. "I will use a tissue to clean my eye and then throw the tissue away."
3. "I will use my own washcloth and towel, and not use my brother's."
4. "I will carry a handkerchief with me so that I can wipe my eyes during the day."

10 A 4-month-old infant has severe nasal congestion, nasal mucous drainage, and crusting in and around the nares. What is the best way for the nurse to clear the infant's nasal passages?

1. Administer vasoconstrictive nose drops every three hours.
2. Place the infant in a mist tent.
3. Administer saline drops in the nose and suction with bulb syringe.
4. Instruct the client to blow the nose and keep disposable tissues handy.

➤ *See pages 65–66 for Answers and Rationales.*

I. DISORDERS OF THE EYE

A. *Conjunctivitis*

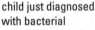

Practice to Pass

Parents of a 2-year-old child just diagnosed with bacterial conjunctivitis with antibiotic ophthalmic ointment prescribed ask the nurse when the child can return to daycare. What is the nurse's correct response?

1. Description: inflammation of conjunctiva, also known as "pink eye"
2. Etiology and pathophysiology
   a. Conjunctiva is a clear membrane lining inside of eyelids and sclera; it is normally pink and clear, smooth and moist
   b. Bacteria, viruses, allergens, trauma, or other irritants can cause conjunctiva to become reddened (erythematous) and edematous
   c. A yellow, white, or green purulent exudate may be present in affected eye; there is excessive tearing of affected eye
   d. Bacterial conjunctivitis is contagious
3. Assessment
   a. Conjunctiva reddened and edematous
   b. Yellow, white, or green purulent exudate
   c. Crusting present on eyelids and lashes
4. Priority nursing diagnoses
   a. Pain
   b. Deficient Knowledge: Safe Administration of Eye Drops and Ointments

5. Planning and implementation
   a. Nursing care focuses on measures to prevent spread of infection
   b. Despite feeling itchy, children should avoid rubbing the eye(s); careful attention to handwashing and avoiding shared items is important
   c. Cleanse eye with warm water and remove any crusting or exudate before instilling eye drops or eye ointment
6. Medication therapy: antibiotic drops or ointment will be ordered if infection is bacterial
7. Client and family education
   a. Teach caregivers to instill antibiotic drops or ointment into conjunctival sac
   b. Give instructions on prevention measures to limit spread of infection to other eye or people; client is not contagious 24 hrs after medication is begun
8. Evaluation: parents demonstrate safe and effective administration of eye drops/ointment; infection does not spread to other family members

B. *Amblyopia*

   1. Description

      a. Also known as "lazy eye"

      b. Reduction of central vision in an eye that is normal

   2. Etiology and pathophysiology

      a. Results from untreated strabismus, and causes decreased vision in one or both eyes

      b. Visual loss is caused by suppression of signals by brain

   3. Assessment

      a. Diagnosed with assessment and vision testing by an optometrist or ophthalmologist

      b. Nursing assessments depend upon age of child

      c. Manifestations of visual impairment for infants include lack of tracking objects or lights with eyes, and poor or no eye contact

      d. Signs of visual impairment in toddlers and older children are excessive tearing, rubbing and squinting of eyes, frequent blinking, and holding objects close to eyes to see them or to read

   4. Priority nursing diagnoses

      a. Impaired Sensory Perception

      b. Disturbed Body Image

   5. Planning and implementation

      a. Medical treatment options include corrective lenses in eyeglasses, occluding unaffected eye with a patch (occlusion therapy), eye muscle exercises

      b. Treatment is discontinued when vision has improved; however, 20/20 visual acuity is rarely attained

      c. Treatment of amblyopia is most successful when accomplished by age 7 to 8 years of age

      d. Untreated amblyopia can lead to permanent visual impairment

      e. Nursing care involves educating parents and child about necessity of completing treatment

   6. Child and family education

      a. Teach parents means of patching unaffected eye while maintaining skin integrity

      b. Child and parents need explanation of therapy and long-term benefits

   7. Evaluation: child completes treatment as prescribed

C. *Strabismus*

   1. Description: misalignment of eyes

      a. Most common type is esotropia (crossed eyes)

      b. Eyes appear misaligned to the examiner

   2. Etiology and pathophysiology

      a. Caused by lack of coordination of the eye muscles

      b. Positive family history occurs in about 50% of cases

      c. Pseudostrabismus or false appearance of crossed eyes due to lack development of facial features or wide epicanthal folds is common in young infants and is not an indicator of strabismus in older child

   3. Assessment: screening tests include cover-uncover test and corneal light reflex (Hirschberg test)

      a. Cover-uncover test: ask client to fix his or her gaze straight ahead, focusing on a distant object; cover one eye with an opaque card; as eye is covered, observe uncovered eye for movement; remove card while observing eye just uncovered for movement; this test screens for deviation in eye alignment and eye muscle weakness; eye muscle weakness is seen as movement of "lazy eye" when it attempts to refocus during the cover test

Figure 3-1

Corneal light reflex results
showing strabismus

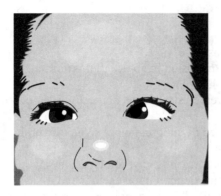

Figure 3-1

Corneal light reflex results
showing strabismus

    b. Corneal light reflex (Hirschberg test): assesses parallel symmetry of eyes; examiner shines a penlight directly onto corneas of both eyes, holding penlight about 12 inches away from client's nasal bridge while client focuses on a distant object; examiner should see light reflected at same spot in both eyes; an asymmetric light reflex indicates a deviation in alignment of client's eyes (see Figure 3-1)

4. Priority nursing diagnoses

    a. Impaired Sensory Perception (visual)

    b. Disturbed Body Image

    c. Risk for Injury related to visual impairment

    d. Risk for Impaired Growth and Development related to visual impairment

    e. Risk for Ineffective Family Coping related to caring for child with visual impairment

5. Planning and implementation: treatment of strabismus includes occlusion therapy ("good eye" is patched forcing client to focus with weaker eye, thus strengthening eye muscles), corrective lenses in eyeglasses, eye drops to cause blurred vision in "good eye," eye muscle exercises

6. Surgical treatment

    a. Strabismus can be corrected surgically if conservative treatment has failed to correct condition; surgery on rectus muscles of eyes can achieve normal eye alignment

    b. Congenital strabismus should be corrected before 24 months of age to prevent amblyopia (decreased vision of one or both eyes)

7. Client and family education: explanation of eye patching is given to parents; preoperative teaching includes benefits and risks of surgery, as well as maintaining NPO status prior to surgery

8. Evaluation: parents maintain eye patching as ordered; client and parents are prepared for surgical procedure

Practice to Pass

The nurse is assessing a 14-month-old client brought to the clinic by the mother who states, "I'm concerned about her crossed eyes." What assessments can the nurse perform to screen the child for strabismus?

II. DISORDERS OF THE EAR

    A. *Otitis media*

      1. Description

        a. Inflammation of middle ear

        b. One of the most common childhood illnesses; occurs more frequently in boys and children who attend child care centers

      2. Etiology and pathophysiology

        a. Greatest incidence is between 6 and 36 months of age during winter months

        b. Is related to dysfunction of Eustachian tube, which provides drainage and ventilation of middle ear; when it is blocked because of edema from an upper respiratory infection, fluid can accumulate in middle ear and act as a medium for bacterial growth leading to middle ear infection (see Figure 3-2)

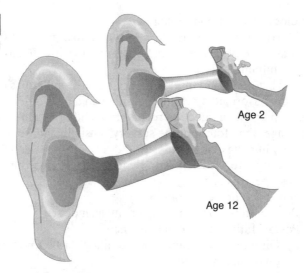

Figure 3-2

Eustachian tube in a child

Age 2

Age 12

Position of eustachian tube is at a lesser angle in the young child, resulting in decreased drainage.

End of eustachian tube in nasal pharynx opens during sucking.

Eustachian tube equalizes air pressure between the middle ear and the outside environment and allows for drainage of secretions from middle ear mucosa.

    c. Children with facial malformations such as cleft palate and Down syndrome have anatomic variations of their Eustachian tubes, which can make them more vulnerable to otitis media

    d. Causative organisms: most common organisms in otitis media are *Streptococcus pneumoniae*, *Haemophilus influenzae*, *Neisseria catarrhalis*, and *Moroxella catarrhalis*

3. Assessment

    a. Ear pain, irritability, diarrhea, fever, and vomiting are common

    b. Pulling at the affected ear may be noted; some children are asymptomatic

    c. Diagnosis is based on an examination of tympanic membrane using an otoscope; a red, bulging, nonmobile tympanic membrane indicates otitis media

4. Priority nursing diagnoses

    a. Pain

    b. Hyperthermia

    c. Risk for Injury

5. Planning and implementation

    a. Teach parents that as child grows older, position of Eustachian tube changes to facilitate drainage of middle ear

    b. Recurrent infections will eventually cease

    c. Parents should avoid smoking around child, as exposure to secondhand smoke increases incidence of otitis media; wood burning stoves should be limited

6. Medication therapy: analgesics (acetaminophen or ibuprofen) for discomfort and hyperthermia; administer antibiotics as ordered for bacterial infections

    a. Acute otitis media is treated with antibiotic therapy for 10 days in children less than 6 years

    b. Children over age 6 years are treated with antibiotics for five to seven days

7. Child and family education: teach parents that otitis media is a bacterial infection and requires a full course of treatment with antibiotics; caution parents to avoid discontinuing antibiotic when symptoms subside, but do complete full course of antibiotic therapy, usually 5 to 14 days

8. Evaluation: child recovers from otitis media without sequelae; child completes antibiotic therapy as ordered

B. Myringotomy and insertion of tympanostomy tubes

    1. Description: surgical incision of tympanic membrane with insertion of pressure-equalizing tympanostomy ear tubes to drain fluid from middle ear

2. Etiology and pathophysiology
   a. Myringotomy and insertion of tympanostomy tubes may be indicated for recurrent acute otitis media and otitis media with effusion (fluid in middle ear without inflammation)
   b. Myringotomy and insertion of tympanostomy tubes is a common surgical procedure performed on children, usually in a day surgery center
3. Assessment: if an infection recurs frequently (six times) or has a persistent effusion for longer than four months, surgery is usually indicated
4. Priority nursing diagnoses
   a. Preoperative: Deficient Knowledge (surgical procedure), Anxiety (parents and child)
   b. Postoperative: Pain
5. Planning and implementation
   a. Preoperative nursing management: includes client and family preoperative teaching
   b. Postoperative nursing management
      1) Offer pain medication (acetaminophen) as ordered for discomfort and at bedtime; encourage rest
      2) Encourage intake of generous amounts of fluids; encourage regular diet
      3) Place drops in child's ears if prescribed
6. Client and family education
   a. In addition to pain relief management, parents should follow physician's directions for postoperative care of ear; often eardrops are prescribed
   b. Some physicians require parents to insert earplugs for bathing and swimming, and avoid water in ear canal; others do not
   c. Teach parents that ear tubes will spontaneously extrude and fall out; they may note presence of spool-shaped tube in child's ear canal; ear tubes usually fall out in about one year
7. Evaluation: parents are able to observe for pain and administer ear drop or oral medication; parents insert ear plugs for bathtub and swimming if ordered

C. Hearing impairment

1. Description
   a. Condition that interferes with ability to receive auditory communications from environment
   b. There are three types of hearing impairment: conductive hearing loss, sensorineural hearing loss, and mixed hearing loss
   c. Hearing impairment is one form of **sensory impairment**, while visual impairment would be another
2. Etiology and pathophysiology
   a. Conductive hearing loss: occurs when tympanic membrane cannot vibrate freely, or when sounds cannot reach middle ear; common causes are otitis media, impacted cerumen, and foreign body in the ear canal
   b. Sensorineural hearing loss: occurs with damage to cochlea or auditory nerve; sensorineural hearing loss may be congenital (as in congenital rubella syndrome) or acquired (ototoxic drugs); hearing loss may also be genetic in origin, as in hearing loss of those affected with Tay-Sachs disease
   c. Mixed hearing loss: mixed hearing loss involves a combination of conductive and sensorineural hearing losses
3. Assessment of hearing loss/impairment
   a. In infants and young children: language development is affected; hearing loss should be diagnosed as early as possible to promote optimal language development
   b. In infancy: does not startle to loud noises, arouses to touch and not noise, does not turn head to sounds or localize sounds, little or no babbling or vocalizations

  c. In toddlers and preschoolers: communicates through gestures; little or no speech; unintelligible speech; developmental delay; no response to doorbell, telephone

  d. In school-age children and adolescents: sits close to speaker or turns up TV volume loudly, poor school performance, speech problems, cannot correctly respond except when able to view speaker's face

  e. Diagnosis: type of hearing loss is diagnosed by otoscopic examination, tympanography, and audiography

 4. Priority nursing diagnoses

  a. Impaired Sensory Perception (auditory)

  b. Impaired Verbal Communication

  c. Risk for Impaired Growth and Development

  d. Risk for Ineffective Family Coping

 5. Planning and implementation

  a. If hearing loss is correctable, treatment of cause underlying hearing loss is accomplished, for example, removal of a foreign body in conductive loss

  b. If hearing loss cannot be corrected, a multidisciplinary team consisting of otolaryngologist, audiologist, pediatrician, nurse, and speech-language pathologist should work with child and family to obtain appropriate therapies and enhance communication

  c. Hearing aids may be prescribed

  d. Cochlear implants may be used for children who have significant sensorineural hearing loss or profound deafness

   1) Minimum age to receive a cochlear implant is 12 months old; most are 2–6 years old

   2) Aids with development of speech foundations

   3) Follow-up includes speech therapy

   4) Increased risk of bacterial meningitis; all children who receive implant must receive pneumococcal vaccine (PCV) prior to surgery

  e. Nurses function in preventing acquired hearing loss through educating others to avoid exposure to loud noises

  f. Advocate prompt treatment of otitis media

  g. Nurses should be skilled in developmental assessment to aid in early identification of infants and children with hearing loss; early identification is important to prevent significant delays in developmental progress and school performance

  h. Nurses should act as advocates for clients with hearing impairment and their families; nurses can provide support and appropriate referrals to child and family dealing with this disability

 6. Client and family education

  a. Teach parents means of communicating with their children

  b. Encourage parents to enroll their child in early intervention to promote speech development

 7. Evaluation: child develops communication skills; hearing evaluations do not deteriorate

▶ **Practice to Pass**

An 18-month-old client with a history of chronic otitis media is scheduled for bilateral myringotomy with placement of tympanostomy tubes. What content will you plan to include in your preoperative and postoperative teaching sessions with the parents?

III. DISORDERS OF THE THROAT

 A. *Pharyngitis*

  1. Description: an infection of pharynx, often involving tonsils

  2. Etiology and pathophysiology

   a. A common disorder in children 4 to 7 years of age

   b. Pharyngitis is rare in infancy

      c. Approximately 80% of pharyngitis is of viral etiology, and relief of symptoms is indicated

      d. Bacterial pharyngitis is most often caused by *group A beta-hemolytic streptococcus* and requires antibiotic therapy

  3. Assessment

      a. Symptoms include sore throat, difficulty swallowing, drooling caused by sore throat, and inability to swallow saliva secretions; inflammation of pharynx and enlargement of tonsils (with or without exudate), fever, vomiting, cough, lymphadenopathy, and headache; hoarseness or a change in voice quality may be noted

      b. A throat culture is necessary to diagnose viral or bacterial etiology of pharyngitis; streptococcal infections can be diagnosed within minutes using a rapid strep test

  4. Priority nursing diagnoses

      a. Pain

      b. Deficient Fluid Volume

      c. Risk for Hyperthermia

      d. Risk for Injury (seizures secondary to high temperature)

  5. Planning and implementation

      a. In viral pharyngitis, relief of symptoms is indicated; offer diet that is easy to swallow (soft or liquids) and soothing to sore throat (no citrus juices or other foods that could cause burning or increased irritation)

      b. Saltwater gargles, throat lozenges, or anesthetic sprays can be used to promote pain relief

  6. Medication therapy

      a. Administer analgesics (acetaminophen) as ordered

      b. Administer antibiotics as ordered for bacterial infections

  7. Child and family education

      a. Stress to parents importance of completing full course of antibiotic therapy to eradicate infectious organisms

      b. Untreated or inadequately treated streptococcal infections can result in acute rheumatic fever, glomerulonephritis, or other serious sequelae

  8. Evaluation: child recovers from pharyngitis without sequelae; child completes antibiotic therapy

B. *Tonsillitis*

  1. Description: inflammation of tonsils located in posterior pharynx

  2. Etiology and pathophysiology

      a. Inflammation occurs as a result of viral or bacterial infection

      b. Causative organism in bacterial infection can be *group A beta-hemolytic streptococcus*, which is particularly virulent

  3. Assessment

      a. Diagnosis of bacterial or viral etiology is made by throat culture

      b. Streptococcal infection can be diagnosed within minutes using a rapid strep test

      c. Symptoms

         1) Enlarged, reddened tonsils, with or without exudate

         2) Sore throat, difficulty swallowing because of severe sore throat

         3) Drooling, caused by the inability to swallow saliva secretions

         4) Lymphadenopathy

         5) Mouth breathing

  4. Priority nursing diagnoses

      a. Pain

      b. Deficient Fluid Volume

    c. Risk for Hyperthermia

    d. Risk for Injury (seizures secondary to hyperthermia)

5. Planning and implementation

    a. Management for viral tonsillitis is symptom relief, i.e., promoting comfort, pain relief with acetaminophen (Tylenol); management is similar to that of viral pharyngitis

    b. Management for bacterial tonsillitis is antibiotic therapy as well as symptom relief

     c. Nursing management: offer diet that is easy to swallow (soft or liquids) and soothing to sore throat (no citrus juices or other foods that could cause burning or increased irritation)

    d. Use of saltwater gargles, throat lozenges, or anesthetic sprays can promote pain relief

6. Medication therapy: analgesics (acetaminophen) for discomfort and hyperthermia; administer antibiotics as ordered for bacterial infections

7. Child and family education: stress to parents importance of completing full course of antibiotic therapy to eradicate infectious organisms; explain how to manage symptoms

8. Evaluation: child recovers from tonsillitis without sequelae; child completes antibiotic therapy as ordered

C. Tonsillectomy

1. Description: surgical removal of tonsils to prevent recurrent tonsillitis

2. Etiology and pathophysiology

    a. Tonsillectomy may be indicated for recurrent tonsillitis, peritonsillar abscess, or respiratory compromise from airway obstruction; adenoidectomy is possible too

    b. Tonsillectomy is one of the most common childhood surgical procedures

    c. Tonsillectomy is commonly performed in a day-surgery setting, ambulatory surgical setting, or may require an overnight stay in the hospital

3. Assessment: children should be free from symptoms of tonsillitis for at least one week prior to surgery

4. Priority nursing diagnoses

    a. Preoperative

        1) Deficient Knowledge (surgical procedure)

        2) Anxiety (parents and child)

    b. Postoperative

        1) Risk for Aspiration

        2) Ineffective Airway Clearance

        3) Risk for Deficient Fluid Volume

        4) Pain

5. Planning and implementation

    a. Preoperative nursing management: includes client and family preoperative teaching and baseline lab data, including bleeding and clotting times

     b. Postoperative nursing management

        1) Provide pain control with analgesic medications and ice collar

        2) One of the most common complications is excessive bleeding or hemorrhaging from operative site; observe child for frequent or continual swallowing, vomiting bright red blood, and changes in vital signs

        3) Offer clear, chilled fluids when awake and alert; avoid red-colored fluids because emesis of these fluids could be mistaken for blood

        4) Teach child and parents that a sore throat is to be expected for approximately one week postoperatively

6. Client and family education

    a. Discharge teaching includes teaching about analgesic medications to be given at home

    b. Instruct parents to assess child for signs of complications, such as hemorrhage from the operative site

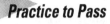

Practice to Pass

The nurse is evaluating a child who was seen in the clinic six days ago for streptococcal pharyngitis. The child complains of a sore throat today, and reports that the oral antibiotic medication prescribed was finished "a few days ago." How should the nurse proceed with assessment?

      c. Instruct parents to ensure adequate fluid intake (necessary to prevent dehydration), advance child's diet as tolerated to include soft, nonirritating and non-acidic foods, and avoid strenuous activity for about 7 to 10 days

      d. The child may return to school in 10 days, when operative site is adequately healed

  7. Evaluation: parents describe signs and symptoms of bleeding; parents state fluids and foods appropriate for postoperative child

IV. DISORDERS OF THE NOSE: EPISTAXIS

A. Description: epistaxis is also known as nosebleed

B. Etiology and pathophysiology

  1. Very common in children, especially boys

  2. Superficial veins in nares are a common source of bleeding

  3. Bleeding can occur from irritation, drying of mucosa from low humidity, or from picking the nose

C. Assessment

  1. Assess vital signs of child brought to emergency department or clinic with uncontrolled epistaxis while simultaneous efforts to control bleeding are being performed

  2. If child has experienced significant blood loss, hemoglobin and hematocrit may be measured

D. Priority nursing diagnoses

  1. Risk for Impaired Tissue Perfusion

  2. Risk for Ineffective Airway Clearance

E. Planning and implementation

  1. Teach parents and child to humidify air (especially during winter months and nighttime hours) and have child sleep with head elevated to prevent recurrence

  2. Following an episode of nosebleed, child is prone to rebleeding; child should not bend forward, drink hot liquids, exercise excessively, or take hot baths or showers for three to four days following an episode of nosebleed

F. Medical management

  1. If bleeding cannot be controlled by applying pressure, topical vasoconstrictive agents may be used, such as Neo-Synephrine, epinephrine, or thrombin

  2. Cautery may be required with silver nitrate or electrocautery

  3. If bleeding cannot be stopped, nose may be packed with absorbent packing material by health care provider to stop bleeding

G. Child and family education

  1. Teach parents how to stop a nosebleed at home by applying steady pressure to both nostrils just below nasal bone for 10 to 15 minutes

  2. Instruct parents to have child sit upright and slightly forward to be best able to apply pressure to nostrils and prevent excessive swallowing of blood

  3. Instruct parents to seek health care if bleeding cannot be stopped

  4. Teach child to avoid picking at nose or forcefully blowing nose; teach to release sneezes through mouth

H. Evaluation: parents describe appropriate means of controlling bleeding; parents identify ways they can reduce the likelihood of recurrence; parents describe symptoms that necessitate physician intervention

Practice to Pass

Following an emergency department visit for epistaxis, the parent of an 11-year-old child with a history of recurrent epistaxis states, "I wish we could prevent these nosebleeds." What teaching regarding home care can the nurse provide?

Case Study

A 7-year-old child has experienced recurrent tonsillitis for the past year. He is scheduled for a tonsillectomy later in the day. The nurse is assessing the child to obtain a database and is providing preoperative teaching and a tour of the recovery area and day surgery area to the child and parents.

1. What health history data is important to elicit from the family?

2. What laboratory tests can the nurse anticipate that will need to be completed prior to surgery?

3. What content should the nurse emphasize in pre-operative teaching directed toward the parents?

4. What content should the nurse emphasize in preoperative teaching that is directed toward the child undergoing surgery?

5. What physical assessments of the child are indicated?

For suggested responses, see pages 351–352.

POSTTEST

1 A child is to receive eye drops that have been ordered to treat conjunctivitis. Indicate on the picture where the nurse should place the drops. Draw an "X" in the correct area on the image shown.

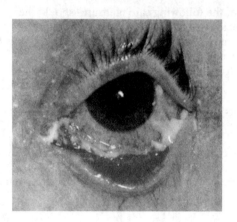

2 The nurse is caring for a 6-year-old child who just returned to the day-surgery recovery area following a tonsillectomy, adenoidectomy, and bilateral myringotomy with insertion of tympanostomy tubes. Which assessment data indicates to the nurse that the child is experiencing active, uncontrolled bleeding at the operative site?

1. Tachycardia, hypertension, and hemoptysis
2. Bradycardia, hypotension, and increased swallowing
3. Tachycardia, hypotension, and decreased swallowing
4. Tachycardia, hypotension, and increased swallowing

3 The nurse caring for a pediatric client following tonsillectomy considers which of the following unique to pediatric assessment and nursing care?

1. A child's behavioral response to pain is affected by age and developmental level.
2. Recovery from a painful procedure occurs at a faster rate in children as compared to adults.
3. Opioid analgesic use in children is dangerous because of increased risk of addiction and respiratory depression.
4. The immaturity of the nervous system in young children provides them with an increased pain threshold.

4 The nurse is beginning an otoscopic examination of the ear of a 2-year-old child. The child cries, kicks, and pulls away from the nurse. The nurse should take which of the following actions?

1. Explain to the child why the ear must be examined.
2. Postpone the examination until the next clinic visit in one year.
3. State, "I thought you were going to be grown up for me today."
4. Get assistance to gently restrain the child to proceed with the exam.

5 During a day-surgery hospitalization experience for tonsillectomy for a 4-year-old child, the nurse anticipates that the child will most likely be fearful of which of the following?

1. Intrusive procedures
2. Immobilization
3. Premature death
4. Unfamiliar caregivers

6 The nurse is performing an assessment of a 14-month-old toddler admitted to the day surgery unit for bilateral myringotomy and placement of tympanostomy tubes. To take an accurate temperature, the nurse should use which of the following? Select all that apply.

1. A tympanic thermometer with disposable speculum
2. An oral thermometer with disposable plastic sheath
3. A rectal thermometer with disposable plastic sheath
4. A temporal thermometer slid across the forehead to the top of the ear
5. A temperature strip placed on the child's forehead

7 Which of the following care measures should the nurse include when providing discharge teaching instructions for the pediatric client who has bilateral bacterial conjunctivitis? Select all that apply.

1. Use of warm, moist disposable compresses to remove crusting
2. Use of oral antihistamine medication to relieve eye itching
3. Use of topical anesthetics applied to relieve discomfort
4. Teach the parents to administer the antibiotic eye medication
5. Teach the child to wash hands frequently throughout the day

8 The nurse should teach the parent of an infant diagnosed with viral nasopharyngitis to notify the health care provider if which of the following occurs?

1. Increased fussiness
2. Cough
3. Temperature greater than 98.6°F
4. Signs of ear infection

9 A mother asks how to use saline nasal drops for her infant's nasopharyngitis. What is the appropriate response by the nurse?

1. "Do not use the drops or dropper for any other family member."
2. "Save any remaining medication for the next time the child is congested."
3. "Administer the drops frequently, until the nasal congestion subsides."
4. "Insert the dropper tip as far into the infant's nose as is possible."

10 The nurse teaches the importance of finishing the full course of oral antibiotic therapy to the caregivers of a toddler who has streptococcal pharyngitis. The nurse explains that a potential complication of inadequately treated streptococcal infection is which of the following?

1. Otitis media
2. Diabetes insipidus
3. Nephrotic syndrome
4. Acute rheumatic fever

➤ *See pages 66–67 for Answers and Rationales.*

ANSWERS & RATIONALES

Pretest

1 **Answer: 1** **Rationale:** Amoxicillin is given only by the oral route. Because of this, the nurse cannot give the dose and must question the order. There is no problem with the dosage or the frequency. **Cognitive Level:** Applying **Client Need:** Pharmacological and Parenteral Therapies **Integrated Process:** Nursing Process: Implementation **Content Area:** Child Health **Strategy:** Critical words are *amoxicillin* and *IVPB*. The question identifies an error in ordering amoxicillin. Focus on route, dose, and timing to determine the right answer. **Reference:** Potts, N., & Mandleco, B. (2012). *Pediatric nursing: Caring for children and their families* (3rd ed.). Clifton Park, NY: Delmar, pp. 614–615.

2 **Answer: 3** **Rationale:** Candida infections are a common side effect of antibiotic therapy due to alteration of the normal bacterial flora by the antibiotic agent. The white patches in the mouth do not represent allergic reaction, herpes simplex infection, or mumps. **Cognitive Level:** Analyzing **Client Need:** Physiological Adaptation **Integrated Process:** Nursing Process: Assessment **Content Area:** Child Health **Strategy:** Critical words are *cefprozil* and *patches of white on the child's oral mucosa that cannot be removed*. Recalling side effects of antibiotic therapy is necessary to answer the question correctly. This question asks for an association between antibiotics and the development of thrush infection due to loss of normal flora. **Reference:** Ball, J., Bindler, R., & Cowen, K. (2010). *Child health nursing: Partnering with children & families* (2nd ed.). Upper Saddle River, NJ: Pearson/Prentice Hall, p. 1501.

3 **Answer: 2** **Rationale:** To prevent antibiotic resistance, it is imperative to complete the full course of antibiotic therapy, even though symptoms may have resolved before the antibiotic is finished. Medicating with ear drops is not indicated unless the child had ear or tympanostomy tubes with access to the middle ear. The client may not be a candidate for a myringotomy and insertion of tympanostomy tubes. Eliminating allergens is not the focus of teaching for the client with otitis media. **Cognitive Level:** Analyzing **Client Need:** Physiological Adaptation **Integrated Process:** Teaching and Learning **Content Area:** Child Health **Strategy:** Critical words are *otitis media* and *highest priority*. Consider the item of information that would be relevant and important for all cases. **Reference:** Ball, J., Bindler, R., & Cowen, K. (2010). *Child health nursing: Partnering with children & families* (2nd ed.). Upper Saddle River, NJ: Pearson/Prentice Hall, p. 811.

4 **Answer: 2, 5** **Rationale:** The nurse must observe the post-tonsillectomy client for signs of excessive bleeding or hemorrhage from the operative site. In the posterior pharynx, the bleeding can be concealed by the child swallowing the blood. Applying heat to the neck, warm liquids, or giving a straw would be contraindicated, as this could cause bleeding. **Cognitive Level:** Analyzing **Client**

Need: Physiological Adaptation **Integrated Process:** Nursing Process: Planning **Content Area:** Child Health **Strategy:** Critical words are *nursing care of a child who is postoperative for a tonsillectomy*. Note that two options seem to be opposites, increasing the likelihood that one of them is correct. **Reference:** Potts, N., & Mandleco, B. (2012). *Pediatric nursing: Caring for children and their families* (3rd ed.). Clifton Park, NY: Delmar, pp. 796–797.

5 **Answer: 3** **Rationale:** The common cold is a viral infection. It is self-limiting, with symptoms lasting about 4 to 10 days. Therefore, emphasis is on symptom management. Nutritional intake may be decreased but is not priority in this situation. Antibiotics are not indicated for a viral infection. Injury prevention is a general concern for a child, but does not relate to the question. **Cognitive Level:** Analyzing **Client Need:** Physiological Adaptation **Integrated Process:** Nursing Process: Planning **Content Area:** Child Health **Strategy:** Critical words are *common cold* and *primary goal of nursing care*. The core concept is the medical diagnosis and, therefore, focus on determining the purpose of nursing interventions. **Reference:** Potts, N., & Mandleco, B. (2012). *Pediatric nursing: Caring for children and their families* (3rd ed.). Clifton Park, NY: Delmar, pp. 794–795.

6 **Answer: 3** **Rationale:** Turning up the volume loudly is a behavioral indicator suggesting hearing impairment. The other options are behaviors that may be consistent with the preschool developmental level and not indicative of hearing impairment. **Cognitive Level:** Analyzing **Client Need:** Physiological Adaptation **Integrated Process:** Nursing Process: Assessment **Content Area:** Child Health **Strategy:** Critical words are *sign* and *possible hearing impairment*. Knowledge of hearing impairment and behavioral indicators at the preschool developmental level helps to answer the question correctly. The only symptom that relates to hearing is turning volume up. **Reference:** Potts, N., & Mandleco, B. (2012). *Pediatric nursing: Caring for children and their families* (3rd ed.). Clifton Park, NY: Delmar, p. 1159.

7 **Answer: 2** **Rationale:** Development of parent-infant attachment is important in promoting developmental progress. Parents are encouraged to talk, sing, and interact with their baby to learn about their infant's response, and to provide appropriate stimulation at 1 month of age. The other options are incorrect statements to the parents. **Cognitive Level:** Analyzing **Client Need:** Physiological Adaptation **Integrated Process:** Teaching and Learning **Content Area:** Child Health **Strategy:** Critical words are *1-month-old client who is blind* and *promote development*. Use knowledge of normal interventions for parents of 1-month-olds to promote normal development. Then identify those that do not require vision. **Reference:** Potts, N., & Mandleco, B. (2012). *Pediatric nursing: Caring for children and their families* (3rd ed.). Clifton Park, NY: Delmar, pp. 1180–1182.

8 **Answer: 4** **Rationale:** Purulent exudate and crusting are characteristics of conjunctivitis. Conjunctivitis associated with foreign body can cause severe eye pain. Serous drainage and periorbital edema are not associated with conjunctivitis. **Cognitive Level:** Applying **Client Need:** Physiological Adaptation **Integrated Process:** Nursing Process: Assessment **Content Area:** Child Health **Strategy:** Critical words are *child with conjunctivitis* and *most likely assess*. Note that in this question, two choices describe discharge from the eye. That indicates that one of these choices is probably the right answer. **Reference:** Potts, N., & Mandleco, B. (2012). *Pediatric nursing: Caring for children and their families* (3rd ed.). Clifton Park, NY: Delmar, p. 1179.

9 **Answer: 4** **Rationale:** The infected area should be cleansed with a disposable tissue after a single use. Handwashing is important to prevent the spread of infection. Items that come in contact with the infected eye are considered contaminated. **Cognitive Level:** Analyzing **Client Need:** Physiological Adaptation **Integrated Process:** Nursing Process: Evaluation **Content Area:** Child Health **Strategy:** Critical words are *measures to prevent the spread* and *further teaching is needed*. This indicates the correct option is one that is an incorrect response from the child. Consider which of the options fails to uphold principles of infection control to choose correctly. **Reference:** Potts, N., & Mandleco, B. (2012). *Pediatric nursing: Caring for children and their families* (3rd ed.). Clifton Park, NY: Delmar, p. 1179.

10 **Answer: 3** **Rationale:** Administration of saline nose drops followed by suction with a bulb syringe is appropriate treatment for loosening and removing nasal congestion. Parents or caregivers should be reminded to wash the bulb syringe daily and rinse between uses. Administration of vasoconstrictive nose drops is contraindicated for infants. A mist tent is not the treatment for nasal congestion. The 4-month-old infant is not able to follow directions. **Cognitive Level:** Analyzing **Client Need:** Physiological Adaptation **Integrated Process:** Nursing Process: Implementation **Content Area:** Child Health **Strategy:** Critical words are *infant has severe nasal congestion* and *best way to clear the nasal passages*. Consider the age of the child to aid in choosing correctly. **Reference:** Potts, N., & Mandleco, B. (2012). *Pediatric nursing: Caring for children and their families* (3rd ed.). Clifton Park, NY: Delmar, p. 622.

Posttest

1 **Answer:**

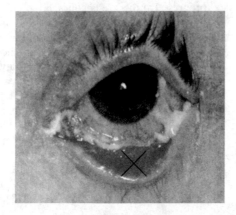

Rationale: The procedure for instilling eye drops begins with washing hands and applying clean gloves. After ensuring the medication is at room temperature and removing any discharge from the eye, the lower lid is pulled down to make a sac and the drops are applied there. The tip of the dropper should never touch the eye surface. **Cognitive Level:** Applying **Client Need:** Pharmacological and Parenteral Therapies **Integrated Process:** Nursing Process: Implementation **Content Area:** Child Health **Strategy:** The core concept is safe administration of eye drops. Recall that ointment needs to be administered in the lower conjunctival sac to follow correct administration procedure. **Reference:** Ball, J., Bindler, R., & Cowen, K. (2010). *Child health nursing: Partnering with children & families* (2nd ed.). Upper Saddle River, NJ: Pearson/Prentice Hall, p. 795.

2 **Answer: 4** **Rationale:** The nurse observes increased swallowing rather than decreased swallowing when there is bleeding following tonsillectomy. The child may also spit out red blood from the mouth at this time. Tachycardia and hypotension are late signs of significant blood loss, and these would be consistent with active uncontrolled bleeding. The child would not exhibit hypertension or bradycardia. **Cognitive Level:** Analyzing **Client Need:** Physiological Adaptation **Integrated Process:** Nursing Process: Diagnosis **Content Area:** Child Health **Strategy:** The choices here have multiple responses; consider each option individually. When considering postoperative bleeding, differentiate early signs from later signs, as well as those that are not related to blood loss. **Reference:** Ball, J., Bindler, R., & Cowen, K. (2010). *Child health nursing: Partnering with children & families* (2nd ed.). Upper Saddle River, NJ: Pearson/Prentice Hall, p. 831.

3 **Answer: 1** **Rationale:** Age and developmental level affect the pain response of a child. Infants are less able to communicate their feelings than an older child and usually demonstrate restlessness and crying behaviors. Adolescents are able to describe their pain sensations. Children do not generally recover from painful procedures more quickly than adults. Children do not have higher pain thresholds than adults Opioids are effective analgesics in the pediatric population. **Cognitive Level:** Applying **Client Need:** Physiological Adaptation **Integrated Process:** Nursing Process: Planning **Content Area:** Child Health **Strategy:** Consider the two core concepts in this question—response to pain and children as they differ from adults. Use knowledge of postoperative care and appropriate developmental considerations to choose the correct answer. **Reference:** Ball, J., Bindler, R., & Cowen, K. (2010). *Child health nursing: Partnering with children & families* (2nd ed.). Upper Saddle River, NJ: Pearson/Prentice Hall, pp. 526–527.

4 **Answer: 4** **Rationale:** Uncooperative pediatric clients may need to be gently restrained long enough to accomplish the assessment or procedure that is necessary. Parents may be able to assist with this effectively. A 2-year-old will not listen to explanations and is not likely to respond to pleas for acting maturely. The exam should not be postponed until the next yearly exam. **Cognitive Level:** Analyzing **Client Need:** Health Promotion and Maintenance **Integrated Process:** Nursing Process: Implementation **Content Area:** Child Health **Strategy:** Critical words are *2-year-old* and *cries, kicks, and pulls away*. This child, at the age of 2, is too young to understand. Reason that the answer is an intervention that allows for the exam to proceed. **Reference:** Ball, J., Bindler, R., & Cowen, K. (2010). *Child health nursing: Partnering with children & families* (2nd ed.). Upper Saddle River, NJ: Pearson/Prentice Hall, p. 211.

5 **Answer: 1** **Rationale:** One of the greatest fears of preschoolers is fear of mutilation. Immobilization and premature death are not developmentally appropriate concerns of a preschooler. Unfamiliar caregivers could be a concern for any child, but is less so than the fear of mutilation for a child of this age. **Cognitive Level:** Applying **Client Need:** Psychosocial Integrity **Integrated Process:** Nursing Process: Planning **Content Area:** Foundational Sciences **Strategy:** Knowledge of normal stress reaction to hospitalization for the developmental stage is necessary to answer the question. Compare each response with the age of the child to determine which behavior is developmentally appropriate. **Reference:** Potts, N., & Mandleco, B. (2012). *Pediatric nursing: Caring for children and their families* (3rd ed.). Clifton Park, NY: Delmar, p. 532.

6 **Answer: 1, 4** **Rationale:** Tympanic temperature readings are usually not affected by earwax, ear infections, or tympanostomy tubes. The temporal artery temperature is a non-invasive accurate method of measuring temperature at all developmental levels. A 14-month-old is not able to hold the thermometer under the tongue appropriately. Rectal temperatures should only be taken when other routes are unavailable. The temperature strip is not as accurate as other methods. **Cognitive Level:** Analyzing **Client Need:** Basic Care and Comfort **Integrated Process:** Nursing Process: Assessment **Content Area:** Child Health **Strategy:** Consider the age of the child and safety to eliminate the rectal and oral temperatures. Then consider the need for accuracy to eliminate the forehead strip. **Reference:** Potts, N., & Mandleco, B. (2012). *Pediatric nursing: Caring for children and their families* (3rd ed.). Clifton Park, NY: Delmar, pp. 442–443.

7 **Answer: 1, 4, 5** **Rationale:** Crusting of dried exudate is common with bacterial conjunctivitis. The parents will need to know how to administer the eye drops or ointment. Washing the hands frequently will reduce the spread of the infection, which is hand-to-eye and spreads easily to other children. The use of antihistamines and topical anesthetics is not indicated in the management of bacterial conjunctivitis. **Cognitive Level:** Applying **Client Need:** Physiological Adaptation **Integrated Process:** Nursing Process: Implementation **Content Area:** Child Health **Strategy:** Critical words are *home-care measures* and *bacterial conjunctivitis*. Knowledge of conjunctivitis as a contagious disease and management will help to answer the question correctly. Consider both medical and nursing interventions as

necessary to treat this infection. **Reference:** Ball, J., Bindler, R., & Cowen, K. (2010). *Child health nursing: Partnering with children & families* (2nd ed.). Upper Saddle River, NJ: Pearson/Prentice Hall, p. 795.

8 **Answer: 4** **Rationale:** Increased fussiness and elevated temperature are expected symptoms of viral pharyngitis in infants. A cough may occur because of local irritation. Symptoms of ear infection can occur because of secondary infection and should be reported to the health care provider. **Cognitive Level:** Analyzing **Client Need:** Physiological Adaptation **Integrated Process:** Teaching and Learning **Content Area:** Child Health **Strategy:** The core concept is that the illness is viral. Viral infections are usually treated symptomatically, but complications should always be noted. Knowledge of the complications of nasopharyngitis is then necessary to answer correctly. **Reference:** Ball, J., Bindler, R., & Cowen, K. (2010). *Child health nursing: Partnering with children & families* (2nd ed.). Upper Saddle River, NJ: Pearson/Prentice Hall, p. 807.

9 **Answer: 1** **Rationale:** Decongestant nose drops or spray use is contraindicated in the infant population, however normal saline is considered safe. For the older child, eliminating contact or sharing of items with the infected person can reduce the potential spread of infection to other family members. Medication should be used as specifically ordered. Medication should not be saved for use during future illness. The dropper should not be inserted "as far as possible" due to risk of injury to the infant. **Cognitive Level:** Analyzing **Client Need:** Pharmacological and Parenteral Therapies **Integrated Process:** Nursing Process: Implementation **Content Area:** Child Health **Strategy:** Critical words are *nasal drops are prescribed for an infant*. Specific knowledge of use of medication in this developmental level and the correct method to administer nasal drops will help to answer this question correctly. **Reference:** Ball, J., Bindler, R., & Cowen, K. (2010). *Child health nursing: Partnering with children & families* (2nd ed.). Upper Saddle River, NJ: Pearson/Prentice Hall, pp. 826–827.

10 **Answer: 4** **Rationale:** Rheumatic fever can follow an infection of certain strains of group-A beta-hemolytic streptococci. Otitis media is an ear infection that can be caused by many organisms, but is not the priority concern related to a strep infection. Diabetes insipidus and nephrotic syndrome are pituitary and renal disorders, respectively, but are not related to sequelae of strep infection. **Cognitive Level:** Applying **Client Need:** Physiological Adaptation **Integrated Process:** Teaching and Learning **Content Area:** Child Health **Strategy:** The core question is *what is a sequela of untreated streptococcus infection?* Knowledge of antibiotic resistance and complications from strep help to answer the question correctly. **Reference:** Ball, J., Bindler, R., & Cowen, K. (2010). *Child health nursing: Partnering with children & families* (2nd ed.). Upper Saddle River, NJ: Pearson/Prentice Hall, p. 956

References

Ball, J., Bindler, R., & Cowen, K. (2010). *Child health nursing: Partnering with children and families* (2nd ed.). Upper Saddle River, NJ: Pearson Education.

Hockenberry, M., & Wilson, D. (2009). *Wong's essentials of pediatric nursing* (8th ed.). St. Louis, MO: Elsevier.

Hockenberry, M., & Wilson, D. (2011). *Wong's nursing care of infants and children* (9th ed.). St. Louis, MO: Elsevier.

Jarvis, C. (2012). *Physical examination and health assessment* (6th ed.). St. Louis, MO: Elsevier.

Kee, J. (2010). *Laboratory and diagnostic tests* (8th ed.). Upper Saddle River, NJ: Pearson Education, Inc.

London, M., Ladewig, P., Ball, J., Bindler, R., & Cowen, K. (2011). *Maternal & child nursing care* (3rd ed.). Upper Saddle River, NJ: Pearson Education.

Respiratory Health Problems

4

Chapter Outline

Overview of Anatomy and Physiology of Respiratory System

Diagnostic Tests of the Respiratory System

Congenital Respiratory Health Problems

Acquired Respiratory Health Problems

Infectious Respiratory Health Problems

Accidents and Injuries Causing Respiratory Health Problems

Objectives

➤ Identify data essential to the assessment of alterations in health of the respiratory system in a child.

➤ Discuss the clinical manifestations and pathophysiology of alterations in health of the respiratory system of a child.

➤ Discuss therapeutic management of a child with alterations in health of the respiratory system.

➤ Describe nursing management of a child with alterations in health of the respiratory system.

NCLEX-RN® Test Prep

Use the accompanying online resource, NursingReviewsandRationales, to test yourself with hundreds of NCLEX®-style practice questions.

Review at a Glance

alveoli small, saclike dilatations of terminal bronchioles where oxygen–carbon dioxide gas exchange takes place

atelectasis incomplete expansion or collapse of lung caused by obstruction of airway from secretions or a foreign body

barrel chest anteroposterior diameter of chest is increased to give chest a rounded appearance; caused by air trapping and hyperinflation of alveoli, resulting in skeletal changes

bronchopulmonary dysplasia (BPD) chronic obstructive pulmonary disease occurring in infants after prolonged exposure to mechanical ventilation and oxygen therapy

digital clubbing increased rounding of nails of fingers and toes with a loss of normal angle at base of nail; an indication of hypoxia

dyspnea difficult breathing

epiglottis structure that covers larynx during swallowing to prevent food from entering trachea

foreign body aspiration inhalation, intentional or otherwise, of an object into respiratory tract

hypercapnia excessive carbon dioxide in blood

hypoxemia deficiency of oxygen in blood

laryngotracheobronchitis a viral infection that causes inflammation,

edema, and narrowing of larynx, trachea, and bronchi

peak expiratory flow rate maximum amount of air that can be forcibly exhaled

surfactant phospholipid produced by alveoli that reduces surface tension of fluids and aids in lung expansion

sweat test measures sweat sodium and chloride concentrations; sample is collected from child's forearm on absorbent material; a level greater than 60 mEq/L is diagnostic for cystic fibrosis

tachypnea rapid respirations

trigger initiator of an asthmatic episode

PRETEST

1 The mother of an infant who has had recurrent respiratory infections asks the nurse why infants are at increased risk for complications from respiratory infections. What information should the nurse include when formulating a response?

1. Airway structures are larger, allowing for entry of larger numbers of organisms.
2. Respiratory rate is slower than in adults.
3. Parents are unable to accurately assess respiratory problems.
4. Airways are narrower and more easily obstructed.

2 The mother of a neonate hospitalized with an upper respiratory tract infection asks why her baby will not take her bottle. The nurse's best answer would be which of the following?

1. "She's probably not hungry."
2. "It's okay because we're giving her intravenous fluids; therefore, she is not hungry."
3. "Newborns breathe through their noses. Congestion may be interfering with her breathing and eating at the same time."
4. "She might need a different type of formula. We'll call the physician to get a new order."

3 A 4-year-old female child presents to the emergency department with a sore throat, difficulty swallowing, and a suspected diagnosis of acute epiglottitis. Initial assessment of the child should include which of the following? Select all that apply.

1. Throat culture
2. Vital signs
3. Past medical history
4. Auscultation of chest
5. Observation of swallowing ability

4 The nurse is providing homecare instructions to the parents of a child with cystic fibrosis. Which statement by the parents indicates that they do not understand the treatment regimen? Select all that apply.

1. "We will perform chest physiotherapy and postural drainage four times a day."
2. "We will keep her away from the church nursery if any of the children are coughing and have fever or runny noses."
3. "If her bowel movements are normal and her appetite is good, she does not need her pancreatic enzymes."
4. "The relay races and swimming at our Sunday school picnic next week will be good exercise for her."
5. "My child will not need any special dietary intake."

5 A 2-year-old child is being discharged after bronchoscopy for removal of a coin from his esophagus. The most important topic of discharge teaching would be the importance of which of the following?

1. Reassuring the child that he is fine
2. Proper nutrition for the next few days
3. Restricting his access to small toys or objects
4. Administering acetaminophen for his sore throat

6 A 15-year-old child with a history of cystic fibrosis is admitted to the pediatric unit with assessment findings of crackles, increased cough, and greenish sputum. A two-week hospitalization is anticipated. Which nursing intervention holds the highest priority?

1. Referral to Child Life Services for school lesson plans
2. Arranging for liberal visitation from peers
3. Taking a diet history
4. Gaining intravenous access

7 A 7-year-old child is brought to the emergency department for an acute asthma attack. He is wheezing, tachypneic, diaphoretic, and looks frightened. The nurse should prepare to administer which of the following?

1. IV methylprednisolone
2. Albuterol
3. Oral prednisone
4. Cromolyn sodium

8 The nurse would select which of the following as an appropriate nursing diagnosis for the family of a toddler being treated for acute laryngotracheobronchitis?

1. Anticipatory Grieving
2. Impaired Growth and Development related to acute onset of illness
3. Impaired Social Interaction related to confinement in hospital
4. Fear/Anxiety related to dyspnea and noisy breathing

9 A 3-year-old child with bacterial pneumonia is crying and says it hurts when he coughs. The nurse would teach the child to do which of the following?

1. Hug his teddy bear when he coughs
2. Ask for pain medicine before he coughs
3. Take a sip of water before coughing
4. Try very hard not to cough

10 An infant with chronic bronchopulmonary dysplasia (BPD) and a tracheostomy is being discharged on home oxygen therapy. Which statement by the mother indicates that further teaching is needed before discharge?

1. "I will call my pediatrician if she gets a fever or has more secretions than usual from her tracheostomy."
2. "I have a cute bib to loosely cover her tracheostomy when she eats and when we go outside in the wind."
3. "We are so glad the baby will get to go with us on our camping trip to Yellowstone National Park. We have been waiting for her to get well so we can go."
4. "We have already notified Alabama Power Company that our baby is coming home today."

➤ *See pages 88–90 for Answers and Rationales.*

I. OVERVIEW OF ANATOMY AND PHYSIOLOGY OF RESPIRATORY SYSTEM

A. Structures

1. Upper airways: nose, pharynx, and larynx provide pathway for air to enter body and ultimately lungs; **epiglottis** covers larynx, which is located between pharynx and trachea, and keeps food from entering lower respiratory tract; these upper structures also warm, humidify, and filter inspired air
2. Lower airways: trachea, bronchi, bronchioles, and **alveoli** conduct air and produce surfactant; alveoli are small, saclike extensions of terminal bronchioles where gas exchange takes place and blood is reoxygenated; hairlike projections called cilia provide mucus to upper airway to aid in trapping of debris and foreign particles; **surfactant** is a phospholipid that aids in lung elasticity and alveoli expansion

B. Physiology

1. Prenatal development
   a. Development of respiratory system should be complete prior to birth to establish breathing and exchange of oxygen (O_2) and carbon dioxide (CO_2) at birth; premature infants lack sufficient surfactant and have many underdeveloped and uninflatable alveoli, which compromise gas exchange
   b. Oxygenation is responsibility of placenta in utero; fetal pulmonary blood flow is minimal, there is little lung movement, and collapsed lungs are filled with fluid excreted through alveoli; pulmonary vascular resistance is increased and most blood is shunted away from lungs by foramen ovale and ductus arteriosus

 2. Postnatal changes
   a. The birth process and delivery stimulate breathing and inflation of lungs; a decreased O_2 level in blood (**hypoxemia**), an increased CO_2 level (**hypercapnia**), and acidosis stimulate respiratory center in medulla of brainstem and cause initiation of breathing

    b. Compression of chest through birth canal squeezes fetal lung fluid from lungs, and abrupt coolness of outside environment sends impulses to respiratory center in medulla

    c. Surfactant reduces surface tension of fluid lining the alveoli to facilitate entry of air into lungs; inspiration causes diaphragm to contract, lengthen, and decrease intrapulmonic pressure; gases then move from an area of higher to lower concentration; O_2 and CO_2 exchange that occurs in alveoli and blood provides body tissues with O_2 needed for survival

C. Pediatric differences

    1. Size

        a. There is a shorter distance between structures in young children

        b. Lumen of young child's respiratory tract is smaller and, thus, more easily obstructed; diameter of trachea is approximately the size of child's little finger

        c. There are fewer alveoli at birth; numbers, size, and shape continue to increase until puberty

        d. Eustachian tubes are shorter and more horizontal, facilitating transfer of pathogens into middle ear; lymphoid and tonsillar tissue is normally enlarged and may obstruct passage of air

    2. Function

        a. Neonates are nose-breathers; therefore, any obstruction in nasal passages interferes with breathing and eating

        b. Narrower airways increase airway resistance and child's risk for obstruction by edema, mucus, or foreign objects

        c. Infant's airway walls have less cartilage, and are more flexible and more prone to collapse; intercostal muscles are immature; chest wall is less stable, and retractions are more common

        d. Newborns have less respiratory mucus to function as a cleaning agent

        e. Increased respiratory and metabolic rates increase need for oxygen

II. DIAGNOSTIC TESTS OF THE RESPIRATORY SYSTEM

Practice to Pass

A 12-month-old child returns to the pediatric unit after a bronchoscopy. His mother is concerned that he has not eaten today and starts to prepare a bottle of formula. How will you respond to her?

A. Chest x-ray: visualization of size and shape of airways, lungs, heart, diaphragm, and rib cage; posterior, anterior, lateral, and oblique views may be taken; no preparation or discomfort occurs other than wearing lead apron if repeated x-rays are taken; female adolescents should be protected with a lead apron if there is any possibility of pregnancy

B. Computed tomography (CT scan): visualization of tumors or lesions; contrast medium may be used, necessitating that child not eat or drink for three to four hours prior to procedure; this procedure requires immobilization and possibly sedation

C. Bronchoscopy: a bronchoscope is utilized to visualize trachea and bronchi directly; lesions can be located and sized; secretions and foreign bodies can be cleared from airway

    1. Preprocedure care

        a. Witness signature on informed consent: procedure is done under local or general anesthesia; assess client and family's understanding and anxiety level

        b. Child should be NPO to guard against aspiration when gag reflex is suppressed

        c. Administer prescribed sedative or narcotic as premedication; observe for bradycardia and hypotension

    2. Postprocedure care

        a. Assess for return of swallow and gag reflexes; keep NPO until reflexes return; position flat and side-lying if not fully alert

        b. Observe for signs of airway obstruction: dyspnea, cyanosis, stridor

        c. Expect blood-streaked sputum for several hours; report any frank blood (may indicate hemorrhage)

D. **Pulmonary function tests** measure child's respiratory ability, response to treatment, and degree of lung disease; a child as young as 5 or 6 years is usually able to follow commands and cooperate; **peak expiratory flow rate** (PEFR), the maximum amount of air that can be exhaled after a normal inspiration, is a very useful test of function; a spirometer is used and child is allowed to become familiar with equipment; instructions include practice in breathing normally through mouth and blowing into spirometer

E. **Sputum culture**
   1. Isolates pathogens and identifies sensitivities for antibiotic selection if needed
   2. Best collected in early morning as secretions accumulate during sleep and thus contain most organisms
   3. Young children are unable to produce sputum; nasal or gastric washing with sterile saline is performed to obtain a sample; maintain standard precautions and wear protective eyewear and masks if splashing is a possibility

F. **Arterial blood gases (ABGs)**
   1. Determine level of O_2 and CO_2 circulating in an arterial blood sample
   2. Provide information about acid–base balance
   3. Collect in a heparinized syringe; place on ice and transport to lab immediately; apply pressure to puncture site for at least five minutes and monitor for hematoma formation and adequacy of peripheral circulation

G. **Pulse oximetry** measures O_2 saturation and need for O_2 therapy; it is noninvasive and measures amount of infrared light waves absorbed as they travel through perfused areas of body

III. CONGENITAL RESPIRATORY HEALTH PROBLEMS

A. **Cystic fibrosis (CF)**
   1. Description
      a. Multisystem disorder of exocrine glands, leading to increased production of thick mucus in bronchioles, small intestines, and pancreatic and bile ducts
      b. Increased viscosity of secretions obstructs small passageways of these organs and interferes with normal pulmonary and digestive functioning
         1) Lung problems are most serious threat to life; thick, sticky secretions pool in bronchioles, cause **atelectasis** (collapse of alveoli) and serve as a medium for bacterial growth
         2) Pancreatic ducts become clogged with thick secretions and prevent pancreatic enzymes from reaching duodenum, impairing digestion and absorption
         3) Small intestines, in the absence of pancreatic enzymes, are unable to absorb fats and protein; thus, growth and puberty are retarded
   2. Etiology and pathophysiology
      a. Inherited as an autosomal recessive trait; gene on chromosome 7 responsible for functioning of cystic fibrosis transmembrane regulator (CFTR) is defective; absence of CFTR as a chloride channel interferes with sodium-chloride transport, prohibiting movement of water across cell membranes; the most common cystic fibrosis gene mutation ΔF508 (delta 508) causes the most common CF symptoms
      b. Usually diagnosed in infancy and early childhood; affects white children primarily; rarely seen in blacks and children of Asian descent; males and females are affected equally
      c. Life expectancy has increased to median age of 30 years, but disease is terminal; death usually results from resistant pulmonary organisms and fibrosis and destruction of lung tissues

3. Assessment
   a. Diagnostic
      1) **Sweat test** (pilocarpine iontophoreses) analyzes sodium and chloride content in sweat; a chloride concentration greater than 60 meq/L is diagnostic of cystic fibrosis (gold standard for diagnosis); parents often report that infants taste salty when kissed
      2) 72-hour fecal fat
      3) Chest x-ray
      4) Prior to delivery, prenatal DNA analysis of amniotic fluid shows intestinal alkaline phosphatase is reduced in a fetus with CF
   b. Nursing
      1) History usually reveals frequent bouts of respiratory infections
      2) Observe for any respiratory impairment, i.e., cough, presence and color of sputum, **dyspnea** (difficulty breathing), color of nailbeds and mucous membranes, pulse oximetry; auscultate breath sounds for equality, crackles, wheezes, or any increased respiratory effort, observe for clubbing of fingers and toes; **digital clubbing** (indicating hypoxia) produces nails with increased rounding and a loss of normal angle at base of nail
      3) Assess nutritional status by obtaining height and weight and plot on growth charts; skin turgor and mucous membranes reveal hydration status; record diet history and activity tolerance; signs of malabsorption include bulky, frothy, foul-smelling stools called steatorrhea, and unusually protuberant abdomen and thin extremities; often first sign of CF is meconium ileus, where intestine is blocked with thick, tenacious secretions in newborn period and neonate is unable to pass first meconium stool
4. Priority nursing diagnoses
   a. Ineffective Airway Clearance
   b. Impaired Gas Exchange
   c. Risk for Infection
   d. Imbalanced Nutrition: Less Than Body Requirements
   e. Activity Intolerance
   f. Fear/Anxiety
   g. Deficient Knowledge
   h. Risk for Ineffective Family Coping
5. Planning and implementation
   a. Respiratory: monitor for retractions, dyspnea, cyanosis, color of sputum, quality of cough; ensure bronchial hygiene is performed, auscultate breath sounds before and after treatments; encourage coughing and deep breathing exercises and physical activity as tolerated; administer prescribed antibiotics and bronchodilator
   b. Digestive: provide high-calorie (150% above normal recommendations), high-protein diet and snacks; give infants a predigested formula such as Pregestimil or Nutramigen; administer pancreatic enzymes with all meals and snacks; individualize to achieve stools as near normal as possible; administer fat-soluble vitamins; determine food preferences to encourage acceptance of diet; weigh daily; avoid pulmonary treatments immediately after meals to decrease risk of vomiting
6. Medications: antibiotics for treatment of pulmonary infection and purulent secretions, pancreatic enzymes for fat absorption, vitamin supplementation, mucolytics to decrease viscosity of sputum, bronchodilators to improve lung function; see Table 4-1 for overview of commonly ordered respiratory care medications
7. Client and family education
   a. Avoid exposure to respiratory infections; report immediately any fever, increase in cough, or change in sputum

Table 4-1	Medications Commonly Used to Treat Respiratory Problems		
Medication	**Use**	**Action**	**Nursing Considerations**
Bronchodilators **Includes short and long-acting beta$_2$ agonists** Albuterol (Proventil) Epinephrine (Adrenalin) Metaproterenol (Alupent) Terbutaline (Brethaire) Levalbuterol (Xopenex) Pirbuterol (Maxair) Salmeterol (Serevent) Formoterol (Foradil)	May be used for acute and daily therapy; routes of administration include oral, inhaled, and parenteral	Relax smooth muscles in the airways	Tachycardia, restlessness, and increased activity may be side effects; reduction in dose usually lessens the undesired effects; inhaled drugs have more rapid onset; to prevent exercise-induced asthma episode, give drug at least 15 minutes before sustained activity
Anti-inflammatory corticosteroids Prednisone (Deltasone and others) Methylprednisolone (Medrol) Beclomethasone (Vanceril) Budesonide (Pulmicort) Fluticasone (Flovent) Fluticasone propionate (Advair)	Used to reduce the inflammatory response during or to prevent an asthmatic attack; oral, inhaled, IV preparations are available	Reduce inflammation and mucosal edema in airways	Lowest possible dose of steroids to avoid side effects of growth retardation, fluid retention, increased appetite, mood changes; inhaled steroids have fewer side effects than oral administration; rinse mouth after inhalation to prevent oral candidiasis; take oral drug with food or milk to minimize stomach upset; give at least 15 minutes before prolonged exercise to prevent exercise-induced asthma episode
Nonsteroidal anti-inflammatory drugs (NSAIDs) Cromolyn sodium (Intal) Nedrocromil sodium (Tilade)	Used as prophylaxis or treatment of asthma; oral, nasal, and inhaled preparations are available (cromolyn); inhaled preparation only (nedrocromil)	Used prophylactically and for prevention of exercise-induced asthma episode	Should be taken regularly for proper effect
Diuretic Furosemide (Lasix) available	Diuretic; oral, IV preparations are available	Removes excess fluid from lungs	Monitor for electrolyte changes; maintain strict intake and output; advise clients to take drug in morning to avoid sleep disturbances from increased urination
Mucolytics Dornase alfa (Pulmozyme) Acetylcysteine (Mucomyst)	Used in cystic fibrosis as inhalation drug	Loosen and thin pulmonary secretions to facilitate removal by coughing	Teach proper use of inhaler
Antibiotics Penicillins Cephalosporins Aminoglycosides Fluoroquinolones	Used for bacterial infections in pneumonia, epiglottis after cultures to determine sensitivities; available in oral or parenteral forms	Kill bacteria to cure infection	Obtain specimens for cultures and sensitivities; ascertain client allergies and drug reactions; administer drugs as scheduled; course of drug therapy may be prolonged, teach family to complete the entire antibiotic dose for the time prescribed; family should observe for signs of superinfection, such as thrush or monilial diaper dermatitis
Pancreatic enzymes Pancrelipase (Creon, Pancrease, Pancrecarb, Cotazym, Ultrase)	Used in cystic fibrosis to aid in digestion and absorption of nutrients; supplied in capsule form that can be opened and the powder sprinkled on a small amount of food	Pancreatic enzyme replacement	Enzymes must be consumed before or with every meal or snack; capsules can be swallowed whole or mixed with applesauce for infants and small children; if taken apart do not add powder to hot foods or enzyme activity will be compromised; enzyme dosage is adjusted based on number and consistency of stools and whether or not adequate weight gain is maintained

---

Box 4-1

Chest Physiotherapy (CPT)

- Child is dressed in a lightweight shirt.
- Percussion is performed with a cupped hand striking the chest over a portion of the lung; if done properly, a popping sound will be heard.
- Some children, especially older children and adolescents, use an oscillating vest to mobilize secretions instead of chest physiotherapy.
- Postural drainage facilitates removal of secretions that are loosened during percussion; for drainage, various head-down positions drain all lung segments.
- Positioning for bronchial drainage can be achieved by child standing on his head, hanging upside down on monkey bars, and other playground activities that are fun for the child.
- Avoid performing CPT immediately after eating.

Practice to Pass

A 6-year-old child has cystic fibrosis and is hospitalized for an acute respiratory infection. The play-room has scheduled a puppet show and the child's mother asks you if he can get his antibiotics later so he will not miss the show. What facts will you consider as you decide how to respond?

   b. Chest percussion and postural drainage must be performed three to four times daily; noncompliance will result in increased hospitalizations and infections; see Box 4-1 for instructions on chest physiotherapy and postural drainage
   c. High-calorie, high-protein diet is essential; give pancreatic enzymes with all meals and snacks; may need extra salt in hot weather
   d. Physical activity and exercise loosen secretions and promote lung expansion
   e. Provide information on community resources, such as Cystic Fibrosis Foundation, American Lung Association; provide social service consults, home-health referrals with visiting nurses and respiratory therapists
   f. Genetic counseling will help guide future childbearing decisions
   g. Provide written information on medications, breathing exercises, chest physiotherapy, and postural drainage
   h. Suggest clergy, mental health services, respite care, and families of other children with CF to assist with psychologic and emotional coping with chronic, progressive illness
8. Evaluation: family demonstrates and verbalizes intent to adhere to home care regimen of pulmonary treatments, medications, diet, and exercises; child gains weight consistently, participates in self-care and age-appropriate activities; child demonstrates ability to clear secretions from airway by productive cough, O_2 saturation greater than 94% and decreased respiratory distress

IV. ACQUIRED RESPIRATORY HEALTH PROBLEMS

   A. *Bronchopulmonary dysplasia (BPD)*
   1. Description
   a. Chronic obstructive pulmonary disease occurring in infants after prolonged O_2 therapy and mechanical ventilation
   b. Premature infants with BPD have usually survived respiratory distress syndrome; term infants generally have serious respiratory problems, also requiring ventilatory assistance
   2. Etiology and pathophysiology
   a. High oxygen concentrations and mechanical ventilation damage bronchial epithelium and alveoli; thickened alveolar walls, scarring, and fibrosis lead to atelectasis, poor airway clearance of mucus, and poor gas exchange; chronic low oxygenation results in decreased lung compliance and altered function
   b. Lung immaturity is a major contributor to occurrence of BPD, and improved survival rates of premature infants have increased incidence of BPD; as little as three days of positive pressure ventilation can increase an infant's risk of developing BPD
   c. There may be a genetic predisposition; males have increased morbidity

Figure 4-1

Barrel chest

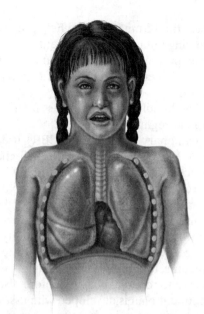

3. Assessments
   a. Diagnosed by chest x-ray, which reveals lung changes and air trapping with or without hyperinflation
   b. ABGs reveal hypercapnia and respiratory acidosis
   c. Respiratory observations include **tachypnea** (rapid respirations), tachycardia, increased work of breathing, retractions, wheezing, and **barrel chest** (rounding of chest caused by trapped air) (Figure 4-1)
   d. Pallor, activity intolerance, and poor feeding result from chronic hypoxia
4. Priority nursing diagnoses
   a. Impaired Gas Exchange
   b. Ineffective Airway Clearance
   c. Imbalanced Nutrition: Less Than Body Requirements
   d. Impaired Growth and Development
   e. Caregiver Role Strain
   f. Risk for Infection
   g. Anxiety/Fear
5. Planning and implementation
   a. Infants with BPD are cared for in intensive care units and require an artificial airway; avoid pressure or trauma to endotracheal tube and infant's airway
   b. Suction, turn, and weigh carefully to ensure O_2 saturations are maintained
   c. Monitor respiratory status continuously; infant's condition can worsen in a short period of time
   d. Monitor for fluid overload; infants are at increased risk for pulmonary edema; weigh daily; maintain strict intake and output
   e. Strict handwashing; avoid exposure to respiratory infections
   f. Cluster nursing care to minimize O_2 requirements and caloric expenditure
   g. Plan quiet stimulation and activities to foster normal infant development and parental bonding given the extended, and often repeated, hospitalizations of infants with BPD
6. Medications (see Table 4-1)
   a. Bronchodilators open airways and increase lung compliance
   b. Corticosteroids reduce edema and inflammation in airways

    c. Diuretics remove excess fluid from lungs and help prevent pulmonary edema; may require accompanying potassium supplementation

    d. Antibiotics may be given prophylactically; palivizumab (Synagis) injections 15 mg/kg are given monthly from October through April for high-risk infants to prevent RSV

7. Client and family education

    a. Infants are discharged with multiple needs; assess family's understanding and ability to follow treatment regimen

    b. Teach parents cardiopulmonary resuscitation (CPR), use of home monitoring equipment, and oxygen therapy; infants are usually discharged with a tracheostomy when oxygen concentration requirements are low

    c. Review infection control practices, i.e., handwashing, avoidance of family members with respiratory infections; teach warning signs of illness

    d. Teach safety precautions regarding O_2 therapy and tracheostomy care; see Box 4-2 for instructions on home tracheostomy care; contact utility companies, emergency services, and telephone companies before discharge of a technology-dependent child

    e. Review basic care—feeding, bathing, playing, holding—with parents; allow parents opportunities to care for child in hospital before discharge; after basic care is mastered, medical treatment plan is developed with assistance of parents

    f. Make referrals to community agencies for supplies, medications, nutrition, parental support, and stimulation programs to foster growth and development

---

Box 4-2

Tracheostomy Home Care and Oxygen Therapy

Discharge instructions for a child with a tracheostomy should include the following:

- Keep small toys, talcum powder, plastic bibs and bedding, and any small particles away from child to decrease risk for aspiration or occlusion of trachea.
- Be sure child wears cloth bib loosely over tracheostomy when eating to prevent food particles from entering tube.
- Be careful when bathing to keep water from entering trachea; showers are not recommended.
- Cover tracheostomy loosely when outside in strong wind and cold to prevent tracheal spasms.
- Observe skin around tracheostomy daily for redness, breakdown, or any signs of infection.
- Change tracheostomy ties weekly or more frequently if needed; be sure to use non-fraying material; always have assistance to change ties.
- Clean area around tracheostomy daily with half-strength saline or diluted soap and water. When dry, place a notched gauze pad under and around the tube.
- Suction tracheostomy tube when needed to remove secretions from the child's airway; use sterile gloves and limit suctioning to five seconds. Insert suction catheter only to the length of the tracheostomy tube and apply intermittent suction while withdrawing the catheter. Some hospitals use a closed suction system with colored dots on the suction catheter used for suction limits.
- Be sure child is allowed to rest between suctioning if catheter is passed more than once.
- Notify physician if tracheal secretions are increased or become purulent, or if child develops a fever.
- Keep written instructions available at all times.
- Keep emergency bag with extra suction catheters and tracheostomy tubes available.
- Notify utility companies and emergency medical services that child in the home requires emergency equipment.
- Do not allow smoking in the home of child with oxygen therapy; avoid friction-type toys.
- Keep oxygen tanks away from any heat source; keep a fire extinguisher nearby.

Practice to Pass

What are the risk factors contributing to the development of bronchopulmonary dysplasia (BPD)?

8. Evaluation: family demonstrates ability to care for child and seek medical attention when needed; infant maintains ABGs within normal range; infant demonstrates ability to clear airway by respiratory rate and rhythm within normal limits; infant demonstrates consistent growth and performs age-appropriate developmental tasks

B. Asthma

1. Description
   a. Chronic inflammatory disorder in which airways narrow and are hyperreactive to stimuli that do not affect nonasthmatic individuals
   b. Exposure to an irritant causes bronchial muscles to go into spasm, leading to increased respiratory effort; increased airway resistance, air trapping, and exhaustion results

2. Etiology and pathophysiology
   a. Exposure to an irritant causes constriction of bronchial smooth muscle, edema, increased secretion of thick mucus, and airway narrowing; expiration through the narrowed lumen is impaired, resulting in air trapping and hyperinflation of alveoli
   b. The initiator of an asthmatic episode, called a **trigger**, can be any number of stimuli, including inhalants, airborne pollens, stress, weather changes, exercise, viral or bacterial agents, food additives, etc.
   c. It is unclear exactly how heredity factors into occurrence of asthma, but there is a familial tendency
   d. Although incidence of asthma has risen, severity of attacks may lessen as child grows and airway increases in size

3. Assessments
   a. Diagnostic
      1) Chest x-ray reveals hyperinflation of airways
      2) Pulmonary function tests reveal reduced peak expiratory flow rate (PEFR); using peak flow meter daily warns of impending attack
   b. Wheezing and dry cough indicate an asthma episode; prolonged expiration, restlessness, fatigue, and tachypnea are observed as child struggles to breathe despite hyperinflated, poorly ventilated alveoli
   c. Chronic use of accessory muscles for respiration leads to a barrel chest in children with frequent exacerbations

4. Priority nursing diagnoses
   a. Ineffective Airway Clearance
   b. Impaired Gas Exchange
   c. Activity Intolerance or Fatigue
   d. Ineffective Family Processes
   e. Deficient Knowledge

5. Planning and implementation
   a. Assess for cyanosis or marked respiratory distress; administer humidified oxygen if needed; monitor pulse oximetry
   b. Maintain IV access to ensure sufficient intake of fluids to replace insensible losses from hyperventilation and for medication administration; avoid cold liquids to decrease risk of bronchospasm
   c. Monitor airway response to treatment; sudden cessation of wheezing and decreased breath sounds with increased respirations may indicate worsening of child's condition
   d. Position in high-Fowler's and cluster nursing care to conserve child's energy

6. Medications for asthma include bronchodilators and anti-inflammatory agents administered orally, parenterally, or by inhalation (see Table 4-1)

7. Client and family education
   a. Explain that goal is to prevent acute asthma episodes and to ensure optimal physical and psychologic health; check status daily with peak flow meter
   b. Teach family to identify and avoid potential triggers
   c. Assess family's coping skills and ability and willingness to care for child and adhere to therapy
   d. Review parents' understanding of asthma and how to recognize signs and symptoms of an impending attack
   e. Teach parents to monitor PEFR: 80–100% green; 50–80% yellow; <50% red
   f. Arrange for additional support and continuous education through special camps, clinics, schools, and community agencies such as the American Lung Association
8. Evaluation: family verbalizes accurate knowledge of asthma and plans to adhere to therapy; child engages in age-appropriate activities; child maintains clear airway with normal respiratory effort; child maintains adequate ventilatory capacity as evidenced by PEFR at personal best

V. INFECTIOUS RESPIRATORY HEALTH PROBLEMS

A. Acute *laryngotracheobronchitis* (LTB)

1. Description
   a. Viral infection that causes inflammation, edema, and narrowing of larynx, trachea, and bronchi; usually LTB is preceded by a recent upper respiratory infection
   b. LTB is most common in infants and toddlers and affects boys more often than girls; it is the most common of the croup syndromes
2. Etiology and pathophysiology
   a. LTB is usually caused by parainfluenzae virus, influenzae A and B, respiratory syncytial virus (RSV) and *Mycoplasma Pneumoniae*
   b. Inflammation and narrowing of airways cause inspiratory stridor and suprasternal retractions as child struggles to inhale air; increased production of thick secretions and edema further obstruct airway and cause hypoxia and CO_2 accumulation; leads to respiratory acidosis and respiratory failure
3. Assessments
   a. Onset is gradual after upper respiratory infection

   b. Child awakens at night with low-grade fever, barking seal-like cough, and acute stridor; noisy breathing and the use of accessory muscles increase
   c. Child is agitated, restless, has a frightened appearance, sore throat, and rhinorrhea
   d. Pulse oximetry is used to detect hypoxemia; anteroposterior (AP) and lateral upper airway x-rays are ordered
4. Priority nursing diagnoses
   a. Ineffective Breathing Pattern
   b. Fear/Anxiety
   c. Deficient Knowledge
   d. Risk for Deficient Fluid Volume
5. Planning and implementation
   a. Monitor child's respiratory effort continuously to ensure a patent airway; observe for diminished breath sounds, circumoral cyanosis, cessation of noisy breathing, and drooling; may use Clinical Scoring System for Assessing Children with Stridor, which assigns rating of 0 to 3 each on categories for stridor, retractions, air entry, color, and level of consciousness
   b. Quiet respiratory effort is a sign of physical exhaustion and impending respiratory failure

    c. Provide humidity and supplemental O_2; intravenous (IV) fluids prevent dehydration and help liquefy secretions; increased humidity may not affect overall symptoms

    d. Assist child to assume upright position or any position of comfort; promote a calm, quiet environment; keep parents nearby to decrease child's stress and to lessen crying

    e. Keep emergency intubation equipment available at bedside; nurse is also immediately available

    f. Assess parental and child's anxiety level; provide emotional support

6. Medications (see Table 4-1)

    a. Bronchodilators and nebulized racemic epinephrine are used less frequently with croup because they do not reduce symptoms and may provide only temporary relief

    b. Corticosteroids, especially oral or IM dexamethasone (Decadron), three times daily for 72 hours, decrease inflammation and edema

7. Client and family education

    a. Assess parental anxiety and ability to adhere to medical recommendations

    b. Symptoms are usually worse at night and may recur for several nights; instruct parents that child can be cared for at home if able to take fluids by mouth and has no stridor at rest

    c. Cool mist humidifier and presence of parents can be initial treatment of crisis; comforting measures include cuddling, rocking, singing, and any calming measures until breathing becomes easier

    d. Instruct parents to seek medical attention immediately if breathing becomes labored, child seems exhausted or very agitated, or if symptoms do not improve after cool air humidity treatment

    e. Teach parents that LTB is a viral illness; avoid contact with large groups of people and practice infection control measures

8. Evaluation: parents demonstrate understanding of home care and need for medical attention; child breathes without difficulty; breath sounds are clear; heart and respiratory rates are within normal limits for age

B. Epiglottitis

1. Description

    a. Inflammation and swelling of epiglottis, primarily affecting children between ages of 2 and 8 years

    b. Site of obstruction is supraglottic and is life threatening because edema in this area can obstruct airway and occlude trachea within minutes

2. Etiology and pathophysiology

    a. Bacteria, usually *Haemophilus influenzae*, cause epiglottis to become cherry red, swollen, and so edematous that it obstructs airway; secretions pool in pharynx and larynx; child has a sore throat and is unable to swallow; complete airway obstruction can occur within two to six hours; considered a medical emergency

    b. Onset is sudden, in a previously healthy child; the Hib vaccine has reduced incidence of epiglottitis to rarely occurring, although the causative organisms may also be streptococcus and staphylococcus

3. Assessments

    a. Child awakens with sudden onset of high fever (102.2°F), extremely sore throat, and pain on swallowing

    b. Child is very anxious, restless, looks ill, and insists on sitting upright leaning on arms, with chin thrust out and mouth open (tripod position)

    c. Dysphonia (muffled voice), dysphagia (difficulty swallowing), drooling of saliva, and distressed respiratory effort are classic signs of epiglottitis

    d. Edematous, cherry-red epiglottis is most reliable diagnostic sign

    e. Examination of throat is contraindicated, however, unless emergency intubation equipment and trained personnel are available; physical manipulation of hypersensitive and irritated airway muscles may result in spasm and complete obstruction

    f. Lateral neck x-ray confirms an enlarged epiglottis; x-rays are portable and completed in examination room with child on parent's lap to minimize stress and maximize child's comfort and calm behavior

    g. Complete blood count and blood cultures are taken once child is intubated and stabilized

4. Priority nursing diagnoses

    a. Fear

    b. High Risk for Suffocation

    c. Ineffective Breathing Pattern

    d. Ineffective Airway Clearance

5. Planning and implementation

    a. Assess continuously for respiratory distress and decrease in respiratory effort; report changes in status

    b. Never leave child unattended; support child in position of comfort; encourage parents to hug and cuddle their child

    c. All invasive procedures, including starting an IV infusion, ABGs, and blood cultures are performed in operating room; do not attempt to casually examine throat

    d. Keep endotracheal and tracheotomy tubes and suction equipment at bedside; assist with emergency ventilation if needed before child is taken to operating room for airway insertion

    e. Child is usually intubated for 24 hours; restraints may be necessary to prevent dislodgment of tube, as swelling of the epiglottis may prohibit reintubation

    f. Provide support for child and family and alleviate anxiety; explain all procedures clearly and calmly

    g. Keep child NPO; IV fluids provide hydration; administer antipyretics and antibiotics as prescribed

    h. After extubation, monitor child closely in intensive care unit to ensure immediate assessment if respiratory effort is compromised

6. Medications

    a. Antibiotics treat bacterial infection and are usually given for 7 to 10 days; child is discharged in about three days on oral antibiotics

    b. Antipyretics treat fever and manage the pain of sore throat

    c. Dexamethasone (Decadron), a corticosteroid, may be given for 24 hours before extubation to decrease edema

7. Child and family education

    a. Provide emotional support and explain all procedures calmly; encourage parents to cuddle and comfort child

    b. Prepare child and parents for airway insertion in operating room

    c. Teach parents importance of completing antibiotic regimen after discharge; explain medications, how to administer, and any side effects to be expected

    d. Discuss importance of Hib vaccine and reassure parents that recurrence of epiglottitis is uncommon

8. Evaluation: parents describe home care and completion of antibiotics; child breathes without difficulty and maintains pink mucous membranes and nail beds; child demonstrates relaxed posture and sleeps quietly

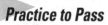

Practice to Pass

You are the nurse in the emergency department. The mother of a 2-year-old with epiglottitis tells you that she has to call her husband to come to the hospital. She saw a telephone down the hall and informs you that she will be right back. What are your concerns? How will you respond?

C. Pneumonia

1. Description
   a. Inflammation of lungs that occurs most often in infants and young children; bronchioles and alveolar spaces are affected
   b. Pneumonia may be a primary condition or can occur secondary to another illness

2. Etiology and pathophysiology
   a. Viruses from upper respiratory tract are usual cause; virus invades alveoli and bronchial mucosa, causing sloughing and debris; respiratory syncytial virus (RSV) is common organism and causes severe illness in immunocompromised infant
   b. Bacterial pneumonia occurs when organisms circulating in bloodstream travel to lungs, increase in number, and damage pulmonary cells; alveoli are filled with fluid and exudate and may involve one segment or entire lung; a history of a viral infection usually precedes bacterial pneumonia
   c. *Mycoplasma pneumoniae* infection is most common in older children (over 5 years) in fall and winter, and occurs in crowded living conditions

3. Assessments
   a. Viral pneumonia
      1) Child usually presents with mild fever, nonproductive cough, and rhinitis
      2) Disease is self-limiting and lasts five to seven days; high-risk infants with RSV invasion may demonstrate wheezing, tachypnea, and increased respiratory distress
   b. Bacterial pneumonia
      1) Children with bacterial pneumonia usually present with high fever, productive cough, and ill appearance
      2) There may be retractions, grunting respirations, chills, and chest pain; respiratory distress is significant and accompanied by restlessness and anxiety
   c. Chest x-ray reveals density of lung tissue, patchy infiltrates, and increased fluid; pulse oximetry and ABG measurements determine oxygenation; complete blood count and blood cultures determine if causative agent is viral or bacterial; consolidation or patchy infiltrate occur regardless of type and may cause diminished breath sounds upon auscultation

4. Nursing diagnoses
   a. Ineffective Airway Clearance
   b. Ineffective Breathing Pattern
   c. Risk for Deficient Fluid Volume
   d. Anxiety
   e. Activity Intolerance/Pain

5. Planning and implementation
   a. Monitor breath sounds, respiratory rate, use of accessory muscles, color, O_2 saturation levels, and level of activity and restlessness every two hours
   b. Encourage child to assume position of comfort, usually upright; assist child to cough, deep breathe, and change position often; teach splinting to ease discomfort with coughing; lying on affected side may also splint chest and decrease discomfort
   c. Ensure chest physiotherapy is performed as ordered; administer O_2 if needed; encourage child to use incentive spirometer
   d. Administer antipyretics and analgesics for temperature control and pain relief
   e. Administer oral and/or IV fluids as ordered to ensure hydration; keep strict intake and output records; weigh daily; assess for signs of dehydration
   f. Provide cool mist to aid in temperature reduction; change linens and bedclothes often to prevent chilling from dampness

      g. Assist infants and young children with clearing secretions by bulb syringe and/or deep suction as needed

      h. Provide emotional support to parents

      i. Cluster nursing care to allow for periods of undisturbed rest and a quiet environment

  6. Medications

      a. Antibiotics treat bacterial infection after culture and sensitivity reports indicate causative organism

      b. Acetaminophen and ibuprofen reduce fever and promote comfort

  7. Client and family education

      a. Explain all treatments and procedures to child and family; encourage parents to stay and participate in child's care

      b. Assess ability of parents to care for child at home

      c. Teach parents to take child's temperature; discuss importance of oral fluids and inform parents of recommended amounts appropriate to child's age

      d. Child may go home on oral antibiotics; explain actions, dosage, times, and importance of continuing until entire prescription is completed; discuss any expected side effects

      e. Discuss infection control and prevention measures; explain importance of avoiding ill contacts and adhering to immunization schedule; the *Haemophilis influenzae* type b vaccine, pneumococcal conjugate vaccine with *Streptococcus pneumoniae* coverage, and 23-valent pneumococcal vaccine (recommended for children >2 years or who are immunosuppressed) have greatly decreased the incidence of pneumonia

      f. Child will need additional rest periods after discharge

      g. Lungs may not be completely healed when symptoms disappear; follow-up chest x-ray may be needed to determine status of lung tissue

  8. Evaluation: parents verbalize knowledge and ability to adhere to treatment regimen regarding medications, oral fluids, assistance with clearing of secretions; child is afebrile, and respiratory rate and O_2 saturation levels are within normal limits for age; child participates in activities of daily living and consumes adequate hydration; child receives appropriate immunizations

D. Bronchiolitis

  1. Description

      a. Inflammation of bronchioles with edema and excess accumulation of mucus; air trapping and atelectasis result from increased airway resistance because of small obstructed bronchioles

      b. A major cause of hospitalization of high-risk infants

  2. Etiology and pathophysiology

      a. Respiratory syncytial virus (RSV) is primary causative organism; virus is spread by contact with contaminated objects; RSV is not airborne but can live for several hours on nonporous surfaces

      b. RSV bronchiolitis is most prevalent during first 2 years of life, with most occurrences in spring and winter; bronchiolitis usually begins with a mild upper respiratory infection; as disease progresses, gas exchange is compromised, hypoxemia results, and metabolic acidosis develops

  3. Assessments

      a. Clinical manifestations include worsening of an upper respiratory tract infection with tachypnea, retractions, low-grade fever, anorexia, thick nasal secretions, and increasingly labored breathing; older infants may have a frequent, dry cough

      b. Auscultation of lungs reveals wheezing or crackles

      c. Nasopharyngeal washing to obtain respiratory secretions identifies causative virus; chest x-ray may be normal or indicate hyperinflation or nonspecific inflammation

4. Priority nursing diagnoses

      a. Ineffective Airway Clearance related to increased airway secretions

      b. Impaired Gas Exchange related to lack of oxygen

      c. Parental Anxiety related to child's respiratory distress

      d. Deficient Fluid Volume related to decreased intake

5. Planning and implementation

      a. Complete a respiratory assessment hourly; provide humidified O_2 to ease respiratory effort; pulse oximetry to assess O_2 levels

      b. Clear nasal passages with bulb syringe or small French catheter; elevate head of bed

      c. Cluster nursing care to allow for rest; assess anxiety level of parents and provide support; maintain a calm environment

      d. IV fluids may be needed if oral intake is compromised; monitor strict intake and output; weigh daily to assess fluid loss

      e. Maintain strict handwashing and contact precautions; caregivers should not care for other high-risk children

6. Medications

      a. Palivizumab (Synagis) is used to prevent RSV for high risk clients under the age of 2 years

      b. Bronchodilators and steroids are sometimes used

7. Client and family education

      a. Explain disease process and provide support to lessen anxiety

      b. Encourage parents to assist in care of their infant; explain all procedures and treatments

      c. Teach parents to use bulb syringe as needed to keep nasal passages clear

      d. Teach parents to provide frequent oral fluids; notify physician if child demonstrates symptoms of dehydration, including crying without tears, sunken eyes, lethargy, or "acts sick"

      e. Instruct parents to notify physician if child refuses to eat or breathing becomes worse

      f. Instruct parents to use humidifier in child's bedroom and to clean humidifier to decrease risk of fungus and mold growth

      g. Teach parents to avoid smoking in child's vicinity

      h. Teach parents to practice strict handwashing; keep child away from individuals with upper respiratory infections; RSV can reoccur

8. Evaluation: child demonstrates clear breath sounds and regular respirations; child consumes adequate oral fluids and has moist mucous membranes; parents verbalize understanding of disease and participate in child's care

VI. ACCIDENTS AND INJURIES CAUSING RESPIRATORY HEALTH PROBLEMS

A. Foreign body aspiration

    1. Description

      a. Inhalation of an object into respiratory tract, intentional or otherwise

      b. Peak age for **foreign body aspiration** is children less than 3 years of age; it is a leading cause of death in children under 1 year

    2. Etiology and pathophysiology

      a. Foreign bodies usually lodge in right main bronchus because it is shorter and wider than left; obstruction may be partial or complete and causes atelectasis, air trapping, and hyperinflation distal to site of obstruction

b. The type and shape of object, as well as small diameter of an infant's airway, determines severity of problem; round objects such as hot dogs, round candy, nuts, and grapes do not break apart and are more likely to occlude the airway; latex balloons are particularly hazardous; objects with irregular shapes may irritate airway and partially obstruct airflow

    c. Failure to remove a foreign object is usually fatal; a delay in removal may cause aspiration pneumonia

3. Assessments

    a. Sudden coughing and gagging is first sign and objects in upper airway may be expelled

    b. Partial obstruction may cause symptoms of respiratory infection for days or even weeks; child may have hoarseness, croupy cough, wheezing, and dyspnea

    c. If obstruction is worsening, child will demonstrate stridor, cyanosis, and difficulty swallowing and speaking

    d. A child who cannot speak, is cyanotic, and collapses requires immediate attention for complete airway obstruction

    e. Fluoroscopy and chest x-ray reveal foreign body in respiratory tract

4. Priority nursing diagnoses

    a. Ineffective Airway Clearance

    b. Ineffective Breathing Pattern

    c. Fear/Anxiety

    d. Deficient Knowledge related to child safety

5. Planning and implementation

    a. Respiratory assessment to determine severity of problem and degree of obstruction; continuous monitoring to provide assistance if obstruction worsens

    b. If total airway obstruction occurs, perform back blows and chest thrusts for infants, and Heimlich maneuver in children older than 1 year

    c. Keep NPO; foreign body is usually removed in surgery

    d. Position for comfort and to optimize airway; provide emotional support to parents and child and alleviate anxiety

    e. After removal of object, assess for additional obstruction that may be caused by laryngeal edema and tissue swelling

6. Medications

    a. Antibiotics may be administered if secondary infection is suspected

    b. They may also be used if purulent secretions are present in airway, with or without signs of pneumonia

7. Client and family education

    a. Teach parents about hazards of aspiration and importance of child-proofing the home

    b. Review age-appropriate foods and discuss most frequently aspirated objects: coins, hot dogs, balloons, nuts, popcorn, grapes, round candy, peanut butter

    c. Discuss toy safety and avoidance of toys with small, removable parts; caution against allowing child to run and play with objects in his or her mouth

    d. Teach parents CPR and techniques of chest thrusts, back blows, and abdominal thrusts

8. Evaluation: child maintains a patent airway and has normal breath sounds; parents verbalize an understanding of needed child safety precautions

Practice to Pass

The father of a 3-year-old child is feeding him peanut butter on a spoon at snack time. What information would be appropriate for this dad?

Case Study

A 7-year-old child is being discharged after initial diagnosis and treatment of acute asthma. You are the pediatric asthma educator completing the final education session with his parents.

1. What instructions regarding the peak expiratory flow meter will you discuss?

2. How will you respond when the child's parents tell you they plan to restrict him from physical education at school in order to prevent another attack?

3. What information will assist the child's parents in avoiding an exacerbation by recognizing subtle signs of an asthma episode?

4. What is the purpose of a spacer with the metered dose inhaler?

5. What is the overall goal of asthma education discharge teaching?

For suggested responses, see page 352.

POSTTEST

POSTTEST

① The mother of an infant diagnosed with bronchiolitis asks the nurse what causes this disease. The nurse's response would be based on the knowledge that the majority of infections that cause bronchiolitis are a result of which of the following?

1. *Klebsiella* infection
2. *Mycoplasma pneumoniae*
3. Respiratory syncytial virus (RSV)
4. *Hemophilus influenzae*

② The nurse is educating the parents of a child who was recently diagnosed with asthma. When reviewing the medications, the nurse focuses on which anti-inflammatory corticosteroid used to prevent an asthma attack?

1. Terbutaline (Brethaire)
2. Levalbuterol (Xopenax)
3. Cromolyn sodium (Intal)
4. Budesonide (Pulmicort)

③ An 18-month-old male client, who was seen in the emergency department with respiratory distress, is admitted to the nursing unit with a diagnosis of pneumonia. Following the initial workup, the client is still short of breath but is rubbing his eyes as if he is sleepy. The mother wants to lie the client down for his nap, but he refuses. The nurse suggests which of the following as the most effective strategy to promote rest?

1. Rock the client until he is asleep and then lay him down.
2. Hold him in a supine position while he sleeps.
3. Allow him to sleep in an upright position.
4. Give him an over-the-counter sleeping pill.

④ Which statement by an 8-year-old female client who has asthma indicates that she understands the use of a peak expiratory flow meter?

1. "My peak flow meter can tell me if an asthma episode might be coming, even though I might still be feeling okay."
2. "When I do my peak flow, it works best if I do three breaths without pausing in between breaths."
3. "I always start with the meter reading about halfway up. That way I don't waste any breath."
4. "If I use my peak flow meter every day, I will not have an asthma attack."

5 A child with cystic fibrosis is hospitalized for a respiratory infection. Which documentation in the chart would indicate the need for counseling regarding nutrition and gastrointestinal complications?

1. Frothy, foul-smelling stools
2. Weight unchanged from yesterday
3. Consumed 80% of breakfast
4. Eats three snacks every day

6 An adolescent was diagnosed with cystic fibrosis as an infant. At this time, the nurse anticipates that the adolescent will need additional teaching related to which of the following?

1. Obtaining a sweat chloride test
2. The effect of pancreatic enzymes on sex hormones
3. Increased need for a weight reduction diet
4. Reproductive ability

7 A 10-month-old child is being admitted with laryngotracheobronchitis in the middle of the night. The child has a loud stridor and moderate respiratory distress. In planning care for this child, the nurse will identify which of the following as appropriate nursing diagnoses? Select all that apply.

1. Fear / Anxiety
2. Ineffective Breathing Pattern
3. Risk for Deficient Fluid Volume
4. Deficient Knowledge
5. Anticipatory Grieving

8 A 9-month-old infant has been admitted to the pediatric unit with respiratory syncytial virus infection. The nurse assigned to provide care to this infant will need to be assigned to care for other clients as well. The charge nurse should assign the nurse to which other children as an appropriate assignment? Select all that apply.

1. A toddler with neuroblastoma undergoing chemotherapy
2. A 10-year-old with a fractured femur in traction
3. An infant with immunodeficiency
4. A preschooler with impetigo
5. A 2-year-old with aplastic anemia

9 The nurse is teaching home tracheostomy care to the parents of a toddler. What information would be essential for the nurse to include?

1. The importance of changing the tracheostomy every day
2. How to recognize signs of infection and obstruction
3. How to remove the tracheostomy so the child can talk
4. Teaching the child to keep large objects away from the tube

10 A child with a respiratory infection is scheduled to have a sweat test. After the physician discusses the test with the mother, the mother approaches the nurse and asks the purpose of this diagnostic test. Which response by the nurse would best reinforce the physician's explanation?

1. "This will determine if your child is dehydrated."
2. "This will assess whether your child's sweat glands are functioning."
3. "This will help us to identify the infectious organism."
4. "This will diagnose whether the child has cystic fibrosis."

➤ *See pages 90–92 for Answers and Rationales.*

ANSWERS & RATIONALES

Pretest

1 **Answer: 4** **Rationale:** Infants and young children have narrower airways, and shorter distance between structures; accessory muscles generally used for breathing are immature. The respiratory rate of infants is faster than adults and parents can be taught to assess the child for respiratory problems. **Cognitive Level:** Analyzing **Client Need:** Physiological Adaptation **Integrated Process:** Nursing Process: Implementation **Content Area:** Child Health **Strategy:** Critical words are *why infants are at increased risk for complications from respiratory infections*. The core knowledge is the physiological differences between infants and older children. **Reference:** Ball, J.,

Bindler, R., & Cowen, K. (2010). *Child health nursing: Partnering with children & families* (2nd ed.). Upper Saddle River, NJ: Pearson/Prentice Hall, pp. 840–841.

2 Answer: 3 Rationale: Newborns are unable to coordinate breathing and sucking simultaneously. They are nose-breathers, and anything that interferes with nasal patency impairs feeding as well. The difficulty with sucking does not relate to hunger or selection of formula. **Cognitive Level:** Analyzing **Client Need:** Physiological Adaptation **Integrated Process:** Communication and Documentation **Content Area:** Child Health **Strategy:** Critical words are *neonate hospitalized with an upper respiratory tract infection* and *baby won't take her bottle*. The core concept is a neonate with an upper respiratory infection (URI) and refusal to suck. The knowledge of normal coordination of breathing that is hampered by the nasal congestion will help to guide the correct answer. **Reference:** Ball, J., Bindler, R., & Cowen, K. (2010). *Child health nursing: Partnering with children & families* (2nd ed.). Upper Saddle River, NJ: Pearson/Prentice Hall, p. 840.

3 Answer: 2, 3, 4, 5 Rationale: In epiglottitis, any manipulation of the throat can cause stimulation of the gag reflex. The inflamed, edematous epiglottis could then completely obstruct the airway. All other assessments should be made cautiously to keep the child from experiencing anxiety and irritability. **Cognitive Level:** Applying **Client Need:** Physiological Adaptation **Integrated Process:** Nursing Process: Assessment **Content Area:** Child Health **Strategy:** Critical words are *epiglottitis* and *initial assessment should include*. Knowledge of epiglottitis and its care and management is needed to determine which assessment should not be done. **Reference:** Ball, J., Bindler, R., & Cowen, K. (2010). *Child health nursing: Partnering with children & families* (2nd ed.). Upper Saddle River, NJ: Pearson/Prentice Hall, p. 860.

4 Answer: 3, 5 Rationale: Children with cystic fibrosis require pancreatic enzymes with every meal and snack to counter malabsorption and nutritional problems. They require well-balanced diets with 120–150% of RDA calories and 200% protein. Normal bowel movements indicate that enzyme dosage is appropriate. It is important to avoid other children with infections, but physical activity is encouraged within the child's capability. Chest percussion is a normal part of health maintenance for this child. **Cognitive Level:** Analyzing **Client Need:** Physiological Adaptation **Integrated Process:** Nursing Process: Evaluation **Content Area:** Child Health **Strategy:** Critical words are *child with cystic fibrosis* and *indicates the parents do not understand*. This leaves the two choices that illustrate a lack of understanding of the needed home care. **Reference:** Ball, J., Bindler, R., & Cowen, K. (2010). *Child health nursing: Partnering with children & families* (2nd ed.). Upper Saddle River, NJ: Pearson/Prentice Hall, pp. 898–900.

5 Answer: 3 Rationale: Toddlers put many small objects into their mouths causing risk for aspiration. Reassuring the client is important but not the most important focus of

discharge teaching. Due to discomfort from the bronchoscopy, the client may not feel like eating the first few days after the procedure. The pediatric client may have a transient sore throat from the bronchoscopy procedure but pain is not the focus of the question. **Cognitive Level:** Analyzing **Client Need:** Health Promotion and Maintenance **Integrated Process:** Teaching and Learning **Content Area:** Child Health **Strategy:** Critical words are *removal of a coin* and *most important topic*. Knowledge of foreign body aspiration and teaching about prevention of future aspirations and removal of potential hazards is essential to prevent future problems. **Reference:** Ball, J., Bindler, R., & Cowen, K. (2010). *Child health nursing: Partnering with children & families* (2nd ed.). Upper Saddle River, NJ: Pearson/Prentice Hall, p. 603.

6 Answer: 4 Rationale: Gaining intravenous access is of great importance so the pediatric client can receive IV antibiotics for CF lung infection. It is important for the client to keep up with school assignments during hospitalization but not a priority when newly admitted for antibiotic therapy. Socialization with peers is important but not priority when the adolescent client is admitted for antibiotic therapy. Review and discussion of diet may be discussed at some point during the admission to the hospital. **Cognitive Level:** Analyzing **Client Need:** Physiological Adaptation **Integrated Process:** Nursing Process: Planning **Content Area:** Child Health **Strategy:** Knowledge of cystic fibrosis and illness management of the disease to prevent complications is essential to answer the question. The highest priority for the client will be related to respiratory function. Therefore, planning for IV access allows for rapid implementation of the medical plan of care. **Reference:** Ball, J., Bindler, R., & Cowen, K. (2010). *Child health nursing: Partnering with children & families* (2nd ed.). Upper Saddle River, NJ: Pearson/Prentice Hall, p. 899.

7 Answer: 2 Rationale: Albuterol is a short acting beta2-agonist given via inhalation for relaxation of the smooth muscle in the airway leading to rapid bronchodilation. It should not be used to control asthma on a long term basis. Methylprednisolone is a corticosteroid to decrease airway inflammation and obstruction while enhancing the bronchodilating effects of the beta2-agonists. It does not give immediate relief for an asthma attack. Oral prednisone is a corticosteroid that reduces airway inflammation. While it is used for short-term therapy, the medication does not provide immediate relief. Cromolyn sodium is an anti-inflammatory mast cell inhibitor used to prevent exercise induced asthma. It does not provide immediate relief. **Cognitive Level:** Applying **Client Need:** Pharmacological and Parenteral Therapies **Integrated Process:** Nursing Process: Planning **Content Area:** Pharmacology **Strategy:** The critical word here is *acute* asthma attack. Knowledge of the medications used to treat asthma emergencies is necessary to answer the question correctly. Select the medication that would be utilized during an acute attack. **Reference:** Ball, J., Bindler, R., & Cowen, K. (2010). *Child health* *nursing: Partnering with children & families* (2nd ed.). Upper Saddle River, NJ: Pearson/Prentice Hall, p. 881.

8 **Answer: 4** **Rationale:** The sudden onset of severe respiratory distress is frightening and very stressful for the family and child. There is no prolonged hospital confinement. There is not an anticipated permanent loss for grieving and growth and development is not likely to be affected. **Cognitive Level:** Analyzing **Client Need:** Psychosocial Integrity **Integrated Process:** Nursing Process: Diagnosis **Content Area:** Child Health **Strategy:** Critical words are *toddler* and *laryngotracheobronchitis*. Consider the symptoms of acute laryngeotracheobronchitis since the diagnosis is frightening but not fatal and has no long-term sequelae. **Reference:** Ball, J., Bindler, R., & Cowen, K. (2010). *Child health nursing: Partnering with children & families* (2nd ed.). Upper Saddle River, NJ: Pearson/Prentice Hall, p. 859.

9 **Answer: 1** **Rationale:** Splinting the client's affected side when coughing will lessen the pain. Providing a developmentally appropriate option such as a teddy bear may increase compliance with the intervention. Coughing occurs throughout the day and night. It is not feasible to time the coughing episodes. The cough reflex cannot be prevented or delayed to allow for a sip of water. Coughing should be encouraged to remove the secretions from the lungs. **Cognitive Level:** Applying **Client Need:** Physiological Adaptation **Integrated Process:** Nursing Process: Implementation **Content Area:** Child Health **Strategy:** The child is complaining of pain during coughing, so look for a choice that would reduce pain without suppressing the cough reflex. **Reference:** Ball, J., Bindler, R., & Cowen, K. (2010). *Child health nursing: Partnering with children & families* (2nd ed.). Upper Saddle River, NJ: Pearson/Prentice Hall, p. 870.

10 **Answer: 3** **Rationale:** Tracheostomy care requires access to oxygen and emergency equipment generated by electricity, sometimes not available at camping sites. If the child is receiving oxygen, campfires should be avoided. Camping is not an optimal vacation venue. Increased secretions may indicate infection. The pediatrician should be notified. A non-confining bib will prevent food particles and debris from entering the tracheostomy. Notifying the electric company of a needed back up electrical source in the event of a power failure is essential. **Cognitive Level:** Analyzing **Client Need:** Safety and Infection Control **Integrated Process:** Nursing Process: Evaluation **Content Area:** Child Health **Strategy:** Critical words are *home oxygen therapy* and *statement indicates that further teaching is needed*. Because wording of the question guides you to select an incorrect statement, eliminate all responses that are appropriate for home care of a child with a tracheostomy and receiving oxygen. **Reference:** Ball, J., Bindler, R., & Cowen, K. (2010). *Child health nursing: Partnering with children & families* (2nd ed.). Upper Saddle River, NJ: Pearson/Prentice Hall, pp. 867–868.

Posttest

1 **Answer: 3** **Rationale:** At least one-half of all cases of bronchiolitis are attributed to respiratory syncytial virus. The majority of cases of bronchiolitis are not attributable to *klebsiella*, *mycoplasma pneumoniae*, or *hemophilus influenzae*. **Cognitive Level:** Applying **Client Need:** Physiological Adaptation **Integrated Process:** Teaching and Learning **Content Area:** Child Health **Strategy:** This question asks for basic information related to causation of bronchiolitis. Critical words are *majority* and *bronchiolitis*. Use knowledge of the etiology of the disease to choose the correct answer. **Reference:** Ball, J., Bindler, R., & Cowen, K. (2010). *Child health nursing: Partnering with children & families* (2nd ed.). Upper Saddle River, NJ: Pearson/Prentice Hall, p. 864.

2 **Answer: 4** **Rationale:** Budesonide is an inhaled corticosteroid used to reduce inflammation and mucosal edema in the airways. Budesonide and other corticosteroids are not rescue drugs and will not provide immediate relief. Terbutaline is a short-acting beta agonist (SABA) used to relax smooth muscle in the airway leading to rapid bronchodilation and mucus clearing. Levalbuterol is a short-acting beta agonist (SABA) used for the treatment of acute exacerbations and for the prevention of bronchospasm. Cromolyn sodium is a non-steroidal anti-inflammatory (NSAID) used for asthma. It stabilizes mast cell membranes and inhibits the acute airway narrowing after exposure to cold air and exercise. **Cognitive Level:** Applying **Client Need:** Pharmacological and Parenteral Therapies **Integrated Process:** Nursing Process: Planning **Content Area:** Child Health **Strategy:** The critical words are *anti-inflammatory corticosteroid*. Knowledge of the groups of medications commonly used to treat asthma is necessary to answer the question correctly. Select the medication that belongs to the corticosteroid group. **Reference:** Ball, J., Bindler, R., & Cowen, K. (2010). *Child health nursing: Partnering with children & families* (2nd ed.). Upper Saddle River, NJ: Pearson/Prentice Hall, pp. 886–887.

3 **Answer: 3** **Rationale:** The upright position promotes oxygenation and decreases respiratory distress. Laying the client in the supine or prone position causes more discomfort and respiratory distress. The client should be held or placed in a semi or high Fowler's position. Holding the client in a supine position may cause more discomfort and distress. Over-the-counter sleeping pills are contraindicated for an 18-month-old client. **Cognitive Level:** Analyzing **Client Need:** Physiological Adaptation **Integrated Process:** Nursing Process: Implementation **Content Area:** Child Health **Strategy:** The core concept is positioning for respiratory distress. Determine the correct answer by analyzing which choice best promotes oxygenation. **Reference:** Potts, N., & Mandleco, B. (2012). *Pediatric nursing: Caring for children and their families* (3rd ed.). Clifton Park, NY: Delmar, p. 804.

4 **Answer: 1** **Rationale:** The peak flow meter provides a quantitative measurement of the maximum flow of air that the cooperative client can push forcefully out of the lungs. Consistent readings between 50–80% or less of the client's "personal best" indicate an asthma episode may be imminent. When using the peak flow meter, it is essential to pause and recover between breaths to ensure optimal peak expiratory flow. The meter is set according to the pediatric client's height and personal best after reviewing the recorded peak expiratory flow readings (PEFRs) measured twice daily for two to three weeks. The peak expiratory flow meter is a screening tool for asthma. It is not a treatment. **Cognitive Level:** Analyzing **Client Need:** Physiological Adaptation **Integrated Process:** Teaching and Learning **Content Area:** Child Health **Strategy:** Critical words are *understands* and *peak expiratory flow meter*. Knowledge of this device and how it helps to manage asthma helps to answer the question. **Reference:** Potts, N. & Mandleco, B. (2012). *Pediatric nursing: Caring for children and their families* (3rd ed.). Clifton Park, NY: Delmar, p. 814.

5 **Answer: 1** **Rationale:** Frothy, foul-smelling stools reflect malabsorption and indicate that pancreatic enzymes are not being consumed or dosages may need adjustment. Maintenance of weight and consuming meals and snacks are positive nutrition goals for children with cystic fibrosis. **Cognitive Level:** Applying **Client Need:** Physiological Adaptation **Integrated Process:** Nursing Process: Assessment **Content Area:** Foundational Sciences **Strategy:** Eliminate normal findings to determine which documentation indicates the need for nutrition intervention. **Reference:** Ball, J., Bindler, R., & Cowen, K. (2010). *Child health nursing: Partnering with children & families* (2nd ed.). Upper Saddle River, NJ: Pearson/Prentice Hall, pp. 898–900.

6 **Answer: 4** **Rationale:** The developmental task of adolescence is to set future goals, including marriage and family. Men are usually sterile, and women may have decreased fertility as thick cervical mucus interferes with mobility of sperm. The difference between sterility and impotence should also be addressed. The client does not need information about a sweat chloride test (diagnostic test for the disease) or weight reduction. There is no adverse effect of pancreatic enzymes on sex hormones. **Cognitive Level:** Applying **Client Need:** Health Promotion and Maintenance **Integrated Process:** Nursing Process: Planning **Content Area:** Child Health **Strategy:** The critical word is *adolescent*. Consider the changes that occur with adolescence to determine the needs at this time. **Reference:** Ball, J., Bindler, R., & Cowen, K. (2010). *Child health nursing: Partnering with children & families* (2nd ed.). Upper Saddle River, NJ: Pearson/Prentice Hall, p. 902.

7 **Answer: 1, 2, 3, 4** **Rationale:** The child and the parents will be anxious about the child's condition and the need for emergency admission to the hospital. Respiratory distress is an obvious sign and defining characteristic of ineffective breathing pattern. The child will need extra fluids due to increased insensible fluid loss and inability to take fluids due to respiratory distress. The parents will want to know the cause of the disease and interventions for future episodes. The outcome for this disease is usually positive anticipatory grieving would not be appropriate. **Cognitive Level:** Applying **Client Need:** Respiratory **Integrated Process:** Nursing Process: Planning **Content Area:** Strategy: Appropriate nursing diagnoses are based on the clinical picture of the disease. With this in mind, select nursing diagnoses that relate to breathing, effects of dyspnea on fluid and food intake, and the need for information about the disease. **Reference:** Ball, J., Bindler, R., & Cowen, K. (2010). *Child health nursing: Partnering with children & families* (2nd ed.). Upper Saddle River, NJ: Pearson/Prentice Hall, pp. 856–860.

8 **Answer: 2, 4** **Rationale:** If the nurse and health care providers wash their hands between contacts with the pediatric clients, the nurse may care for the client with RSV and the fractured femur. Both pediatric clients have communicable illnesses, making it an acceptable assignment; however, the nurse should follow isolation procedures carefully. The administration of chemotherapy causes neutropenia, causing the toddler to become more susceptible to disease. The immunodeficiency precludes the same nurse carrying for the client with RSV and the one who has an immunodeficiency. Aplastic anemia causes a decrease in all cell levels in the blood causing neutropenia. It would be an incorrect decision to assign the nurse to both clients. **Cognitive Level:** Applying **Client Need:** Safety and Infection Control **Integrated Process:** Nursing Process: Planning **Content Area:** Child Health **Strategy:** The core concept is risk of transmission of infection from an infant with RSV. The correct choices would avoid infants and clients who are immunocompromised. **Reference:** Ball, J., Bindler, R., & Cowen, K. (2010). *Child health nursing: Partnering with children & families* (2nd ed.). Upper Saddle River, NJ: Pearson/Prentice Hall, p. 864.

9 **Answer: 2** **Rationale:** Accumulating mucopurulent secretions may provide a medium for bacterial growth or can obstruct the lumen of the tube. Suctioning is another risk for introduction of bacteria. Early recognition of signs of infection is important. The tube does not need to be changed every day and cannot be removed. Small objects, not large objects, pose a risk to aspiration and would need to be avoided. **Cognitive Level:** Applying **Client Need:** Physiological Adaptation **Integrated Process:** Teaching and Learning **Content Area:** Child Health **Strategy:** The core concept is the most essential information for home tracheostomy care. Recall that infection and obstruction are key concerns related to artificial airways. **Reference:** Hockenberry, M., & Wilson, D. (2009). *Wong's essentials of pediatric nursing* (8th ed.). St Louis, Missouri: Mosby, pp. 741–745.

ANSWERS & RATIONALES

10 **Answer: 4** **Rationale:** Children with cystic fibrosis have elevated chloride concentrations of sweat because of the dysfunction of the exocrine glands. The sweat chloride test does not determine degree of dehydration, sweat gland function, or aid in microorganism identification. **Cognitive Level:** Analyzing **Client Need:** Reduction of Risk Potential **Integrated Process:** Nursing Process: Implementation **Content**

Area: Child Health **Strategy:** The critical word in this question is *purpose*. Consider the reason for the test in making a selection. **Reference:** Ball, J., Bindler, R., & Cowen, K. (2010). *Child health nursing: Partnering with children & families* (2nd ed.). Upper Saddle River, NJ: Pearson/Prentice Hall, pp. 895–896.

References

Ball, J., Bindler, R., & Cowen, K. (2010). *Child health nursing: Partnering with children and families* (2nd ed.). Upper Saddle River, NJ: Pearson, pp. 839–907.

Bindler, R., & Ball, J. (2008). *Clinical skills manual for pediatric nursing: Caring for children* (4th ed.). Upper Saddle River, NJ: Pearson, pp. 112–119.

Hockenberry, M., & Wilson, D. (2009). *Wong's essentials of pediatric nursing* (8th ed.). St. Louis, MO: Elsevier.

Hockenberry, M., & Wilson, D. (2011). *Wong's nursing care of infants and children* (9th ed.). St. Louis, MO: Elsevier.

Jarvis, C. (2012). *Physical examination and health assessment* (6th ed.). St. Louis, MO: Elsevier.

London, M., Ladewig, P., Ball, J., Bindler, R., & Cowen, K. (2011). *Maternal & child nursing care* (3rd ed.). Upper Saddle River, NJ: Pearson Education.

Smith, S., Duell, D., & Martin, B. (2012). *Clinical nursing skills: Basic to advanced skills* (8th ed.). Upper Saddle River, NJ: Pearson Education, Inc.

Cardiac Health Problems

5

Chapter Outline

Overview of Anatomy and Physiology of Cardiac System

Congenital Cardiac Health Problems

Acquired Cardiac Health Problems

Objectives

➤ Identify data essential to assessing alterations in health of the cardiac system in a child.
➤ Discuss the clinical manifestations and pathophysiology of alterations in health of the cardiac system of a child.
➤ Discuss therapeutic management of a child with alterations in health of the cardiac system.
➤ Describe nursing management of a child with alterations in health of the cardiac system.

NCLEX-RN® Test Prep

Use the accompanying online resource, NursingReviewsandRationales, to test yourself with hundreds of NCLEX®-style practice questions.

Review at a Glance

acyanotic heart defect a heart condition that does not cause deoxygenation, or low oxygen levels; color of skin and mucous membranes are usually normal pink

cardiac catheterization a test that examines heart by placing a catheter into a vein or artery and advancing it to heart in order to sample oxygen levels and take pressure measurements in heart chambers

cyanotic heart defect a heart condition that causes blood to contain less oxygen than required; skin and mucous membrane color is usually pale to blue

echocardiogram a graphic record of walls, valves, and vessels of heart produced by ultrasound

Jones Criteria guidelines for diagnosis of initial attack of rheumatic fever developed by Jones in 1992

left to right shunt movement of blood from left side of heart to right side through an abnormal opening

lymphadenopathy a condition that causes swollen glands and can be caused by infection or cancer

murmur a heart sound resembling running water through a tight space; usually indicates a malfunctioning valve or an abnormal opening in cardiac septum

polycythemia a condition of more red blood cells than normal; often indicates hypoxemia and body's compensatory response

prostaglandin E1 a hormone that reopens ductus arteriosus; it is used in cases where blood is not oxygenating properly and patent ductus arteriosus allows for mixing of saturated and unsaturated blood

right to left shunt movement of blood from right side of heart to left side of heart through an abnormal opening in septum; this results in deoxygenated blood because systemic blood bypasses lungs and is ejected into aorta

vasculitis inflammation of tunica intima (inner lining) of arteries and veins

PRETEST

1 An infant is admitted with an acyanotic heart defect. Which assessment finding should be discussed with the physician?

1. Heart murmur
2. Dyspnea
3. Weight gain
4. Eupnea

2 The nurse is caring for an infant with a cyanotic heart defect. Symptoms that would indicate risk for congestive heart failure include which of the following? Select all that apply.

1. Respiratory crackles and frothy secretions
2. Increased blood pressure
3. Oxygen saturation increase
4. Hepatomegaly
5. Rapid weight gain

3 A child admitted with a diagnosis of "rule out rheumatic fever" has all of the following laboratory findings. Which finding supports the diagnosis of rheumatic fever?

1. Elevated antistreptolysin-O (ASO)
2. Elevated hematocrit
3. Blood cultures negative
4. White blood cell count within the normal range

4 A child is admitted with possible coarctation of the aorta. The admitting nurse reviews the medical orders for the child and should question which of the following orders?

1. Regular diet
2. BP of upper and lower extremities every four hours
3. Intake and output every shift
4. Vital signs on admission, then daily

5 A child with tetralogy of Fallot becomes acutely ill with an increase in cyanosis, tachycardia, and tachypnea. To relieve the cardiac load, the nurse will do which of the following?

1. Place the child in Trendelenburg position.
2. Place the child in knee–chest position.
3. Have oxygen equipment available.
4. Have suction equipment available.

6 A child with a cyanotic heart defect is being discharged home to await surgical repair. In the discharge teaching, the nurse instructs the parents to do which of the following?

1. Prevent the child from crying at all.
2. Observe the child for signs of increased intracranial pressure.
3. Obtain training in cardio-pulmonary resuscitation.
4. Identify growth and development milestones.

7 A child with rheumatic fever is admitted to the nursing unit. The nurse's most important intervention at this time is to do which of the following?

1. Prevent spread of rheumatic fever.
2. Provide comfort measures for arthralgia.
3. Evaluate for nervous system complications.
4. Teach parents about cardiopulmonary resuscitation (CPR).

8 A child with Kawasaki's disease is admitted to the pediatric unit. To promote comfort, the nurse should do which of the following?

1. Administer aspirin and immunoglobulins as ordered.
2. Splint extremities to prevent contractures.
3. Keep child NPO for the first 24 hours.
4. Encourage a vigorous exercise program.

9 A pediatric client is discharged after an acute phase of rheumatic fever. The priority discharge instruction given by the nurse is that the child can be expected to do which of the following?

1. Resume regular activities.
2. Take antibiotics as ordered.
3. Maintain complete bedrest.
4. Experience central nervous system (CNS) complications.

10 The nurse is talking with the parents of an infant with patent ductus arteriosus. The nurse uses the accompanying picture to illustrate where the defect occurs. Indicate the spot representing patent ductus arteriosus. Draw an "X" in the correct area on the image shown.

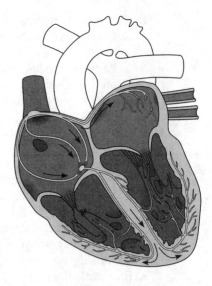

➤ *See pages 109–110 for Answers and Rationales.*

I. OVERVIEW OF ANATOMY AND PHYSIOLOGY OF CARDIAC SYSTEM

A. Heart has four chambers: right and left atria (upper chambers), and right and left ventricles (lower chambers)

B. Heart has four valves: pulmonic (right ventricle to pulmonary artery), aortic (left ventricle to aorta), tricuspid (right atrium to right ventricle) and mitral (left atrium to left ventricle)

C. Fetal circulation

1. Ductus venosus

    a. Umbilical vein carries oxygenated blood from placenta to infant

    b. Blood bypasses liver through ductus venosus

    c. When umbilical cord is clamped and cut, blood flow ceases and ductus venosus closes

    d. Blood flows into liver

2. Foramen ovale

    a. Systemic blood enters right atrium

    b. Oxygenated blood flows from right to left atria through foramen ovale

    c. Blood bypasses lungs which are nonfunctional

    d. Blood flows from left atria to left ventricle and out to aorta

    e. Foramen ovale closes after birth with change in pressure in cardiac chambers

3. Ductus arteriosus

    a. A fistula between aorta and pulmonary artery allows for mixing of blood

    b. Blood flowing through pulmonary artery may enter aorta through a patent ductus arteriosus

    c. Ductus arteriosus closes after birth, sometimes with first few breaths but may take up to three days

D. Oxygenation

    1. Oxygen is bound to hemoglobin on red blood cells

    2. Hematocrit and hemoglobin facilitate oxygenation

    3. Desaturated blood contains more than 5 grams of unoxygenated hemoglobin per 100 mL of blood

E. Cardiac function

    1. Heart rate is sensitive to oxygen level

    2. Cardiac output is dependent on heart rate until child is 5 years old

    3. Child has an increased risk of heart failure

        a. Immature heart is sensitive to volume or pressure overload

        b. Muscle fibers are less developed

    4. Use of cardiorespiratory monitor
      a. Use alcohol swabs to clean skin areas where leads will be applied and allow skin to dry
      b. Place electrodes on child's chest: one on right side, one on left, and one (ground) on lateral side of abdomen; electrode colors may vary
      c. Check connections frequently especially if disconnection occurs due to movement of child

F. Diagnostic tests for cardiac system
    1. Radiography (x-ray)
      a. Reveals size and contour of heart
      b. Visualizes characteristics of pulmonary vascular markings
      c. Nursing: no special care
    2. Echocardiography (ultrasound)
      a. Identifies heart structure
      b. Identifies pattern of movement, hemodynamics
      c. Nursing: no special care
    3. Electrocardiogram (ECG)
      a. Records quality of major electrical activity of heart
      b. Identifies dysrhythmias
      c. Nursing: no special care
    4. Holter monitor: 24 hour monitoring of ECG
    5. Stress ECG: ECG done after exercise
    6. Cardiac catheterization
      a. Description: examines heart by placing a catheter into an artery or vein and advancing it to heart
      b. Measurements
        1) Oxygen levels in each chamber
        2) Pressure in each chamber
      c. Identifies anatomic alterations
      d. Preprocedure care
        1) Age-appropriate teaching including information of what child will feel, see, and hear
        2) Family support
        3) NPO after midnight
        4) Oral sedation is given
        5) Obtain baseline vital signs, hemoglobin, hematocrit, and pedal pulses
      e. Postprocedure care
        1) Monitor for bleeding: hematoma, hemorrhage, thrombus
          a) Maintain direct pressure to insertion site for 15 minutes and a pressure dressing for six hours
          b) Obtain vital signs, neurovascular checks to extremity distal to insertion site every 15 minutes for first hour, then every 30 minutes for one hour or longer until stable
          c) Maintain bedrest for six hours
        2) Monitor for dysrhythmias
        3) Monitor for infection
        4) Assess insertion site and distal extremity
        5) Assess for diuresis related to dye
      f. Discharge teaching
        1) Teach signs of complications to family (bleeding, infection, thrombosis)
        2) Encourage quiet play only for first 24 hours to avoid disturbing insertion site

3) Encourage increased fluid intake to maintain hydration to offset diuretic effect of contrast dye

G. Surgical procedures

    1. Palliative: surgery designed to improve overall condition of child; does not correct disorder; many palliative surgeries may create additional defects that allow for better exchange of blood between chambers

    2. Correction: surgery designed to resolve cardiac problem

II. CONGENITAL CARDIAC HEALTH PROBLEMS

A. *Acyanotic heart defects*: heart conditions that do not cause deoxygenation or low oxygen levels; skin and mucous membrane color is usually normal pink

    1. Atrial septal defect (see Figure 5-1)

        a. Description

            1) Defect between atria

            2) Septal wall defect allowing blood to flow from left atrium to right atrium, called a **left to right shunt**

        b. Etiology and pathophysiology

            1) Opening between atria

            2) Foramen ovale fails to close

            3) Sometimes much of septum is absent

            4) Increased pulmonary blood flow

        c. Assessment

            1) Often asymptomatic if small defect

            2) Dyspnea

            3) Fatigue, poor growth

            4) Soft systolic **murmur** (abnormal heart sound) in pulmonic area, splitting S_2

            5) **Echocardiogram**: a diagnostic test that utilizes ultrasound; shows right ventricular overload and shunt size

            6) Congestive heart failure (CHF)

            7) Cardiac catheterization: visualization of defect

        d. Priority nursing diagnoses

            1) Anxiety

            2) Ineffective Family Coping: Disabling

            3) Risk for Impaired Growth and Development

            4) Risk for Infection

            5) Imbalanced Nutrition: Less Than Body Requirements

            6) Impaired Gas Exchange

Figure 5-1

Atrial septal defect

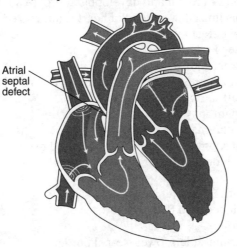

Atrial septal defect

Table 5-1 **Nursing Care of the Child with an Acyanotic Heart Defect**

Nursing Diagnosis	Nursing Care
Anxiety; Ineffective Family Coping: Disabling	1. Assess coping mechanisms of family. 2. Provide family with information about condition. 3. Refer family to American Heart Association or cardiac support group.
Risk for Impaired Growth and Development	1. Treat the child as normally as possible. Teach parents that children are more comfortable when they know what to expect. 2. Promote mental development activities as appropriate for age and condition. 3. Anticipate regression of developmental milestones especially if child is hospitalized frequently.
Risk for Infection	1. Limit exposure to individuals with infections. 2. Promote good pulmonary hygiene—change position, use percussion and postural drainage or oscillating vest if ordered.
Imbalanced Nutrition: Less Than Body Requirements	1. Offer small frequent feedings. 2. Use soft nipple for infant to ease the stress of sucking. Encourage the breastfeeding mother to pump breast milk if infant lacks strength to suck. 3. Organize nursing care to allow for rest.
Impaired Gas Exchange	1. Promote good pulmonary hygiene. 2. Monitor intake and output. Limit fluids as ordered. 3. Administer diuretics as ordered. Monitor potassium level. 4. Change position every two hours.

  e. Planning and intervention
  1) Surgical closure or patch of defect
  2) Transcatheter device closure during cardiac catheterization
  3) Nursing management of child with acyanotic heart disease (see Table 5-1)
  f. Client and family education
  1) Explain to parents the purpose of tests and procedures
  2) Teach parents ways to support nutrition, reduce stress on heart, promote rest, and support growth and development during preoperative period
  3) Teach parents signs of CHF and infection
  4) Prepare parents and child for surgery by visiting intensive care unit, explaining equipment and sounds
  5) Prepare older child for postoperative experience, including coughing and deep breathing and need for movement
  6) Teach need for antibiotic prophylaxis to prevent subacute bacterial endocarditis
  g. Evaluation: child's growth and development progresses regularly; child's gas exchange is maximized; workload of heart is minimized
2. Ventricular septal defect (VSD)
  a. Description (see Figure 5-2)
  1) Defect between ventricles
  2) Septal wall incomplete allowing blood to flow from left ventricle to right ventricle (left to right shunt)
  b. Etiology and pathophysiology
  1) Increased pulmonary blood flow
  2) Left to right shunting of blood flow is caused by higher pressure in left ventricle
  3) Shunting of blood causes an increased workload on right ventricle
  c. Assessment
  1) Tachypnea, dyspnea
  2) Poor growth, reduced fluid intake
  3) Palpable thrill
  4) Systolic murmur at left lower sternal border

Practice to Pass

A child is being discharged after a surgical repair of a ventricular septal defect. What does the nurse include in the discharge teaching plan?

Figure 5-2

Ventricular septal defect

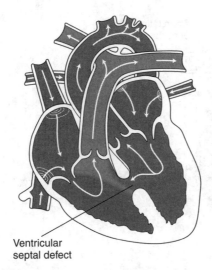

Ventricular
septal defect

     5) ECG and radiology detect larger septal defects
     6) Signs of CHF
  d. Priority nursing diagnoses (see Table 5-1 again)
  e. Planning and intervention
     1) Occasionally, spontaneous closure occurs
     2) Surgical patching if failure to thrive occurs
     3) Prophylactic antibiotics treatment to prevent endocarditis if recommended
     4) Preoperative nursing care involves promoting growth and development and promoting oxygenation (see Table 5-1 again)
     5) Postoperative nursing care continues with activities of preoperative care, while providing analgesics as necessary to provide comfort and using sterile dressings on incision
  f. Client and family education
     1) Explain to parents the purpose of tests and procedures
     2) Teach parents ways to support nutrition, reduce stress on heart, promote rest, support growth and development during preoperative period
     3) Teach parents signs of CHF and infection
     4) Prepare parents and child for surgery by visiting the intensive care unit, explaining equipment and sounds
     5) Prepare older child for postoperative experience including coughing and deep breathing and need for movement
     6) Teach need for antibiotic prophylaxis to prevent subacute bacterial endocarditis
  g. Evaluation: child's growth and development progresses regularly; child's gas exchange is maximized; workload of the heart is minimized
3. Coarctation of aorta
  a. Description (see Figure 5-3)
     1) Narrowing of descending aorta
     2) Restricts blood flow leaving heart
  b. Etiology and pathophysiology
     1) Narrowing or constriction of descending aorta
     2) Often near ductus arteriosus
     3) Progressive disorder that leads to CHF
  c. Assessment
     1) May be asymptomatic
     2) Blood pressure difference of 20 mm between upper and lower extremities, upper extremity pressure higher

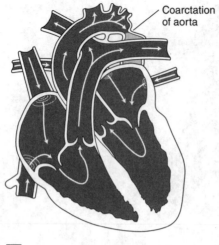

Figure 5-3

Coarctation of aorta

Coarctation of aorta

Decreased blood flow

     3) Brachial and radial pulses full, femoral pulses weak
     4) Headache, vertigo, and epistaxis
     5) Exercise intolerance
     6) Left ventricular hypertrophy
     7) Dyspnea
     8) Cerebrovascular accident (CVA) secondary to hypertension in upper circulation
   d. Priority nursing diagnoses
     1) Ineffective Tissue Perfusion (renal)
     2) Risk for Injury
     3) Activity Intolerance
     4) Deficient Knowledge
     5) Others as previously listed in Table 5-1
   e. Therapeutic management
     1) Balloon cardiac catheterization with insertion of endovascular stents
     2) Surgical resection and patch of coarctation
     3) Possible prophylaxis for endocarditis when undergoing surgical or dental procedures
     4) Prior to correction, monitor BP in upper and lower extremities
     5) Rebound hypertension occurs in immediate postoperative period

Practice to Pass

A pediatric client is being discharged to home following a cardiac catheterization. What are three priority points in the nurse's discharge teaching to the family?

   f. Client and family education
     1) Prepare parents for tests and procedures child will undergo
     2) Teach parents signs and symptoms of worsening condition
     3) Educate parents on administration of cardiac and vasoactive drugs
     4) Child may need prophylactic antibiotics before surgical and dental procedures
   g. Evaluation: child's growth and development progresses regularly; child's gas exchange is maximized; workload of heart is minimized
B. Cyanotic heart defects: heart conditions that cause blood to contain less oxygen than required; skin and mucous membrane color is usually pale to blue
   1. Tetralogy of Fallot (see Figure 5-4)
    a. Description
     1) Four defects that combine to allow blood flow to bypass lungs and enter left side of heart, called a **right to left shunt**
     2) Unoxygenated blood enters body circulation accounting for cyanosis

Figure 5-4

Tetralogy of Fallot

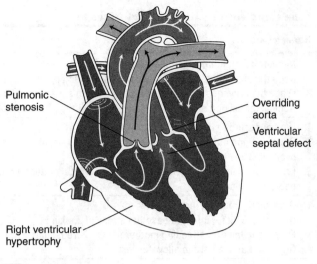

Pulmonic stenosis

Overriding aorta

Ventricular septal defect

Right ventricular hypertrophy

☐ Decreased blood flow

b. Etiology and pathophysiology
  1) Four defects: pulmonic stenosis, right ventricular hypertrophy, ventricular septal defect, and overriding aorta
  2) Atrial septal defect occurs at times
  3) Deficient oxygen in the tissues leads to acidosis
  4) Hypercyanosis (TET) spells occur, which are transient periods when there is an increase in right to left shunting of blood
c. Assessment
  1) TET spells characterized by hypoxia, pallor, and tachypnea; precipitated by crying, defecation, and feeding; older children will assume a squatting position to decrease blood return from the lower extremities; treatment involves placing child in knee–chest position, administering morphine or propranolol and oxygen
  2) Clubbing of digits
  3) **Polycythemia** (excess number of red blood cells), metabolic acidosis
  4) Poor growth, exercise intolerance
  5) Systolic murmur in pulmonic area
  6) Right ventricular hypertrophy
  7) Cardiac catheterization visualizes anomalous structures
d. Priority nursing diagnoses (see Table 5-2)
e. Therapeutic management
  1) **Prostaglandin E1**: to maintain open ductus arteriosus
  2) Palliative surgery to improve oxygenation includes shunting procedures
  3) Corrective surgery includes patching VSD and relieving pulmonary stenosis
  4) See Table 5-2 for associated nursing care
f. Client and family education
  1) Teach parents to promote nutrition in light of weak suck
  2) Discuss activities to promote oxygenation
  3) Describe symptoms of respiratory infections
  4) Describe treatments and procedures child will undergo
g. Evaluation: parents and child describe treatments and procedures; child gains weight steadily; child's mental development progresses; child remains free of symptoms of respiratory infections

Table 5-2 **Nursing Care of the Child with Cyanotic Heart Disease**

Nursing Diagnosis	Nursing Care
Ineffective Cardiopulmonary Tissue Perfusion	1. Monitor hemoglobin and hematocrit levels. 2. Keep the child calm. Do not allow long periods of crying. 3. When hypercyanosis occurs, assist the child to squatting or knee–chest position. 4. Administer oxygen and morphine as ordered during these spells.
High Risk for Infection	1. Limit exposure to individuals with infections. 2. Promote good pulmonary hygiene—change position, percussion and postural drainage or oscillating vest 3. Prophylactic antibiotics when undergoing surgical or dental treatments to prevent subacute bacterial endocarditis.
Risk for Imbalanced Nutrition: Less Than Body Requirements	1. Offer small, frequent feedings. 2. Use soft nipple for infant to ease the stress of sucking. 3. Encourage the breastfeeding mother to pump breast milk if infant lacks strength to suck. 4. Organize nursing care to allow for rest.
Risk for Impaired Gas Exchange	1. Limit activity. 2. Maintain clear airways. 3. Monitor electrolytes.

Risk for Decreased Cardiac Output	1. Assess vital signs.
	2. Monitor for signs of CHF.
	3. Note peripheral edema.
	4. Weigh child daily.
	5. Maintain strict intake and output measurement.
	6. Administer diuretics as ordered.
	7. Administer oxygen as ordered.
	8. Palpate liver every 4 to 12 hours (indicates right-sided failure).
	9. Administer digoxin as ordered:
	   a. Assess for apical pulse for one full minute—monitor for bradycardia or arrhythmias.
	   b. Be consistent in measurement of medication and time of administration.
	   c. Do not repeat dose if child vomits.

Risk for Injury	1. Monitor hemoglobin and hematocrit. 2. Observe for signs of thrombus formation.

Practice to Pass

A child has been given a diagnosis of transposition of the great vessels. How would you explain the disorder to the family? What is the most important point that the family needs to understand and implement prior to surgery?

!

2. Transposition of the great vessels
   a. Description (see Figure 5-5)
      1) Aorta arises from right ventricle, and pulmonary artery arises from left ventricle
      2) Other anomalies exist that increase mixing of blood between two separate circulations; these anomalies promote oxygenation
      3) Right to left shunting of blood occurs
   b. Etiology and pathophysiology
      1) Pulmonary artery originates from left ventricle; blood travels from left ventricle to pulmonary artery, then to lungs, and then back into left atrium
      2) Aorta originates from right ventricle; blood leaves right ventricle by aorta, travels to body cells and returns to right atrium by way of vena cava
      3) There are two closed circulation pathways
      4) Survival depends on foramen ovale remaining open to mix oxygenated and deoxygenated blood
   c. Assessment
      1) Progressive cyanosis → hypoxia → acidosis
      2) Signs and symptoms of CHF
      3) Tachypnea

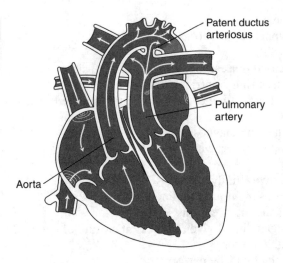

Figure 5-5

Transposition of great vessels

Patent ductus arteriosus

Pulmonary artery

Aorta

4) Poor feeding

5) Failure to grow

6) Echocardiogram identifies misplacement of arteries

d. Priority nursing diagnoses (see Table 5-2 again)

e. Therapeutic management

    1) Prostaglandin E1 to maintain open ductus arteriosus

    2) Palliative surgical interventions

    3) Corrective surgery

    4) Prophylactic antibiotic therapy before routine dental and medical procedures to prevent endocarditis is recommended in selected circumstances (American Heart Association): unrepaired or incompletely repaired cyanotic heart disease (including palliative shunts or conduits); during first six months after complete repair of congenital heart defect with prosthetic material or device (placed either by surgery or catheter intervention); any repaired congenital heart defect with residual defect at or adjacent to site of prosthetic patch or device; cardiac transplant

    5) Nursing activities to promote nutrition and reduce respiratory congestion (see Table 5-2)

f. Child and family education

    1) Home care requirements related to nutrition, rest, and oxygenation

    2) Preparation for procedures and treatments

    3) Safe administration of cardiac drugs and diuretics

g. Evaluation: parents and child describe treatments and surgical procedures; child's growth and development progresses steadily; child maintains adequate gas exchange; parents administer medications effectively and safely

3. Hypoplastic left heart syndrome

  a. Description

    1) Abnormally small left ventricle noted at birth

    2) Inability of heart to supply oxygen needs of body

  b. Etiology and pathophysiology

    1) Absent or stenotic mitral and aortic valves

    2) Abnormally small left ventricle and aortic arch

    3) Major resistance to aortic flow

    4) Hypertrophy of right ventricle

    5) Prognosis poor

      c. Assessment
        1) Tachypnea, chest retractions, dyspnea
        2) Cyanosis
        3) Decreased pulses, poor peripheral perfusion
        4) Increased right ventricular impulse
        5) Echocardiogram indicates small and weak left ventricle
        6) CHF
      d. Priority nursing diagnoses
        1) Anticipatory Grieving
        2) Anxiety
        3) Ineffective Family Coping
        4) Others as previously outlined in Table 5-2
      e. Planning and interventions
        1) Prostaglandin E1 given to prevent closure of patent ductus arteriosus
        2) Palliative surgery
        3) Transplant may be performed
        4) Survival rate currently at or above 50%
      f. Evaluation: parents describe treatments and procedures their child is undergoing; parents accept diagnosis and display appropriate grieving behaviors

III. ACQUIRED CARDIAC HEALTH PROBLEMS

A. Rheumatic fever
  1. Description
    a. Systemic inflammatory disease that involves heart and joints; CNS and connective tissue involvement may also occur
    b. Occurs secondary to infection by group A beta-hemolytic streptococcus; most common in children age 5 years to adolescence
  2. Etiology and pathophysiology
    a. Follows one to three weeks after a group A beta-hemolytic streptococcal infection
    b. It may be an autoimmune reaction against beta-hemolytic streptococcus; strep organisms cannot be cultured out of lesions of rheumatic fever
    c. Acute phase lasts two to three weeks and is characterized by inflammation of connective tissue in heart, joints, and skin
    d. Proliferative phase primarily affects heart with Aschoff bodies developing on heart valves; cardiac valve leaflets scar and lead to valvular stenosis and regurgitation
    e. Episode of rheumatic fever lasts up to three months and is self-limiting
    f. Long-term consequence is rheumatic heart disease, which is often manifested in valvular damage
    g. Is difficult to diagnose as it mimics other diseases; diagnosis is usually based on **Jones Criteria**, which describe frequent symptoms of rheumatic fever; symptoms are listed according to likelihood of rheumatic fever infection as major manifestations and minor manifestations; diagnosis is based on presence of two major or one major and two minor criteria
  3. Assessment using Jones Criteria (1992)
    a. Major criteria include
      1) Multiple joints may be involved in inflammatory process; joints affected are most frequently large joints—knees, elbows, and wrists
      2) Carditis is most severe symptom of rheumatic fever; symptoms of carditis include a new murmur, pericardial friction rub, changes on the ECG; tachycardia may be noted by nurse as a pulse greater than 100 while sleeping

    3) Chorea is the CNS symptom of rheumatic fever and involves involuntary movement of limbs; emotional lability and slurred speech may occur; this symptom tends to have a latent period of two months or more from strep infection

    4) Erythema marginatum is an erythematous, macular rash that occurs primarily on trunk and proximal limbs; this symptom is frequently associated with carditis

    5) Subcutaneous nodules are non-tender nodules that develop on skin over flexor surfaces of joints and vertebrae

  b. Minor criteria

    1) Fever: spiking temperature

    2) Arthralgia

    3) Elevated erythrocyte sedimentation rate (ESR), C-reactive protein, and decreased red blood cell (RBC) count

    4) Prolonged P-R and/or Q-T interval on ECG

  c. Supporting evidence (of recent streptococcal infection)

    1) History of streptococcal infection

    2) History of scarlet fever

    3) Positive throat culture for streptococcus

    4) Elevated anti-streptolysin-O (ASO) titer

4. Priority nursing diagnoses

  a. Risk for Injury—Carditis

  b. Pain

  c. Risk for Diversional Activity Deficit

5. Planning and interventions

  a. Bedrest until ESR returns to normal

  b. Use aspirin and prednisone as ordered anti-inflammatory agents to reduce inflammation; aspirin will also promote comfort from painful joints

  c. Monitor client for cardiac function

  d. Give penicillin as ordered in either an oral daily dose or monthly long-acting injection after recovery from rheumatic heart disease to reduce risk of recurrence of strep infection; erythromycin given if allergic to penicillin

  e. Design nursing activities to promote rest and to encourage diversional activities which do not stress heart; maintain bedrest with bathroom privileges

6. Client and family education

  a. Client and parents need to understand pathology of disease as well as rationale for bedrest

  b. Diversional activities are discussed that allow for mental stimulation without physical activity

  c. Assist parents in planning for home care of child

7. Evaluation: child remains free of cardiac complications; parents and child describe safe and effective administration of prophylactic antibiotic

B. Kawasaki's disease

1. Description

  a. A multisystem disorder involving **vasculitis** (inflammation of tunica intima or inner lining of arteries and veins)

  b. Also called mucocutaneous lymph node syndrome

  c. Leading cause of acquired heart disease in children

2. Etiology and pathophysiology

  a. Acute, systemic inflammatory illness involving arteries

  b. Unknown cause but generally affects young children; most frequently affected are boys under 5 years of age

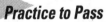
Practice to Pass

The mother of a pediatric client diagnosed with rheumatic fever asks why the client cannot resume activities normal for age. How does the nurse discuss the potential complications?

      c. Three phases of disease

        1) Acute phase characterized by fever, conjunctival hyperemia, swollen hands and feet, rash, and enlarged cervical lymph nodes

        2) Subacute phase is characterized by cracking lips, desquamation of skin on tips of fingers and toes, cardiac disease, and thrombocytosis

        3) Convalescent phase has lingering signs of inflammation

      d. Significantly increased platelet count

      e. Possible cardiac pathology including dysrhythmias, CHF, and myocardial infarction

      f. Coronary artery disease may lead to aneurysms and ischemic heart disease

 3. Assessment

      a. Stage one (one to two weeks): fever lasting longer than five days that is unresponsive to antipyretics, conjunctivitis, crusted and fissured lips, swelling of hands and feet, erythema, **lymphadenopathy** (a condition that causes swollen glands and can be caused by infection or cancer)

      b. Subacute stage (two to four weeks): fever diminishes, irritability, anorexia, desquamation of hands and feet, arthritis and arthralgia, cardiovascular manifestations

      c. Convalescent stage (six to eight weeks): drop in ESR and diminishing signs of illness

4. Priority nursing diagnoses

      a. Risk for Injury

      b. Hyperthermia

      c. Risk for Ineffective Home Health Maintenance

5. Planning and intervention

      a. Administer aspirin 80 to 100 mg/kg/day as antiplatelet agent: child is weaned over time to decrease risk of bleeding

      b. Administer gamma globulin (IVIG) once as ordered to reduce risk of coronary artery lesions and aneurysms; may be repeated if fever does not decrease

       c. Nursing management

        1) Promote comfort

        2) Small frequent feedings

        3) Passive range of motion to extremities

        4) Cool baths

        5) Gentle oral care

        6) Encourage fluids

        7) Monitor for complications

          a) Aneurysms

          b) Side effects of aspirin therapy: bleeding, GI upset

          c) Side effects of IVIG therapy: elevated blood pressure, facial flushing, tightness in chest

        8) Monitor temperature

        9) Monitor eyes for conjunctivitis

6. Client and family education

      a. Safe administration of aspirin therapy

      b. Teach parents to keep skin clean and avoid soaps and lotions

      c. Offer liquids high in calories, low in acids

      d. Low-cholesterol diet

      e. Call physician if child refuses to walk

      f. Monitor temperature in a.m. and p.m. prior to giving aspirin

7. Evaluation: client recovers without serious sequelae; parents describe means to control temperature

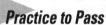

Practice to Pass

The parent of a preschool-age child reports that the child's hands are peeling, eyes are red, and the child has joint pain. What should the school nurse suggest to the parents, and what is the immediate concern?

Case Study

A 1-week-old client is scheduled for palliative surgery for transposition of the great vessels. You are the nurse who is supporting the parents through this illness.

1. What questions will you ask the parents prior to surgery?

2. What assessments do you make preoperatively?

3. What are the priority postoperative nursing interventions?

4. What discharge instructions will you give the parents?

5. The parents ask what emergency situations may arise and how they should respond. What do you say?

For suggested responses, see pages 352–353.

POSTTEST

1 The nurse is teaching a class at an outpatient cardiac clinic held for parents of children with congenital cardiac defects. Before explaining the movement of blood through septal defects, the nurse tells the parents about pressure gradients in the normal heart. The nurse will indicate on this picture of the heart that the pressure is greatest in which chamber? Draw an "X" in the correct area on the image.

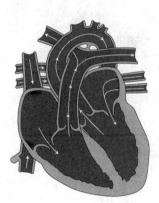

2 An infant who has a congenital heart defect comes into the clinic with irritability, pallor, and increased cyanosis that began quickly over the last 30 minutes. As the nurse assesses the infant, the parent asks why the child's color is bluish. What should the nurse explain related to the infant's skin color?

1. It is caused by a left-to-right shunting of blood.
2. It is associated with liver dysfunction secondary to congestive heart failure.
3. It is related to hemoglobin level and oxygen saturation.
4. It is due to poor iron levels in the child's body.

3 A 14-year-old child is admitted with a diagnosis of "rule out rheumatic fever." Based on Jones Criteria, the nurse assesses for which of the following?

1. Polyarthritis and dental caries
2. Fever, headache, and low red blood cell count
3. Chorea, muscle weakness, and decreased erythrocyte sedimentation rate
4. Erythema, polyarthritis, and elevated antistreptolysin-O (ASO) titer

4 A toddler client is diagnosed with Kawasaki's disease. Upon admission to the pediatric unit, the client's parent asks why the child is receiving aspirin when it has been contraindicated in previous minor illnesses. The nurse explains which of the following? Select all that apply.

1. High doses of aspirin will be given while fever is high.
2. Aspirin dose will be increased after fever is gone.
3. Length of aspirin therapy is related to child's response.
4. Aspirin therapy is not contraindicated and necessary for treatment.
5. Aspirin therapy is frequently not ordered.

5 The nurse has taught the parents of a baby girl client who has congestive heart failure (CHF) about drug therapy with digoxin (Lanoxin) and furosemide (Lasix). The nurse concludes that the parents learned the information when one parent makes which statement about furosemide?

1. "It is given because our baby has a kidney defect."
2. "It helps her heart by reducing the amount of water in her system."
3. "It prevents the digoxin from becoming toxic."
4. "It keeps the potassium levels in her body from getting too high."

6 A 2-year-old boy is being discharged home and will have palliative surgery for tetralogy of Fallot at a later date. The mother wants to know how much physical activity she can allow for the child. What is the nurse's best response?

1. "Allow him to regulate his activity."
2. "Keep him on complete bedrest."
3. "Limit his activities to a few hours per day."
4. "Keep him from crying."

7 After a pediatric client has a cardiac catheterization, which intervention would the nurse consider to be of highest priority during the immediate postprocedure period?

1. Encourage intake of small amounts of fluid.
2. Teach the parents signs of congestive heart failure.
3. Monitor the site for signs of infection.
4. Apply direct pressure to entry site for 15 minutes.

8 A 6-month-old infant is receiving digoxin (Lanoxin) and furosemide (Lasix) for congestive heart failure. The nurse who is evaluating the effectiveness of furosemide would monitor which of the following? Select all that apply.

1. Intake and output
2. Daily weight
3. Hemoglobin and hematocrit levels
4. Pulse rate
5. Partial pressure of oxygen

9 A 2-year-old child has a known cardiac defect and is in congestive heart failure. Which assessment findings best indicate to the nurse a toxic dose of digoxin (Lanoxin)?

1. Tachycardia and dysrhythmia
2. Headache and diarrhea
3. Bradycardia, nausea, and vomiting
4. Tinnitus and nuchal rigidity

10 The home health nurse is monitoring the status of a child with a known cyanotic heart defect. In addition to monitoring cardiac function, the nurse monitors the child's other body systems for problems secondary to the heart defect. Which nursing diagnosis should the nurse write on the client care plan?

1. Imbalanced Nutrition: Less Than Body Requirements
2. Risk for Injury, Seizures
3. Pain
4. Diversional Activity Deficit

➤ *See pages 110–112 for Answers and Rationales.*

ANSWERS & RATIONALES

Pretest

1 **Answer: 2** **Rationale:** Dyspnea may be a sign of congestive heart failure. It should be reported to the physician or health care provider. Heart murmurs are extra noises that blood makes as it flows through the heart. Often, heart murmurs are innocent or not alarming. The presence of a heart murmur should be documented but is not emergent. Weight gain is normal during infancy. It could indicate congestive heart failure, but often is found to be a normal finding. Eupnea is a pattern of normal respiration. **Cognitive Level:** Analyzing **Client Need:** Physiological Adaptation **Integrated Process:** Nursing Process: Assessment **Content Area:** Child Health **Strategy:** Eliminate all normal findings in a client with acyanotic heart disease. Next consider which sign could be a positive developmental sign or a sign of impending heart failure. Without additional information, that option is questionable, so it must be eliminated also. **Reference:** Ball, J., Bindler, R., & Cowen, K. (2010). *Child health nursing: Partnering with children & families* (2nd ed.). Upper Saddle River, NJ: Pearson/Prentice Hall, p. 923.

2 **Answer: 1, 4, 5** **Rationale:** As congestive heart failure progresses, the heart muscle cannot stretch its fibers to accommodate the blood volume, resulting in systemic edema and pulmonary congestion. Auscultating respiratory crackles indicates wet respirations or pulmonary congestion. Right sided heart failure produces blood congestion and enlargement of the liver. Rapid weight gain reflects fluid retention, often seen in congestive heart failure. Caution should be taken not to diagnose CHF on weight gain only. Infants normally gain weight quickly during infancy. Increased blood pressure is not a clinical manifestation of CHF. Oxygen saturation usually decreases when the client has congestive heart failure. **Cognitive Level:** Applying **Client Need:** Physiological Adaptation **Integrated Process:** Nursing Process: Assessment **Content Area:** Child Health **Strategy:** Recall that symptoms of congestive heart failure arise from impaired cardiac output, pulmonary venous congestion, and systemic venous congestion. **Reference:** Ball, J., Bindler, R., & Cowen, K. (2010). *Child health nursing: Partnering with children & families* (2nd ed.). Upper Saddle River, NJ: Pearson/Prentice Hall, pp. 943–944.

3 **Answer: 1** **Rationale:** ASO titers indicate history of streptococcal infection, which is a precursor to rheumatic fever. The other symptoms are not related to this diagnosis. The streptococcus may or may not be present at the time of diagnosis, so the blood culture could be negative or positive and the WBC count normal or elevated. **Cognitive Level:** Analyzing **Client Need:** Physiological Adaptation **Integrated Process:** Nursing Process: Diagnosis

Content Area: Child Health **Strategy:** Recall the purpose of various laboratory tests to choose correctly. Note the association between the syllable -*strep* in the correct option to associate this test with the microorganism that triggered the original precursor infection. **Reference:** Ball, J., Bindler, R., & Cowen, K. (2010). *Child health nursing: Partnering with children & families* (2nd ed.). Upper Saddle River, NJ: Pearson/Prentice Hall, p. 956.

4 **Answer: 4** **Rationale:** Vital sign assessment, especially pulse quality, provides important information to the health care provider. More frequent assessment is necessary. An alternative diet is not indicated for coarctation of the aorta. A regular diet is usually ordered. Reduction of blood flow through the descending aorta causes lower blood pressure in the legs and higher in the arms, neck, and head. Taking the blood pressure in all extremities q4h is appropriate. Intake and output is commonly measured for pediatric cardiac clients. **Cognitive Level:** Analyzing **Client Need:** Physiological Adaptation **Integrated Process:** Nursing Process: Implementation **Content Area:** Child Health **Strategy:** Vital signs include blood pressure. One order says on admission and once a day. The other order says blood pressure every four hours. These orders are in conflict so one is incorrect. Typical clinical manifestation is increased blood pressure in the arms versus the legs. **Reference:** Ball, J., Bindler, R., & Cowen, K. (2010). *Child health nursing: Partnering with children & families* (2nd ed.). Upper Saddle River, NJ: Pearson/Prentice Hall, pp. 941–942.

5 **Answer: 2** **Rationale:** Placing the infant in the knee–chest position relieves cardiac load by increasing pressure on the left side of the heart and decreasing the right to left shunt. Less deoxygenated blood will enter the systemic circulation. The Trendelenburg position offers no benefit to the child with tetralogy of Fallot. Administration of oxygen will increase saturation but will not relieve cardiac load. Suction equipment is needed for management for respiratory secretions but will not relieve cardiac load. **Cognitive Level:** Applying **Client Need:** Physiological Adaptation **Integrated Process:** Nursing Process: Implementation **Content Area:** Child Health **Strategy:** The core concept is to relieve cardiac load. Consider that neither suction nor oxygen will modify cardiac load, so the correct response must have something to do with positioning. Which position will decrease the blood return to the heart? **Reference:** Ball, J., Bindler, R., & Cowen, K. (2010). *Child health nursing: Partnering with children & families* (2nd ed.). Upper Saddle River, NJ: Pearson/Prentice Hall, pp. 932, 935.

6 **Answer: 3** **Rationale:** Parents should be taught cardiopulmonary resuscitation in the event of an emergency. Return demonstration is essential. Crying for short periods provides deep breathing exercises for the client with a cyanotic heart defect. Parents should be taught to monitor for significant cyanosis. Increased intracranial pressure is not related to a cyanotic heart defect. Growth and development may be normal or delayed in a client with a cyanotic heart defect. It would not be the primary concern. **Cognitive Level:** Analyzing **Client Need:** Physiological Adaptation **Integrated Process:** Teaching and Learning **Content Area:** Child Health **Strategy:** Eliminate those responses that do not relate to the heart. Then prioritize the responses that remain. **Reference:** Ball, J., Bindler, R., & Cowen, K. (2010). *Child health nursing: Partnering with children & families,* (2nd ed.). Upper Saddle River, NJ: Pearson/Prentice Hall, p. 938.

7 **Answer: 2** **Rationale:** Arthralgia of two or more joints is a common finding. Providing comfort and relief of pain is a priority. The pediatric client is not infectious. While some clients have an accompanying Sydenham chorea, it is not the most common clinical manifestation. Teaching CPR is usually done at the time of discharge. **Cognitive Level:** Analyzing **Client Need:** Physiological Adaptation **Integrated Process:** Nursing Process: Implementation **Content Area:** Child Health **Strategy:** Consider those responses that relate to rheumatic fever; eliminate options not related to rheumatic fever. Then prioritize the remaining responses, remembering that the stem asks for the most important intervention during hospitalization. **Reference:** Ball, J., Bindler, R., & Cowen, K. (2010). *Child health nursing: Partnering with children & families* (2nd ed.). Upper Saddle River, NJ: Pearson/Prentice Hall, p. 957.

8 **Answer: 1** **Rationale:** Administration of aspirin and immunoglobulins decrease fever and inflammation and thus should promote comfort. The pediatric client has decreased activity during exacerbation of the illness but splinting extremities would not provide comfort. Intake of fluids soothes the clients cracked lips and quenches thirst. The client with Kawasaki disease requires rest to promote comfort, although gentle range of motion will be useful. **Cognitive Level:** Applying **Client Need:** Physiological Adaptation **Integrated Process:** Nursing Process: Implementation **Content Area:** Child Health **Strategy:** Consider activities appropriate for the treatment of a child with this condition. Then consider the options that would promote comfort. **Reference:** Ball, J., Bindler, R., & Cowen, K. (2010). *Child health nursing: Partnering with children & families* (2nd ed.). Upper Saddle River, NJ: Pearson/Prentice Hall, p. 958.

9 **Answer: 2** **Rationale:** Administration of a low dose antibiotic is important to prevent future infections and heart damage. Activities may be limited especially if heart damage is suspected. Complete bedrest is not necessary but limited activity is suggested. Some, not all, clients with rheumatic fever may experience a transient CNS chorea for approximately 5–15 weeks. **Cognitive Level:** Analyzing **Client Need:** Physiological Adaptation **Integrated Process:** Nursing Process: Planning **Content Area:** Child Health **Strategy:** The critical word in

the question is *priority*. This indicates that one option is more important than any others that may also be correct. Use knowledge of the disorder and the process of elimination to make a selection. **Reference:** Ball, J., Bindler, R., & Cowen, K. (2010). *Child health nursing: Partnering with children & families* (2nd ed.). Upper Saddle River, NJ: Pearson/Prentice Hall, p. 957.

10 **Answer:**

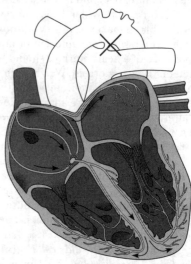

Rationale: The patent ductus is a fetal structure that lies between the aorta and pulmonary artery. In fetal life, the ductus allows blood to bypass the lungs. After birth, because of the change in pressures, oxygenated blood will return to the lungs by the ductus. **Cognitive Level:** Applying **Client Need:** Physiological Adaptation **Integrated Process:** Teaching and Learning **Content Area:** Child Health **Strategy:** The patent ductus arteriosus lies between the aorta and pulmonary artery. **Reference:** Ball, J., Bindler, R., & Cowen, K. (2010). *Child health nursing: Partnering with children & families* (2nd ed.). Upper Saddle River, NJ: Pearson/Prentice Hall, p. 924.

Posttest

1 **Answer:**

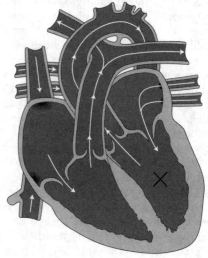

Rationale: The pressure is greatest in the left ventricle because that heart chamber must supply blood throughout the body. The pressure in the other chambers is lower. **Cognitive Level:** Applying **Client Need:** Physiological Adaptation **Integrated Process:** Teaching and Learning **Content Area:** Child Health **Strategy:** Recall that pressure gradients are higher in the ventricles than in the atria. Then recall that the left ventricle has the greatest muscle mass and must push blood throughout the body. **Reference:** Ball, J., Bindler, R., & Cowen, K. (2010). *Child health nursing: Partnering with children & families* (2nd ed.). Upper Saddle River, NJ: Pearson/ Prentice Hall, pp. 913–914.

2 **Answer: 3 Rationale:** If the hemoglobin contains less oxygen, the client's oxygenation saturation will decrease and cyanosis or a bluish color may be apparent. If the cyanosis occurs quickly, the nurse or health care provider should consider it a medical emergency. A left to right shunt is found in acyanotic heart defects. More blood is shunted to the lungs, but cyanosis is not apparent. Liver dysfunction due to right sided congestive heart failure may cause enlargement but not cyanosis. Low or poor iron levels may be exemplified by pallor but cyanosis is not usually present. **Cognitive Level:** Applying **Client Need:** Physiological Adaptation **Integrated Process:** Nursing Process: Implementation **Content Area:** Child Health **Strategy:** Recall that cyanosis is due to unoxygenated hemoglobin. Look at the responses to determine which responses would contribute to unoxygenated hemoglobin. **Reference:** Ball, J., Bindler, R., & Cowen, K. (2010). *Child health nursing: Partnering with children & families* (2nd ed.). Upper Saddle River, NJ: Pearson/Prentice Hall, p. 916.

3 **Answer: 4 Rationale:** Jones Criteria is a protocol to assist in identifying rheumatic fever. It consists of major symptoms, minor symptoms, and supporting evidence. Erythema, polyarthritis, and elevated ASO titer are among the major and minor symptoms and supporting evidence. **Cognitive Level:** Analyzing **Client Need:** Physiological Adaptation **Integrated Process:** Nursing Process: Assessment **Content Area:** Child Health **Strategy:** Recall that the Jones Criteria divides the symptoms of rheumatic fever into major manifestations and minor manifestations based on the frequency seen in the disease. Note that the correct option contains the phrase *strep-*, which is often associated with the term "rheumatic fever." **Reference:** Ball, J., Bindler, R., & Cowen, K. (2010). *Child health nursing: Partnering with children & families* (2nd ed.). Upper Saddle River, NJ: Pearson/Prentice Hall, p. 956.

4 **Answer: 1, 3, 4 Rationale:** Aspirin is indicated and frequently ordered as treatment for Kawasaki disease. It is ordered 80 to 100 mg/kg/day until fever drops. Then aspirin is continued at 10 mg/kg/day until platelet count drops. Aspirin is used as an anti-pyretic and anti-agglutination drug. **Cognitive Level:** Applying **Client Need:** Pharmacological and Parenteral Therapies **Integrated Process:** Teaching and Learning **Content Area:** Child Health **Strategy:** The question requires specific knowledge about the effects of ASA (acetylsalicylic acid or aspirin) on fever and platelets and knowledge of Kawasaki disease. **Reference:** Ball, J., Bindler, R., & Cowen, K. (2010). *Child health nursing: Partnering with children & families* (2nd ed.). Upper Saddle River, NJ: Pearson/Prentice Hall, p. 958.

5 **Answer: 2 Rationale:** Furosemide (Lasix) is considered a loop diuretic. It stops the reabsorption of sodium and chloride in the proximal tubule and loop of Henle, causing diuresis to reduce stress on the heart. The main action of furosemide (Lasix) is to cause diuresis through the kidney. It does not treat a kidney defect. Furosemide (Lasix) does not prevent digoxin from becoming toxic. Furosemide (Lasix) is a potassium-wasting diuretic and is not given for potassium management. **Cognitive Level:** Applying **Client Need:** Pharmacological and Parenteral Therapies **Integrated Process:** Teaching and Learning **Content Area:** Child Health **Strategy:** Recall that Lasix is a diuretic that increases urine output. Next determine which option describes increased urine output. **Reference:** Ball, J., Bindler, R., & Cowen, K. (2010). *Child health nursing: Partnering with children and families* (2nd ed.). Upper Saddle River, NJ: Pearson/Prentice Hall, p. 944.

6 **Answer: 1 Rationale:** The best approach is to allow the pediatric client self-regulated activity. Even a 2-year-old client will rest if fatigued. Complete bedrest is not necessary and prevents normal growth and development. Limiting activity to a few hours per day is usually not necessary and does not allow the client to control the amount of activity. Deliberately attempting to prevent crying should be avoided because it promotes an abnormal parental pattern of relating to the infant. Some crying is therapeutic as deep breathing exercises. **Cognitive Level:** Applying **Client Need:** Physiological Adaptation **Integrated Process:** Nursing Process: Implementation **Content Area:** Child Health **Strategy:** During the toddler years the child begins to explore the environment. Considering the activity level of a 2-year-old as well as the child's need for growth and development, complete bedrest or restricting activity is unrealistic. Controlling infant or toddler crying is unnecessary. **Reference:** Ball, J., Bindler, R., & Cowen, K. (2010). *Child health nursing: Partnering with children and families* (2nd ed.). Upper Saddle River, NJ: Pearson/ Prentice Hall, p. 938.

7 **Answer: 4 Rationale:** Direct pressure on the wound site initially, followed by application of a pressure dressing helps to form a clot and reduce bleeding. Hemorrhage can be life threatening in the immediate post-procedure period. Food intake is a lesser concern than maintaining hemostasis. Infection would not be apparent immediately following the procedure. Signs of congestive heart failure could relate to the original disease process but are not a priority at this time; physiological needs take current priority. **Cognitive Level:** Applying **Client Need:** Reduction of Risk Potential **Integrated Process:** Nursing Process: Implementation **Content Area:** Child Health **Strategy:** Recall key complications after cardiac catheterization, and use the ABCs (airway, breathing,

ANSWERS & RATIONALES

circulation) to determine priorities. **Reference:** Ball, J., Bindler, R., & Cowen, K. (2010). *Child health nursing: Partnering with children & families* (2nd ed.). Upper Saddle River, NJ: Pearson/Prentice Hall, p. 922.

8 **Answer: 1, 2** **Rationale:** Furosemide is a diuretic, so measurements that most directly illustrate output and water loss would be evaluated. With this in mind, intake and output and daily weight would be key assessment parameters, as they typically and accurately reflect fluid balance. The pulse and hemoglobin and hematocrit can be influenced by many variables. Partial pressure of oxygen is measured via arterial blood gases and is unrelated to the question. **Cognitive Level:** Analyzing **Client Need:** Physiological Adaptation **Integrated Process:** Nursing Process: Assessment **Content Area:** Child Health **Strategy:** Recall that furosemide promotes urine output, which indicates that intake and output should be measured. Recall specific tools to measure output to choose correctly. **Reference:** Ball, J., Bindler, R., & Cowen, K. (2010). *Child health nursing: Partnering with children & families* (2nd ed.). Upper Saddle River, NJ: Pearson/Prentice Hall, p. 947.

9 **Answer: 3** **Rationale:** Signs of digoxin toxicity include bradycardia, cardiac dysrhythmias, nausea, vomiting, anorexia, dizziness, headache, weakness, and fatigue. **Cognitive Level:** Applying **Client Need:** Pharmacological and Parenteral Therapies **Integrated Process:** Nursing Process: Evaluation **Content Area:** Child Health **Strategy:** Recall that

the purpose of digoxin is to slow and strengthen the heart so that it can contract more effectively. Reasoning that toxic effects of a drug are often related to excessive effect of its original purpose, select the option that exhibits a change in this direction. **Reference:** Ball, J., Bindler, R., & Cowen, K. (2010). *Child health nursing: Partnering with children & families* (2nd ed.). Upper Saddle River, NJ: Pearson/Prentice Hall, p. 946.

10 **Answer: 1** **Rationale:** Because of activity intolerance and respiratory distress, the child may be unable to take in enough nutrients to meet the body's need for growth. The child is not at risk for seizures or pain because of this health problem. There is no information in the question to support the diagnosis of Diversional Activity Deficit. **Cognitive Level:** Analyzing **Client Need:** Physiological Adaptation **Integrated Process:** Nursing Process: Diagnosis **Content Area:** Child Health **Strategy:** Consider each nursing diagnosis as it would relate to the child with low oxygen levels secondary to a cyanotic heart defect. Eliminate diversional activity deficit as it is a psychosocial need, not a physiological one. Eliminate risk for seizures and pain as unrelated. **Reference:** Ball, J., Bindler, R., & Cowen, K. (2010). *Child health nursing: Partnering with children & families* (2nd ed.). Upper Saddle River, NJ: Pearson/Prentice Hall, p. 948.

References

Ball, J., Bindler, R., & Cowen, K. (2010). *Child health nursing: Partnering with children & families* (2nd ed.). Upper Saddle River, NJ: Pearson Education.

Bindler, R. & Ball, J. (2008). *Clinical skills manual for pediatric nursing: Caring for children* (4th ed.). Upper Saddle River, NJ: Pearson Education.

Hockenberry, M. & Wilson, D. (2009). *Wong's essentials of pediatric nursing* (8th ed.). St. Louis, MO: Elsevier, pp. 862–907.

Pillitteri, A. (2010). *Maternal & child health nursing: Care of the childbearing & childrearing family* (6th ed.). Philadelphia: Lippincott Williams & Wilkins.

New guidelines regarding antibiotics to prevent infective endocarditis (n.d.). Retrieved March 10, 2011, from http://www.americanheart.org/presenter.jhtml?identifier=3047051

Neurologic Health Problems

6

Chapter Outline

Overview of Anatomy and
Physiology of Nervous
System
Diagnostic Tests and
Assessments of Nervous
System

Congenital Neurologic Health
Problems
Acquired Neurologic Health
Problems

Infectious Neurologic Health
Problems
Accidents and Injuries Causing
Neurologic Health Problems

Objectives

➤ Identify data essential to the assessment of alterations in health of
the neurologic system in a child.
➤ Discuss the clinical manifestations and pathophysiology of
alterations in the health of the neurologic system of a child.
➤ Discuss therapeutic management of a child with alterations in
health of the neurologic system.
➤ Describe nursing management of a child with alterations in health
of the neurologic system.

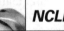

NCLEX-RN® Test Prep

Use the accompanying online resource,
NursingReviewsandRationales, to test
yourself with hundreds of NCLEX®-style
practice questions.

Review at a Glance

Brudzinski's sign noted when
client's head is flexed while in the supine
position, resulting in involuntary flexion
of knees or hips; a positive Brudzinski's
sign is a common sign in meningitis
coma level of unconsciousness in
which client cannot be aroused even
with painful stimuli
Cushing's triad a late sign of
increased intracranial pressure characterized by widening pulse pressure (rising
systolic blood pressure with stable diastolic pressure), bradycardia, and irregular respirations
epidural hematoma bleeding
between the dura and the cranium
intracranial pressure (ICP)
force exerted by brain tissue, cerebrospinal fluid, and blood within cranial vault;
normal ICP is 4 to 12 mm Hg and is
dependent on age in childhood
Kernig's sign demonstrated when
client's leg is raised with knee flexed
and any resistance or pain is felt; it is a

common finding that indicates meningeal
irritation in meningitis
level of consciousness (LOC) a
measure of degree of responsiveness of
mind to sensory stimuli; lower levels indicate decreased neurologic functioning;
levels can be categorized (in order of
decreasing level of function) as confusion, delirium, obtunded, stupor, and coma
meninges fibrous membrane that covers brain and lines vertebral canal; consists of three layers: dura, arachnoid, and
pia mater
myelin a sheath made of a fatty substance that covers axon process of neuron or nerve fibers and increases speed
and accuracy of nerve impulses; myelination process is not complete at birth,
but proceeds in a head to toe direction
and accounts for gradual development
of fine and gross motor skills during
early childhood
neurogenic refers to a lack of innervation to an organ

nuchal rigidity stiffness of neck or
resistance to neck flexion, often seen in
infections of central nervous system
opisthotonus client positions self
with hyperextension of head and neck;
this is seen in meningitis and felt to relieve
some discomfort from meningeal irritation
photophobia sensitivity to light, seen
in some clients with migraine headaches
or viral infections such as measles, meningitis, and encephalitis
pulse pressure difference in systolic and diastolic blood pressure
subdural hematoma bleeding
between dura and cerebrum
spasticity tenseness of muscles,
uncoordinated, stiff movements; can be
seen as scissoring or crossing of legs;
exaggerated reflex reactions
tonic-clonic term frequently used to
describe characteristics of certain seizures; tonic indicates continuous muscle
contraction; clonic indicates alternating
contraction and relaxation of muscles

PRETEST

1 A child with a history of a seizure was admitted two hours ago. The history reports fever, chills, and vomiting for the past 24 hours. In report, the nurse is told that the child has a positive Brudzinski's sign. The nurse considers that which of the following is the most likely cause?

1. Increased intracranial pressure
2. Meningeal irritation
3. Encephalitis
4. Intraventricular hemorrhage

2 A nurse is assessing a new admission. The 6-month-old infant displays irritability, bulging fontanels, and setting-sun eyes. What condition would the nurse suspect based on these manifestations?

1. Increased intracranial pressure
2. Hypertension
3. Skull fracture
4. Myelomeningocele

3 An 8-year-old client with a ventriculoperitoneal shunt was admitted for shunt malfunction. He presents with symptoms of increased intracranial pressure (ICP). The mechanism of the development of his symptoms is most probably related to which mechanism related to the cerebrospinal fluid (CSF)?

1. Increased flow of CSF
2. Increased reabsorption of CSF
3. Obstructed flow of CSF
4. Decreased production of CSF

4 A child with a myelomeningocele is started on a bowel management plan. The child's mother questions why this is being done. What would the nurse use as a basis for a response?

1. Lack of innervation to the colon predisposes the child to diarrhea.
2. Lack of innervation to the anal sphincter predisposes the child to being incontinent.
3. Chronic immobility increases the gastric-colic reflex.
4. Chronic immobility decreases the need for regular bowel movements.

5 A child has just been diagnosed with bacterial meningitis. The parent asks the nurse how long the child will be in isolation. The nurse's reply will be based on a protocol that transmission-based precautions will continue until what point?

1. The organism is identified.
2. The antibiotics are initiated.
3. The antibiotics have been administered for 24 hours.
4. Ten days of antibiotic therapy have been completed.

6 The nurse observes a client with the neck and back arched and extremities severely extended. The mother asks why the child is doing that. The nurse explains that this positioning is known as which of the following?

1. Decerebrate posturing
2. Decorticate posturing
3. Jacksonian seizure
4. Opisthotonos

7 A child is being treated for increased intracranial pressure (ICP). What should the nurse provide as part of the prescribed plan of care to decrease intracranial pressure? Select all that apply.

1. Keep head of bed at a 30-degree angle.
2. Provide supplemental oxygen.
3. Turn head to one side.
4. Administer IV osmotic diuretics.
5. Promote fluid intake.

8 A 10-year-old boy receives a blow to his head with a hard baseball and is admitted to the hospital for observation. If the child were to develop an epidural hematoma, the nurse explains to the parents that the child would most likely display symptoms at which time?

1. In the emergency room or soon after arriving on the unit
2. On the unit at any time over the next few days
3. One or two days after discharge home
4. Anytime over the next two months

9 A 15-year-old client is seen in the emergency department following a head injury from football. During the first few hours after admission, he sleeps unless awakened, but he can be aroused easily and is oriented. In charting assessment findings, how would the nurse describe this level of consciousness?

1. Semicomatose
2. Lethargic
3. Obtunded
4. Stuporous

10 A young child has just been diagnosed with spastic cerebral palsy. The nurse is teaching the parents how to meet their child's dietary needs. The nurse would explain that children with cerebral palsy frequently have special dietary needs or feeding challenges for which reason?

1. The paralysis of their muscles decreases their caloric need.
2. The spasticity of their muscles increases their caloric need.
3. The hypotonic muscles make eating difficult.
4. The child's inactivity increases the risk of obesity.

➤ *See pages 136–138 for Answers and Rationales.*

I. OVERVIEW OF ANATOMY AND PHYSIOLOGY OF NERVOUS SYSTEM

  A. **Several key points** must be remembered when considering nervous system of infants and young children in contrast to adolescents and adults
  B. **Brain and spinal cord develop during first trimester**; they are very susceptible to malformations caused by insults such as infection, substance abuse, or maternal dietary deficiency
  C. **Nervous system is not mature at birth**, but as numbers of glial cells and dendrites increase, refinement continues until about 4 years of age
  D. **Myelination is also incomplete at birth**; *myelin* (a sheath made of a fatty substance that covers axon process of neuron or nerve fibers) is essential to increase speed and accuracy of nerve impulses, providing child with fine and gross motor skills and coordination
  E. **Development is in a cephalocaudal or "head to tail" direction**
  F. **At birth and during early childhood, fontanels are not closed and cranial bones have yet to ossify**; this allows head to expand to accommodate normal growth or increased swelling (or other causes of rising intracranial pressure)
  G. **Young infants have a proportionately large**, heavy head compared to adults and they lack neck strength
  H. **An infant's brain is highly vascular**, and dura can strip away from pericranium; brain is more prone to hemorrhage when shaken or when another force is applied
  I. **Vertebrae are not completely ossified**, placing young children at greater risk for cervical spine injury and compression fractures

II. DIAGNOSTIC TESTS AND ASSESSMENTS OF NERVOUS SYSTEM

  A. **Physical assessment**
    1. **Level of consciousness (LOC)**
      a. This is a measure of responsiveness of brain to stimuli and has two components: alertness and cognitive power

      b. Levels of decreasing consciousness include confusion, delirium, obtunded, stupor, and **coma** (unarousable to painful stimuli)

      c. Glasgow coma scale: an established instrument used to quantify LOC

          1) There are two versions based on child's development level; one for infant and young child (preverbal) and one for older child and adult

          2) Scores on three subscales range from 1 to 4 for eye opening, 1 to 5 for verbal response, and 1 to 6 for motor response

          3) Highest level of functioning would be scored 15, while lowest level of functioning would score a 3 (see Table 6-1)

2. Intracranial pressure (ICP)

      a. Pressure within cranium that surrounds brain, normally 4 to 12 mm Hg

      b. Pressure is caused by volume of brain mass, cerebrospinal fluid (CSF), and blood

      c. An increase in any of these three must be compensated for by the others

      d. Fortunately for a young child whose sutures have not closed, the cranium can expand to a point if there is increased pressure

3. Fontanels

      a. Membranes at juncture of unclosed sutures

      b. Two prominent fontanels: anterior and posterior

4. Developmental milestones

      a. There are specific criteria for comparing fine or gross motor, social, and cognitive skills in children of same age

      b. Most criteria have been validated through cross-sectional and longitudinal studies

      c. Many of these criteria are incorporated into standardized developmental screening instruments such as the Denver II

Table 6-1   **Glasgow Coma Scale**

Assessment	Response	Score*
Eyes open	Spontaneously	4
(Record C if eyes are closed by swelling)	To speech	3
	To pain	2
	No response	1
Best motor response	Obeys commands	6
(Record best upper arm response)	Localized pain	5
	Flexion-withdrawal	4
	Abnormal flexion	3
	Abnormal extension	2
	No response	1
Best verbal response	Oriented	5
(Record T if an endotracheal or tracheostomy tube is in place)	Confused	4
	Inappropriate words	3
	Incomprehensible sounds	2
	No response	1
Total Score:		____

*A higher score indicates a higher level of functioning.

Source: Hogan, MaryAnn; Brancato, Vera; White, Judy; Falkenstein, Kathleen, *Prentice Hall Reviews & rationales: Child health nursing*, 2nd Ed., ©2007. Reprinted and Electronically reproduced by permission of Pearson Education, Inc. Upper Saddle River, NJ.

5. Neurological exam: a specialized physical examination to determine neurologic function; it includes the following criteria:
   a. Description of behavior
   b. Vital signs: pulse, respirations, blood pressure (BP), body temperature
   c. Eyes: pupil size and reactivity, movements, and blinking; additionally, a funduscopic exam may be done to check for papilledema and preretinal hemorrhages
   d. Motor function: presence of spontaneous activity or response to pain; tremors, twitching, or seizures may be observed
   e. Posturing
      1) When cortical control over motor function is lost, primitive posturing reflexes are apparent
      2) Decorticate posturing is seen with a severe dysfunction of cerebral cortex; it includes adduction of arms at shoulders, arms flexed at chest, wrists flexed, hands fisted, and lower extremities flexed (see Figure 6-1A)
      3) Decerebrate posturing is seen with dysfunction at level of midbrain; it includes rigid extension and pronation of arms and legs (see Figure 6-1B)

Figure 6-1

A. Decorticate posturing,
B. Decerebrate posturing.

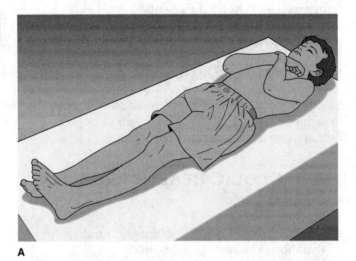

A

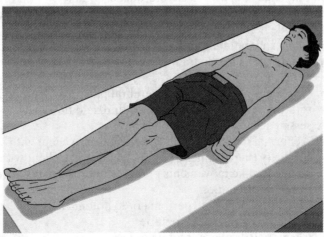

B

     f. Reflexes

      1) Specific reflexes are absent in deep coma such as corneal, pupillary, muscle-stretch, superficial, and plantar

      2) Specific neonatal reflexes such as the Moro, tonic neck, and withdrawal reflexes are evidence of normal neurological functioning, but persistence of these and other neonatal or primitive reflexes after certain ages can indicate areas of dysfunction

    6. Kernig's and Brudzinski's signs: specialized approaches that demonstrate meningeal irritation

     a. Kernig's sign: positive or present when client's leg is raised with knee flexed and any resistance or pain is felt; this is a common finding indicating meningeal irritation in meningitis

     b. Brudzinski's sign: positive or present when client's head is flexed while in supine position, resulting in involuntary flexion of knees or hips; this is a common sign in meningitis

B. Diagnostic tests

    1. Lumbar puncture (LP): insertion of a needle to obtain cerebrospinal fluid (CSF) to assess for blood, glucose, proteins, or bacteria

    2. Magnetic resonance imaging (MRI): a noninvasive procedure usually performed in radiology department that permits visualization of neurologic structures using radio frequency emissions from elements

    3. Computed tomography (CT): radiological procedure where pinpoint x-ray beams are directed on a horizontal or vertical plane which, when entered on a computer, provide "slices" or pictures of cross sections of brain at any axis

    4. Electromyogram (EMG): a procedure that measures electrical potential of individual muscles

    5. Electroencephalogram (EEG): procedure using multiple electrodes placed on head to record changes in electrical potentials or impulses in brain; it can be used to diagnose seizures and determine brain death

III. CONGENITAL NEUROLOGIC HEALTH PROBLEMS

A. Cerebral palsy (CP)

    1. Description

     a. A nonprogressive motor disorder of central nervous system (CNS) resulting in alteration in movement and posture

     b. Classified as spastic, athetoid, ataxic, or mixed

     c. Topographic descriptions explain part(s) of body affected by cerebral palsy and include hemiplegia, diplegia, and quadriplegia

    2. Etiology and pathophysiology

     a. Causes may include trauma, hemorrhage, anoxia, or infection before, during, or after birth

     b. One-third of children with cerebral palsy also have some degree of mental retardation, while the other two thirds do not

    3. Assessment

     a. Abnormal muscle tone and coordination: a client with spastic CP presents with **spasticity** (hypertonicity of muscle groups); a client with athetoid CP presents with wormlike movements of the extremities; ataxic form of CP involves disturbed coordination

     b. Client may display hypertonia or hypotonia and may have varying degrees of tonicity on different extremities

     c. Client may display scissoring of legs

        d. Absence of expected reflexes or presence of reflexes that extend beyond expected age suggest cerebral palsy

        e. Failure to meet developmental norms may be the first indication that "something is wrong"

        f. Physical symptoms include altered speech and difficulty with swallowing; visual and hearing defects may be present; nurse may note scissoring of lower extremities

        g. Seizures may accompany cerebral palsy and may be another indication of brain injury

    4. Priority nursing diagnoses

        a. Impaired Physical Mobility

        b. Self-Care Deficit

        c. Imbalanced Nutrition: Less Than Body Requirements

        d. Risk for Injury related to neuromuscular, perceptual, or cognitive impairments

        e. Impaired Verbal Communication

        f. Fatigue

    5. Planning and implementation

        a. Many clients with CP require increased calorie intake because of spasticity or increased motor functioning

        b. If motor involvement causes client to have poor coordination or if client has seizure activity, there is a need to provide a safe environment, such as protective headgear or a padded bed

        c. Communication can be a problem if there is oral involvement; client may need to use a communication board or computer-assisted communication; the use of touch is an excellent means to communicate caring to a client with limited intelligence

        d. Self-care is a goal for all clients; extensive collaboration with occupational therapists for strategies and devices to assist in this area may be necessary

        e. Risk for aspiration is present if oral muscles are involved; use adaptive feeding devices and positioning during feedings to decrease risk; for some clients with severe spasticity, a gastrostomy tube might be surgically placed for enteral feedings

        f. Collaborate with multidisciplinary team for speech, nutrition, occupational and physical therapies; client and family must be at center of this team

        g. Regional early-intervention consortiums conduct community-based developmental screenings to find clients who might be at risk or have developmental delays from disorders such as cerebral palsy; these clients can then be referred for further assessment so that possible delays can be identified and appropriate early intervention initiated; the most widely used developmental screening test is the Denver II

        h. Provide adequate nutrition and rest

        i. Maintain a safe environment

    6. Surgical procedures and medication therapy

        a. To control spasticity, traditional treatments have included surgery to release tendons and promote mobility, rehabilitation therapies, oral medications, and intramuscular injections of phenol and botulinum toxin

        b. Newer treatment includes use of a surgically implanted intrathecal pump, which administers a continuous infusion of baclofen; potential pump-related problems include infection and overdose; benefits include improved function, gait, and motor control, and generally improved health

7. Client and family education

   a. Teach parents use of physical therapy strategies such as range-of-motion exercises to use at home

   b. Client will need to learn self-care skills such as how to feed and dress self and perform hygiene activities

   c. Teach parents special feeding techniques and use of adaptive devices such as special silverware and dishes; parents may need to learn how to do gastrostomy tube feedings if indicated

8. Evaluation: client establishes optimal physical mobility and self-care skills; client demonstrates adequate nutrition, as evidenced by age-appropriate maintenance or increase in height and weight; client is free from injury; client demonstrates adequate energy level, as evidenced by ability to participate in daily routine; all individuals interacting with client are able to comprehend client's communication; family copes with management of client's health problems

B. Neural tube defects

1. Description: neural tube defects (also known as spina bifida or myelodysplasia) develop during first trimester of fetal development; defects can occur at any place along spinal canal (see Figure 6-2)

2. Etiology and pathophysiology

   a. Etiology is unknown but may be associated with maternal dietary folic acid deficiency; incidence has decreased with emphasis on folic acid supplementation during pregnancy; the degree of disability is determined by location of defect and amount of spinal nerves encased in sac; the higher the defect, the greater the neurologic dysfunction

   b. There are several types of spina bifida or neural tube defects

   1) Spina bifida occulta: posterior vertebral arches fail to fuse, but there is not herniation of spinal cord or **meninges** (fibrous membrane that covers brain and lines vertebral canal); no loss of function

   2) Meningocele: posterior vertebral arches fail to fuse, and there is a saclike protrusion at some point along posterior vertebrae; sac contains meninges and CSF but not spinal cord

Practice to Pass

Describe the multidisciplinary team that will be needed in the rehabilitation of the client with cerebral palsy.

Figure 6-2

Infant with lumbarsacral myelomeningocele

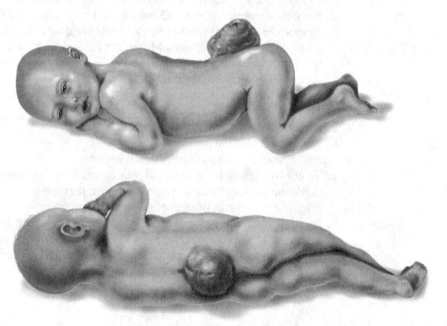

        3) Myelomeningocele: posterior vertebral arches fail to fuse; saclike herniation contains meninges, CSF, as well as a portion of spinal cord or nerve roots; sometimes leakage of CSF occurs

        4) Encephalocele: brain and meninges herniate through defect in skull into a sac

3. Assessment

    a. Prenatal diagnosis of open spinal defects can be determined by elevated levels of alpha-fetoprotein (AFP) in maternal serum and fluid obtained by amniocentesis; can also be assessed on prenatal ultrasound

    b. Meningoceles, myelomeningoceles, and encephaloceles are obvious at birth; spina bifida occulta may have an associated abnormal tuft of hair, dimple, sinus tract or subcutaneous mass at the site

    c. During postnatal period, monitor for leakage of CSF from sac as well as skin integrity of sac; assess for infection around sac and for possible systemic or CNS infection

    d. Assess degree of sensation at or below level of lesion; this can be evidenced by lack of movement or sensation in legs, and a **neurogenic** (lacking innervation) bladder or bowel

    e. Measure head circumference since there is a high risk of hydrocephalus

4. Priority nursing diagnoses

    a. Risk for Infection

    b. Risk for Impaired Skin Integrity

    c. Impaired Urinary Elimination

    d. Bowel Incontinence/Colonic Constipation

    e. Impaired Physical Immobility

5. Planning and implementation

    a. Collaborative management: the defect/sac is surgically repaired during first 48 hours after birth

    b. Focus preoperative care on maintaining skin integrity of sac and keeping it free of infection; position client on side or abdomen to achieve this; keep sac moist with sterile, saline-soaked dressings; avoid contamination of sac area by urine or feces

    c. Clients with myelodysplasia have an increased incidence of latex allergies; monitor for this carefully

    d. Neurogenic bladder: frequent, clean straight catheterization is the preferred method of management; maintain home schedule as much as possible

    e. Neurogenic bowel: work with family to develop a bowel management plan using control of high-fiber diet, adequate fluid intake, and pattern for evacuation of bowels; in some cases, laxatives and enemas are used as prescribed by physician

    f. Collaborate with physical therapy to develop modes of transport, such as wheelchair or using braces with crutches

    g. Since areas with altered sensation are prone to skin breakdown, teach client and family to reposition frequently and inspect affected areas on a regular basis

6. Medication therapy: low-dose antimicrobials may be prescribed to prevent urinary tract infections (UTIs)

7. Client and family education

    a. Teach family about possibility of client developing hydrocephalus and signs/symptoms of increased intracranial pressure (ICP) and what to do if changes develop

    b. Since most children with neural tube defects (except for those with spina bifida occulta) have neurogenic bladder, teaching about clean intermittent straight catheterization is important; work with family to develop a bowel management program also

8. Evaluation: client does not develop CNS or wound infection; client does not develop pressure ulcers; client demonstrates normal renal functioning and adequate urinary elimination by having infrequent UTIs; client evacuates bowels on a routine basis; client becomes physically mobile within limits of neuromuscular potential

C. Hydrocephalus

1. Description: a condition characterized by imbalance between CSF production and absorption resulting in enlarged ventricles and an increase in ICP; if untreated, this condition can cause permanent brain damage

2. Etiology and pathophysiology

   a. Congenital causes include Arnold Chiari malformation associated with myelomeningocele

   b. Can be acquired from meningitis, trauma, or intraventricular hemorrhage in premature infants

   c. Etiology is idiopathic (cause is unknown) in up to 50% of cases

3. Assessment

   a. For infants, increased head circumference, split cranial sutures, high-pitched cry, bulging fontanel, irritability when awake and seizures (see Figure 6-3)

   b. Toddlers and older children may also present with setting-sun eyes, seizures, irritability, papilledema, decreased LOC, and change in vital signs (increased BP and widening **pulse pressure**)

   c. Older children may report headaches and have difficulty with balance or coordination

   d. All children can present with vomiting, lethargy, and Cheyne-Stokes respiratory pattern

   e. Diagnosis confirmed using CT and MRI to reveal location of CSF obstruction

---

Figure 6-3

Development of hydrocephalus in young child. A. Normal ventricles, B. Enlarged ventricles and bulging fontanel.

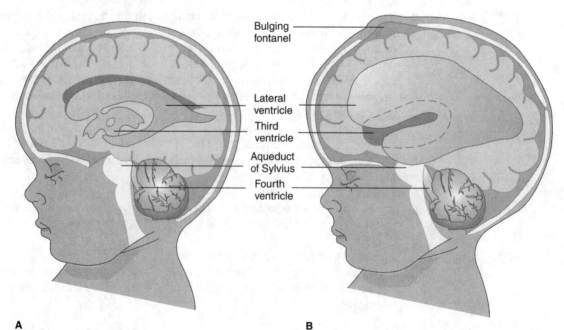

Bulging fontanel

Lateral ventricle

Third ventricle

Aqueduct of Sylvius

Fourth ventricle

A

B

4. Priority nursing diagnoses
   a. Ineffective Tissue Perfusion (cerebral)
   b. Risk for Infection
   c. Risk for Impaired Skin Integrity related to large size of head and inability to move
5. Planning and implementation
   a. Surgical insertion of a tube or "shunt" (with consistency of a piece of spaghetti) into ventricles with other end in either the peritoneum or atrium; the most common version is ventriculoperitoneal; preoperatively monitor client for symptoms of increased ICP; postoperatively position client flat and on unoperative side; if held, it is important not to allow head to be elevated
   b. Postoperatively, monitor client also for symptoms of infection; notify physician if symptoms are present: fever, change in LOC, excessive redness at incision site or along shunt tract, elevated WBC count with leukocytosis or "shift to the left"
6. Medication therapy: client may be on prophylactic antibiotics postoperatively
7. Client and family education
   a. Teach caregiver symptoms of shunt infection and malfunction and what actions to take should symptoms develop
   b. Signs of shunt malfunction
      1) Infant whose cranial suture lines have not fused; signs include increased head circumference, high-pitched cry, bulging fontanel, irritability when awake, and seizures
      2) Toddlers and older children display vomiting, irritability, and headache; as condition persists, setting-sun eyes, seizures, papilledema, decreased LOC, and change in vital signs (increased BP and widening pulse pressure) occur
      3) Older children have difficulty with balance or coordination
      4) All children may have lethargy and Cheyne-Stokes respirations
   c. Some clients with hydrocephalus have brain damage that results in motor, language, perceptual, and intellectual disabilities; parents may need referrals to early-intervention professionals to provide long-term rehabilitation services
   d. Clients with hydrocephalus and myelomeningocele have an increased risk of latex allergies; teach parents to avoid nipples, pacifiers, and toys made of latex products
8. Evaluation: client demonstrates cerebral perfusion as evidenced by age-appropriate response to environment and vital signs within normal limits; client does not demonstrate signs or symptoms of infection; caregivers verbalize purpose of shunt and how to detect infection or malfunction

IV. ACQUIRED NEUROLOGIC HEALTH PROBLEMS

A. Seizures
1. Description
   a. Seizures are alterations in firing of neurons in brain (cortical neuronal discharge); the result of this discharge (seizure activity) depends on where in brain discharge begins and how it spreads
   b. Seizures can be divided into two categories: partial seizures, which begin locally in one hemisphere of brain, and generalized seizures, which begin in both hemispheres of brain
   c. Seizures are the most common alteration in nervous system seen in children; they are present with numerous different conditions involving the CNS
   d. Epilepsy is a chronic disorder characterized by recurrent seizures
   e. Determining type of seizure is done based on history and electroencephalogram (EEG) results

Practice to Pass

Identify the age-related differences in discharge instructions to a parent whose client has a ventriculo-peritoneal shunt.

2. Etiology and pathophysiology
   a. Seizures have many causes; most are idiopathic; somehow seizure threshold has been altered to influence neuronal discharge
   b. Common etiologies of seizures during infancy include perinatal hypoxia, congenital diseases, infections, metabolic or degenerative diseases, drug withdrawal, and neoplasms; common etiologies of seizures during childhood include febrile infections, head injury, lead toxicity, drugs, genetic disorders, and neoplasms
3. Assessment
   a. During actual seizure activity, observe order of events and duration of seizure; for **tonic-clonic** seizures, be certain to time length of seizure until jerking stops; *tonic* indicates continuous muscle contraction; *clonic* indicates alternating contraction and relaxation of muscles; for all other types of seizures, note duration from start of seizure to time that consciousness is regained; describe any precipitating events or unusual behavior; note parts of body involved and if it begins in any particular body part
   b. Observe face for any color change, perspiration, and lack of expression; note if mouth has any deviation to one side or other, teeth clenched, tongue bitten, frothing at mouth, and/or flecks of blood or bleeding; if able to assess pupils, note any change in size, equality, reaction to light, and accommodation
   c. Observe for presence or length of apnea; other general observations might be involuntary urination or defecation
   d. Postictally note duration of postictal period, level of consciousness, orientation (to time, person, place), and any alterations in motor ability or speech
4. Priority nursing diagnoses
   a. Risk for Injury related to type of seizure and possible loss of consciousness
   b. Risk for Aspiration
   c. Ineffective Family Processes related to having child with chronic illness
5. Planning and implementation
   a. Protect client during a seizure: place client on his or her side and protect client from injury; monitor vital signs after seizure ends
   b. Administer antiepileptic medications as ordered
   c. Assist parents or caregivers in understanding and accepting diagnosis
   d. Promote development of a positive self-image for client; talk with client about his or her feelings; plan strategies to promote acceptance and decrease fear among peers
6. Medication therapy
   a. Since seizures are felt to be caused by a heightened sensitivity to neuronal firing, most medication therapy involves using drugs whose actions decrease this sensitivity; 85% of children with epilepsy have seizures that are well controlled by one antiepileptic medication; choice of medication by health care provider will vary depending on type of seizures
   b. Phenobarbital is one of the oldest medications used; carbamazepine (Tegretol) is commonly used at this time
   c. Unfortunately, 15% of children with epilepsy are difficult to manage, and their seizures are not easily controlled; these children can suffer from poor self-esteem, academic failure, and poor social relationships; for some of these children, surgery may be an option to control seizures if focus of epilepsy can be pinpointed
7. Client and family education
   a. Families need to know what to do when client has a seizure; teach safety measures and when to call emergency medical services (EMS); clients with frequent seizures are advised to wear some form of medical alert identification

b. Combination of barbiturates with carbamazepine can potentiate drugs levels; advise parents to not use any over-the-counter medications prior to consulting with client's health care provider (for example, with cold products containing antihistamine, side effects are increased)

c. Educate parents and older clients about type of seizure, medication currently taken and previously taken; teach how to keep a record/history of seizure control or number of seizures experienced and their timing

8. Evaluation: client is free from injury during seizures; client experiences as few seizures as possible; family and client cope with management of seizures; client has a positive self-image

B. Craniosynostosis

1. Description: premature closure of cranial sutures in young children; there is some relationship between craniosynostosis and several inherited syndromes

2. Etiology and pathophysiology

a. Etiology is unknown; craniosynostosis can be diagnosed by clinical exam; diagnosis is confirmed through skull films, CT scan, and MRI

b. Premature closure of skull may lead to increased ICP with subsequent brain damage

3. Assessment: a bony ridge is palpated along a suture line; compensatory growth of skull in directions parallel to closed suture line creates skull deformities; monitor fontanels of all infants for premature closure; measure head circumference to provide additional data related to this diagnosis

4. Priority nursing diagnoses

a. Deficient Knowledge (parental)

b. Risk for Injury

c. Disturbed Body Image

d. Ineffective Family Coping

5. Planning and implementation

a. Medical treatment is surgical correction of skeletal defect

b. Follow all procedures of standard postoperative care: keep incision dry and intact; monitor for signs of increased ICP, changing LOC, and infection during postoperative period

c. Prepare parents and client for client's postoperative appearance; in addition to large, turban-like bandage, client will have orbital edema and bruising; long-term results of surgery should be discussed; "before and after" pictures may assist family in mentally preparing for surgery

d. Fluid restriction may be prescribed in postoperative period; head of bed may be ordered to elevation at 30-degree angle to assist in decreasing facial swelling

6. Client and family education

a. Reassure parents that surgery will improve client's appearance and that most children postoperatively are healthy and have normal brain development

b. Parents may need instructions about how to change dressing at home

7. Evaluation: family verbalizes understanding of perioperative experience; client does not demonstrate any brain injury or infection as evidenced by age-appropriate response to environment, intact sensation/motion to extremities, age-appropriate speech patterns, normal urine output, absence of fever, and no other symptoms of infection

V. INFECTIOUS NEUROLOGIC HEALTH PROBLEMS

A. Meningitis

1. Description: inflammation of meninges; is most common infection of CNS; two primary classifications include viral or aseptic and bacterial

---

Practice to Pass

Parents of a client who has had his or her first seizure have gone through a fairly stressful and frightening experience. Keeping in mind that preparing for discharge can be equally stressful, what are key points the nurse should discuss with the parents in preparation for discharge?

2. Etiology and pathophysiology
   a. Viral etiology includes a wide variety of viral agents or enteroviruses
   b. Bacterial causative organisms include *haemophilus influenzae* (type B), *streptococcus pneumoniae* and *neisseria meningitides* (meningococcal)

3. Assessment
   a. Clinical manifestations of viral meningitis in infants and toddlers are irritability, lethargy, vomiting, and change in appetite; for an older child, infection is usually preceded by a nonspecific febrile illness; client presents with headache, malaise, muscle aches, nausea/vomiting, **photophobia** (sensitivity to light) and nuchal/spinal rigidity
   b. Clinical manifestations of bacterial meningitis in infants and toddlers include poor feeding/suck, vomiting, high-pitched cry, bulging fontanel, fever or hypothermia depending on maturity of infant's neurological system, and poor muscle tone; children and adolescents present with abrupt onset, fever and chills, headache, and **nuchal rigidity** (stiffness of the neck); vomiting, alterations in sensorium, photophobia, delirium, extreme irritability, aggressive or maniacal behavior, seizures and/or drowsiness; positive Kernig or Brudzinski's sign indicates meningeal irritation; **opisthotonus** posture (hyperextension of head and neck) may relieve some discomfort from meningeal irritation; petechial or purpuric rash will be seen if it is a meningococcal infection
   c. Meningitis is diagnosed by laboratory findings; CSF is obtained by lumbar puncture for analysis; findings can differentiate between viral and bacterial meningitis (see Table 6-2); cultures can determine the causative agent

4. Priority nursing diagnoses
   a. Risk for Ineffective Breathing Pattern
   b. Pain
   c. Risk for Injury
   d. Risk for Ineffective Thermoregulation

5. Planning and implementation
   a. Monitor respiratory status and administer oxygen and maintain artificial airway
   b. Provide an environment that will minimize ICP elevation; this can include elevating head of bed 15 to 30 degrees, avoiding neck extension or flexion, and maintaining head in a neutral position; keep environment quiet and subdued, and handle client in a gentle manner
   c. Monitor for cerebral edema; client may be at risk for syndrome of inappropriate antidiuretic hormone (SIADH); suspect this if urine output decreases but serum sodium also decreases; restrict oral fluids and monitor IV fluids to prevent fluid overload
   d. Administer antipyretics as needed for temperature elevation

Table 6-2 | **Comparison of Cerebrospinal Fluid in Meningitis**

	Normal Child Values	**Viral Meningitis**	**Bacterial Meningitis**
Intracranial Pressure	50–100 mm water	Normal or slightly elevated	Elevated
Appearance	Clear	Clear	Cloudy
Leukocytes (mm³)	0–8	Slightly elevated	Elevated
Protein (mg/dL)	14–45	Slightly elevated	Elevated
Glucose (mg/dL)	35–75	Normal or decreased	Decreased

Source: Hogan, MaryAnn; Brancato, Vera; White, Judy; Falkenstein, Kathleen, *Prentice Hall Reviews & rationales: Child health nursing*, 2nd Ed., ©2007. Reprinted and Electronically reproduced by permission of Pearson Education, Inc. Upper Saddle River, NJ.

      e. Assess for evidence of pain with all routine assessments; administer pain medication as prescribed; however, opioid analgesics (narcotics) should be avoided; signs of elevated ICP can be masked by opioids

      f. Clients with bacterial meningitis will need to have transmission-based droplet precautions (in addition to standard precautions) instituted until at least 24 hours of antibiotic therapy have been completed

      g. Monitor client for complications of meningitis (seizures, hearing loss, visual alterations); neurologic sequelae such as mental retardation, cerebral palsy, and hydrocephalus may occur; a complication of meningococcal meningitis is meningococcemia, an overwhelming septic infection that can lead to circulatory collapse and tissue necrosis

      h. Viral meningitis is treated symptomatically; usually only infants are hospitalized for viral meningitis often due to severe dehydration

  6. Medication therapy: bacterial meningitis is treated with intravenous antibiotics sensitive to causative organism; treatment usually continues for 7 to 14 days; preventive care includes Hib vaccine currently available to protect all young children from *haemophilus influenza* B infection; individuals who have close contact with children diagnosed with meningococcal and *H. influenzae* meningitis may receive rifampin (Rifadin) or ciprofloxacin (Cipro) prophylactically

  7. Client and family education

      a. Provide information to parents about disease and its transmission, need for standard and droplet precautions and antibiotic therapy, and need for prophylactic treatment for those in contact with client

      b. Provide parents with information about possible development of sequelae from disease and possible side effects of medications

      c. Share information about follow-up as well as rehabilitation services with family

  8. Evaluation: client demonstrates vital signs within normal limits; client's pain is controlled as evidenced by vital signs within normal limits and relaxed muscle tone; client demonstrates adequate cerebral perfusion; client recovers without sequelae

B. Encephalitis

  1. Description

      a. Encephalitis is an inflammation of brain

      b. Presenting symptoms vary depending on causative organism and location of infection in brain; classic symptoms include an acute febrile illness with neurologic signs

  2. Etiology and pathophysiology

      a. Etiology is usually a viral organism; herpes simplex type 1 is most common cause during neonatal period; enteroviruses are frequently identified as causative agents; nonviral agents include bacteria, parasites, fungi, and rickettsiae

      b. The infectious process usually begins elsewhere in body

      c. Prognosis depends on degree of CNS involvement; permanent neurologic sequelae may result

  3. Assessment

      a. In addition to fever, client may have a severe headache, nausea, or vomiting, and signs of an upper respiratory infection

      b. Neurologic symptoms include those of nuchal rigidity, photophobia, and positive Kernig's and Brudzinski's signs

      c. Client may also be disoriented, confused, with personality or behavior changes; other signs are speech disturbances, motor dysfunction, cranial nerve deficits, and focal or generalized seizures that alternate with periods of screaming, hallucinating, and bizarre movement; LOC can deteriorate from stupor to coma

    4. Priority nursing diagnoses

        a. Risk for Injury related to seizures

        b. Risk for Ineffective Breathing Pattern

        c. Pain

    5. Planning and implementation

        a. Monitor client's vital signs, respiratory status, oxygenation, and urine output

        b. Provide seizure precautions and have resuscitation equipment close to bed; these clients are best managed in intensive care settings during acute phase

        c. Measures must be taken to maintain skin integrity and other complications of immobility; these include proper positioning, frequent turning, and chest physiotherapy

        d. Work with parents in planning for discharge; since many clients have neurologic sequelae, family will need support giving physical and emotional care to child at home; parents will play an active role in rehabilitation process; follow-up visits need to be coordinated; parents may need referral to home care, counseling, social services, and support groups in their community

    6. Medication therapy: if suspected organism is bacterial, appropriate antibiotics will be ordered; acyclovir or other antiviral agents are administered for herpes virus infection

    7. Client and family education

        a. Parents and client need information about causative agent and plan of treatment

        b. Discharge plans need to be started early in hospitalization; because of neurologic sequelae, plans for rehabilitation need to be discussed

    8. Evaluation: client's vital signs are within normal limits; child has no permanent neurologic sequelae; family copes with diagnosis and management of health problem

C. Reye syndrome

    1. Description

        a. An acute metabolic encephalopathy of childhood; fatty degeneration of liver leads to liver dysfunction

        b. Characterized by five stages

            1) Vomiting and lethargy

            2) Combativeness and confusion

            3) Coma, decorticate posturing

            4) Decerebrate posturing

            5) Seizures, loss of deep tendon reflexes, respiratory arrest

    2. Etiology and pathophysiology

        a. While exact etiology is unclear, Reye syndrome usually develops after a mild viral illness such as chickenpox

        b. Research has linked development of Reye syndrome to use of aspirin in children; following the recommendation that parents use only acetaminophen or ibuprofen to medicate children, the incidence of Reye syndrome has significantly decreased

    3. Assessment

        a. Hypoglycemia is one of the earliest signs

        b. Child presents with an abrupt change in LOC; history reveals client recovering from a viral disease with sudden onset of vomiting and mental confusion

        c. Liver enzymes and ammonia levels are elevated; blood glucose levels are below normal and prothrombin time is prolonged; bilirubin levels remain normal; liver biopsy shows small fat deposits

    4. Priority nursing diagnoses

        a. Risk for Injury

    b. Risk for Ineffective Breathing Pattern

    c. Acute Confusion

    d. Risk for Ineffective Family Coping

  5. Planning and implementation

    a. Most clients are monitored in an intensive care unit (ICU) setting; care is focused on support and monitoring of client's physical status; monitoring cerebral edema; fluid restrictions are usually instituted; frequent vital signs and neurological assessments, such as Glasgow Coma Scale, are monitored

    b. Monitor lab values for elevated ammonia, acidosis, or hypoglycemia; note client's intake and output

    c. Provide all standard nursing measures to prevent complications of immobility

    d. Provide emotional support to family; sudden onset and rapid deterioration in client's condition often overwhelm parents' ability to cope

  6. Medication therapy

    a. Controlling cerebral edema is a primary concern; drug management may include corticosteroids to reduce swelling and barbiturates to induce a coma for severe cerebral edema; mannitol (Osmitrol, an osmotic diuretic) may be given

    b. Phenytoin may be used to control seizures

    c. Vitamin K may be given to aid in coagulation

  7. Client and family education

    a. Explain disease and its causality, treatment plan and prognosis; explanations about the ICU and medical equipment in use will help parents cope

    b. Discharge planning will include rehabilitative needs of client as well as follow-up requirements

    c. The public needs to be educated about Reye syndrome and its connection with viral illnesses and administration of salicylates; public needs to be aware that if a client displays symptoms, early medical intervention is associated with a better prognosis

  8. Evaluation: client demonstrates vital signs within normal limits for age; client demonstrates adequate cerebral perfusion; parents display appropriate coping mechanisms

D. Guillain-Barré syndrome

  1. Description

    a. An acute demyelinating disease of nervous system

    b. A polyneuropathy with progressive ascending flaccid paralysis

    c. Paralytic symptoms are usually preceded by mild flu-like illness or sore throat

  2. Etiology and pathophysiology

    a. Etiology is unknown, but Guillain-Barré syndrome is associated with viral illnesses and noninfectious factors such as immunizations, surgery, and trauma

    b. Is thought to be an immune-mediated disease associated with other viral or bacterial infections; characterized by alteration in myelin surrounding peripheral nerves

    c. Inflammation and edema occur in spinal and cranial nerves, with segmented demyelination and compression of nerve roots in dural sheath; conduction is impaired, resulting in ascending partial or complete paralysis of muscles innervated by involved nerves

    d. Nerve involvement may include truncal musculature and cranial nerves leading to respiratory failure or loss of swallow and gag reflexes

    e. Progression of paralysis occurs within one to two weeks

    f. Majority of clients recover over 2 to 15 months with no residual disabilities

  3. Assessment

    a. Muscle weakness, paresthesia, and cramps; paralysis usually ascends from lower extremities; tendon reflexes will be depressed or absent

b. Assess and monitor respiratory function and swallow and gag reflexes

c. Medical diagnosis is confirmed with lumbar puncture and electromyography

  1) Lumbar puncture reveals CSF that has increased protein levels and few WBCs

  2) EMG demonstrates an abnormal pattern of nerve conduction

4. Priority nursing diagnoses

  a. Impaired Physical Mobility

  b. Ineffective Breathing Pattern

  c. Impaired Swallowing

  d. Disturbed Self-Esteem

  e. Risk for Ineffective Family Coping

  f. Diversional Activity Deficit

5. Planning and implementation

  a. Medical treatment includes administration of intravenous immune globulin (IVIG) and immunosuppressive drugs and performing plasmapheresis

  b. Care is supportive and similar to that provided to a tetraplegic client; during initial phase, assess closely for advancement of paralysis to include respiratory area; observe closely for difficulty with breathing or swallowing; place on a cardiac monitor and have all emergency equipment accessible to bedside; clients with respiratory distress usually require mechanical ventilation

  c. Prevent complications using good postural alignment, frequent change of position, and passive ROM exercises; recovery period can last from two weeks to several months depending on degree of paralysis

  d. After the recovery period an extensive rehabilitation process begins; while complete recovery is possible, there is possibility for some permanent disability

  e. Providing emotional support for client and family is an important nursing function; loss of motor functions and control can be very frightening for client; parents need to be encouraged to bring favorite toys from home and provide other comforting activities to help client feel secure

6. Client and family education

  a. Family needs to understand mechanism of disease and treatment strategies being used

  b. Parents need to learn how to provide basic care for client, including proper skin care, turning and positioning

7. Evaluation: client's vital signs are maintained within normal limits for age; client maintains adequate nutritional intake either by mouth, enteral feeding tube, or IV line; client is free of complications of immobility (i.e., maintaining muscle tone through physical therapy); client and family cope with initial loss of function and actively participate in rehabilitation process

VI. ACCIDENTS AND INJURIES CAUSING NEUROLOGIC HEALTH PROBLEMS

A. Head injury

1. Description

  a. Any trauma involving scalp, cranial bones, or structures within skull; injury occurs as a result of force or penetration

  b. Head injury is most common type of childhood injury, with 5% being fatal and 20% being associated with long-term disabilities

  c. Clients with head injury often suffer from side effects of trauma, such as cerebral edema and increased ICP

> **d.** A minor closed head injury is one in which client has normal mental status, no abnormal or focal findings on neurologic examination, and no physical evidence of skull fracture at initial exam shortly after injury; client might have had a temporary loss of consciousness (less than one minute), reported headache, exhibited lethargy, and either vomited and/or had a seizure immediately after injury, but at time of exam has normal findings

2. Etiology and pathophysiology

> **a.** Major cause in young children are falls—from changing tables, beds, sofas, and down stairs, especially in walkers; child abuse or shaken baby syndrome is a possible cause in infants under 1 year of age; other causes include motor vehicle accidents (MVAs), and bicycle, skateboard, snowboard, and skiing accidents, especially where client did not wear any protective helmet; adolescents may also be injured in alcohol- or drug-related MVAs and sports injuries

> **b.** Two categories of head injuries

> > **1)** *Primary injuries* develop at time of trauma when initial tissue damage takes place; this is usually a result of a direct blow to head or acceleration–deceleration movement of brain within skull (contrecoup injury); at time of injury, there is an increase in ICP and arterial pressure; apnea and loss of consciousness may occur

> > **2)** *Secondary brain trauma* develops as a result of body's response to injury; this response can occur from a few hours to a few weeks after injury; brain damage is usually secondary to hypoxia, hypotension, edema, change in blood–brain barrier, or hemorrhage; the resulting increased ICP can cause irreversible brain damage if left untreated

3. Assessment

> **a.** Monitor vital signs and neuro signs frequently; changes can indicate hypoxia, decreased perfusion, shock, or increased ICP; **Cushing's triad** is a late sign of increased ICP, characterized by widening pulse pressure (rising systolic blood pressure with stable diastolic blood pressure), bradycardia, and irregular respirations

> **b.** Monitor neurological signs, cranial nerves, and LOC using Glasgow Coma Scale to detect changes in client's condition

4. Priority nursing diagnoses

> **a.** Ineffective Cerebral Tissue Perfusion

> **b.** Impaired Gas Exchange

> **c.** Ineffective Airway Clearance related to decreased level of consciousness

> **d.** Acute Confusion related to cerebral injury

> **e.** Risk for Ineffective Family Coping

> **f.** Risk for Impaired Growth and Development related to motor, cognitive, and perceptual deficits

5. Planning and implementation

> **a.** To maintain cardiopulmonary function, monitor breathing patterns, check color, and LOC; monitor oxygen saturation with pulse oximeter; it is critical to prevent brain damage, and that oxygen saturation remain over 95%; report any decrease in oxygenation to health care provider immediately; maintain seizure precautions; monitor for any signs of increased ICP and report to health care provider

> **b.** To prevent complications, use good positioning, maintain a quiet environment, and control body temperature

> **c.** To promote optimal recovery, begin rehabilitation while child is still hospitalized; efforts are coordinated between physical, occupational, and speech therapy; teach parents any strategies being used so that they can continue therapy at home; provide emotional support to family

    d. Coordinate services and resources for discharge; clients with major head injury (Glasgow Coma Score less than or equal to 8) have poorer outcomes and significant physical disabilities

6. Medication therapy: for a client who requires hospitalization because of severity of head injury, mannitol may be used to decrease ICP; control of cerebral edema has been shown to be a significant variable in determining outcome for a client with a major head injury

7. Client and family education

    a. For even minor head injuries, teach how to care for client with a head injury; what behaviors to expect from client and symptoms to monitor for should complications develop (mild headache expected; focal deficits are abnormal)

    b. During recovery period of up to six weeks, many clients may tire easily, have memory loss or forgetfulness, are easily distractible, have difficulty concentrating or following directions, irritability or short temper, and need help starting and finishing tasks

8. Evaluation: client's vital signs remain within normal limits for age; client maintains adequate cerebral perfusion; client participates in rehabilitation to attain optimal recovery; family copes with possible long-term disability

B. Skull fractures

1. Description: fracture to any of eight cranial bones

2. Etiology and pathophysiology

    a. A fracture is caused by a considerable force to head; any area of skull with swelling or hematoma should be evaluated as a possible fracture

    b. Types of skull fractures

        1) A linear fracture is a break in continuity of skull, and is usually asymptomatic unless other injury accompanies fracture

        2) A depressed skull fracture occurs when a fragment of skull bone separates from rest of skull and is pushed downward into brain; requires surgical elevation to prevent brain damage; often accompanied by seizures

        3) A basilar fracture involves a fracture at base of skull; common symptoms include leakage of CSF from nose or ears, periorbital ecchymosis (raccoon eyes) and bruising behind the ears (battle sign); because of concern about development of meningitis, client is placed on antibiotics

3. Assessment: diagnosis is made by inspection, palpation, x-rays, and CT scans

4. Priority nursing diagnoses

    a. Risk for Ineffective Cerebral Perfusion

    b. Risk for Infection

5. Planning and implementation

    a. Linear fractures usually heal on their own without intervention; depressed and compound fractures usually require surgical intervention to repair

    b. Routine postoperative care similar to any craniotomy (see craniosynostosis presented earlier)

    c. Monitor for signs of cerebral edema, damage to cranial nerves and infection

6. Medication therapy: often antibiotics are given to prevent infection postoperatively and if scalp was also lacerated a tetanus booster immunization may be indicated

C. Contusion

1. Description: bruising of brain tissue as a result of blunt trauma or coup/contrecoup injuries; it is rare in clients under age of 1 year

2. Etiology and pathophysiology: injury usually involves damage to parenchyma with tears in vessels or tissue, pulling, and subsequent areas of necrosis or infarction

3. Assessment: symptoms will vary depending on site of injury; client may have decreasing LOC

Practice to Pass

The level of growth and development of a client has a direct relationship to the common injuries that occur during that age. Identify the implications of growth and development for head injuries.

    4. Priority nursing diagnoses

      a. Risk for Ineffective Cerebral Tissue Perfusion

      b. Risk for Injury (seizures)

    5. Planning and implementation

      a. Monitor client for signs of complications

      b. Observe for any complications

      c. Observe for sequelae that may result from the injury

    6. Client and family education

      a. Teach parents symptoms of complications that may occur after discharge

      b. Provide written instructions as well as explicit information about when to seek medical care to promote appropriate follow-through

    7. Evaluation: client recovers without sequelae

D. Concussion

    1. Description: concussion or "mild traumatic brain injury" involves some transient loss of consciousness; usually results from blunt head trauma

    2. Etiology and pathophysiology: brain injury is usually related to stretching, compression, or shearing of nerve fibers; postconcussion syndrome occurs after initial head injury; poor concentration and problems with memory may be noted at school; client may complain of headache, dizziness, and photophobia; parents may report a subtle change in personality

    3. Assessment: symptoms include amnesia of event, headache, and nausea; clients are neurologically intact with a Glasgow Coma Score of 13 to 15; there are three levels of concussion severity

      a. Grade 1: client has transient confusion with no loss of consciousness and duration of abnormal mental status for less than 15 minutes

      b. Grade 2: client has transient confusion with no loss of consciousness and duration of abnormal mental status for more than 15 minutes

      c. Grade 3: client has loss of consciousness, for a few seconds or several minutes or longer

    4. Priority nursing diagnoses

      a. Ineffective Cerebral Tissue Perfusion

      b. Ineffective Individual Coping secondary to postconcussion syndrome

    5. Planning and implementation

      a. Treatment is supportive with close observation for 24 hours in an emergency room or at home under certain circumstances

      b. Clients who had loss of consciousness for greater than five minutes or amnesia of event are usually admitted for observation to rule out any other potential injuries

    6. Client and family education: for child discharged home with parents, teach to continue monitoring client and what steps to take if complications arise; teach about postconcussion syndrome; parents should report vomiting and neurologic deficits

E. Subdural hematoma

    1. Description: one of two major sites for bleeding or hemorrhage with a head injury in children; a **subdural hematoma** is bleeding between dura and cerebrum; it is more common than **epidural hematoma** (bleeding between dura and cranium) and is most frequently seen in infants

    2. Etiology and pathophysiology

      a. Subdural hematoma develops slowly, spreads thinly and widely; often results from a fall, birth trauma, or violent shaking

      b. Can be acute (more rapid onset) or chronic (delayed symptoms)

    3. Assessment

      a. Presenting symptoms are caused by increased ICP and include seizures, vomiting, drowsiness, increased head circumference, bulging fontanels, irritability, and other personality changes

b. Older child may report headaches
   c. Acute subdural hematoma is usually symptomatic within 48 hours of injury
   d. Chronic subdural hematoma may take up to two weeks before symptoms are observed
   e. Diagnosis is confirmed by computed tomography (CT) scan
4. Priority nursing diagnoses
   a. Risk for Injury
   b. Ineffective Cerebral Tissue Perfusion
   c. Risk for Ineffective Breathing Pattern
   d. Risk for Acute Confusion
5. Planning and implementation
   a. Monitoring of client's vital signs and LOC is critical for early recognition and intervention following a head injury
   b. A small subdural hematoma may reabsorb itself
   c. Larger acute subdural hematomas require evacuation through burr holes
   d. Craniotomy may be required to evacuate a solid clot
   e. Postoperative nursing care requires continued monitoring of vital signs and LOC
6. Client and family education
   a. Explain to parents why monitoring client is important following head injury
   b. Prepare parents for surgical procedure; remind parents that ecchymosis of eyes will occur following a craniotomy
   c. Discharge instructions include monitoring the client for signs of increased ICP
7. Evaluation: client has early recognition of subdural hematoma; client and parents verbalize that they understand planned surgery; parents restate discharge instructions

F. Epidural hematoma
1. Description: epidural hematoma is bleeding with accumulation between dura and skull; not as common as subdural hematomas
2. Etiology and pathophysiology: accumulation of blood applies force or pressure down onto brain; since bleeding is usually arterial, onset is rapid
3. Assessment
   a. Classic symptoms include initial loss of consciousness, then regaining it, then losing it again; also irritability, headache, and vomiting; symptoms usually evolve within minutes to hours of injury
   b. Can be diagnosed on CT
   c. If left untreated, can be fatal
4. Priority nursing diagnoses
   a. Risk for Injury
   b. Ineffective Cerebral Tissue Perfusion
   c. Risk for Ineffective Breathing Pattern
   d. Risk for Acute Confusion
5. Planning and implementation
   a. Evacuation may be through burr holes or a craniotomy may be required
   b. Rapid recognition and treatment leads to a better prognosis
   c. Nursing care is same as for other types of head injuries and surgical procedures
6. Client and parent education: education for child with an epidural hematoma is same as for other head injuries and cranial surgeries; clients with neurologic sequelae need rehabilitation with parents actively involved in care
7. Evaluation: recognition and intervention of epidural hematoma occurs early and client recovers without sequelae

Practice to Pass

The Glasgow Coma Scale is often used to determine prognosis from a head injury. Compare components of the Glasgow Coma Scale to their relationship with the common symptoms of the minor and major head injury.

Case Study

A 2-week-old white female is admitted to the hospital for high fever and irritability. She is a full-term, vaginal birth to a Gravida 2 para 2 mother. The infant is diagnosed with meningitis. Her parents both work full time and have health insurance. She has a 3-year-old brother. The family does not have any relatives living closer than a three-hour drive.

1. What specific physical parameters should the nurse monitor?

2. Which nursing interventions would have priority during the first 48 hours of her care?

3. What would be the usual medical treatment for this health problem?

4. What developmental implications are there for providing family-centered care for the infant?

5. In planning for discharge, identify specific areas of support for or teaching with the family.

For suggested responses, see page 353.

POSTTEST

1. A 3-month-old infant has been admitted with a diagnosis of encephalitis. What is the priority assessment by the nurse?

1. Pupillary reaction
2. Level of consciousness
3. Ability to maintain airway
4. Response to verbal stimulation

2. The nurse places a young child scheduled for a lumbar puncture in a side-lying position with the head flexed and knees drawn up to the chest. The mother asks why the child has to be positioned this way. How would the nurse explain the rationale for this positioning?

1. Pain is decreased through this comfort measure.
2. Injury to the spinal cord is prevented.
3. Access to the spinal fluid is facilitated.
4. Restraint is needed to prevent unnecessary movement.

3. An 18-month-old child is observed having a seizure. The nurse notes that the child's jaws are clamped. What is the priority responsibility of the nurse at this time?

1. Start oxygen via mask.
2. Insert padded tongue blade.
3. Restrain child to prevent injury to soft tissue.
4. Protect the child from harm from the environment.

4. A 3-year-old child is admitted to the hospital unit with a diagnosis of viral meningitis. The nurse should take which of the following actions in the care of this child? Select all that apply.

1. Allow the child to assume a position of comfort.
2. Keep the lights bright to monitor skin color.
3. Administer acetaminophen for pain.
4. Monitor the child for seizures.
5. Administer antibiotics.

5. The nurse is providing client education for a family whose child has cerebral palsy and is receiving baclofen epidural therapy to control spasticity. Which of the following is most important for the nurse to include in the discussion?

1. The drug acts to inhibit the neurotransmitter GABA.
2. The child should be able to run with normal gait after insertion of the pump.
3. Parents must bring the child back to the clinic on a regular basis to have more medicine added to the pump.
4. Parents can be taught to regulate the dosage on a sliding scale.

6 A 10-year-old client presents with weakness in legs and history of the flu. The medical diagnosis is Guillain-Barré syndrome. It would be imperative for the nurse to inform the physician after assessing which of the following?

1. Weak muscle tone in feet
2. Weak muscle tone in legs
3. Increasing hoarseness
4. Tingling in the hands

7 The nurse is providing discharge instructions for a child who has suffered a head injury within the last four hours. The nurse determines there is a need for additional teaching when the mother makes which statement?

1. "I will call my doctor immediately if my child starts vomiting."
2. "I won't give my child anything stronger than Tylenol for headache."
3. "My child should sleep for at least eight hours without arousing after we get home."
4. "I recognize that continued amnesia about the injury is not uncommon."

8 A 2-year-old child is admitted to the neurosurgical unit following a head injury. The nurse is using the Glasgow Coma Scale to measure neurological functioning. Which assessment finding indicates the lowest level of functioning for this child?

1. Confusion
2. Irritable and cries
3. Eyes open only to pain
4. No response to painful stimuli

9 Upon performing a physical assessment of a 7-month-old child, the nurse notes the following findings. The nurse concludes that which finding is abnormal and could suggest cerebral palsy?

1. No head lag when pulled to a sitting position
2. No Moro or startle reflex
3. Positive tonic neck reflex
4. Absence of tongue extrusion

10 A 4-year-old child is being evaluated for hydrocephalus. The nurse notes which of the following as early signs of hydrocephalus in this child? Select all that apply.

1. Bulging fontanels
2. Rapid enlargement of the head
3. Shrill, high-pitched cry
4. Early morning headache
5. Vomiting upon arising

➤ *See pages 138–139 for Answers and Rationales.*

ANSWERS & RATIONALES
Pretest

1 **Answer: 2** **Rationale:** Brudzinski's sign indicates meningeal irritation. As the head and neck are flexed toward the chest, the legs flex at both the hips and the knees in response. Encephalitis is a rarer condition and thus would be a less common reason for a positive Brudzinski's sign. Increased intracranial pressure and intraventricular hemorrhage may or may not cause meningeal irritation and a positive Brudzinski's sign. **Cognitive Level:** Applying **Client Need:** Physiological Adaptation **Integrated Process:** Nursing Process: Diagnosis **Content Area:** Child Health **Strategy:** Consider how Brudzinski's sign is tested. Flexing the neck is not likely to affect structures in the skull unless the meninges become irritated. **Reference:** Ball, J., Bindler, R., & Cowen, K. (2010). *Child health nursing: Partnering with children and families* (2nd ed.). Upper Saddle River, NJ: Pearson Education, p. 1335.

2 **Answer: 1** **Rationale:** Increased intracranial pressure in infants is characterized by lethargy, irritability, bradycardia, tachycardia, apnea, bulging fontanels, setting-sun eyes, vomiting, and hypertension. Myelomeningocele refers to a neural tube defect, which is obvious on the back. Skull fractures indicate injury to the head and may be asymptomatic or may be accompanied by other pathology that could lead to increased intracranial pressure. Hypertension is not accompanied by the symptom of setting-sun eyes. **Cognitive Level:** Analyzing **Client Need:** Physiological Adaptation **Integrated Process:** Nursing Process: Diagnosis **Content Area:** Child Health **Strategy:** Consider the significance of bulging fontanels as a unique manifestation to help you choose correctly. **Reference:** Ball, J., Bindler, R., & Cowen, K. (2010). *Child health nursing: Partnering with children and families* (2nd ed.). Upper Saddle River, NJ: Pearson Education, pp. 1320–1321, 1335.

3 **Answer: 3** **Rationale:** Initially, the most common mechanisms for development of hydrocephalus include decreased reabsorption (communicating hydrocephalus) and obstruction to the flow of CSF (noncommunicating). Once surgical treatment with shunt placement has been done, obstruction in the shunt (from blockage at either end of the catheter, kinking of catheter, or valve breakdown) can lead to obstructed outflow of CSF. Increased flow of CSF, increased reabsorption of CSF, and decreased production of CSF should lead to decreased ICP. **Cognitive Level:** Analyzing **Client Need:** Physiological Adaptation **Integrated Process:** Nursing Process: Diagnosis **Content Area:** Child Health **Strategy:** Knowledge of shunt function would indicate that a malfunctioning shunt would obstruct the flow of CSF. **Reference:** Ball, J., Bindler, R., & Cowen, K. (2010). *Child health nursing: Partnering with children and families* (2nd ed.). Upper Saddle River, NJ: Pearson Education, pp. 1345, 1347.

4 **Answer: 2** **Rationale:** Most children with spina bifida cystica (myelomeningocele included) have the defect at a level that does affect the innervation to both the colon and anal sphincter. The result is constipation and incontinence. Diarrhea is the opposite of the current concern. Any lack of mobility increases the risk for constipation, and does not increase the gastric-colic reflex. All children need a pattern of regular bowel movements. **Cognitive Level:** Applying **Client Need:** Physiological Adaptation **Integrated Process:** Teaching and Learning **Content Area:** Child Health **Strategy:** Determine if both a lack of mobility and innervation exists. Since they both exist in the child with this spinal defect, consider which would have the most effect on bowel function. **Reference:** Ball, J., Bindler, R., & Cowen, K. (2010). *Child health nursing: Partnering with children and families* (2nd ed.). Upper Saddle River, NJ: Pearson Education, p. 1350.

5 **Answer: 3** **Rationale:** Twenty-four hours of antibiotic therapy usually eliminates the necessity of transmission-based precautions. The client will still be contagious at the time the organism is identified and antibiotics are initiated. It is unnecessary to wait for completion of 10 days of antibiotic therapy to discontinue transmission-based precautions. **Cognitive Level:** Applying **Client Need:** Safety and Infection Control **Integrated Process:** Communication and Documentation **Content Area:** Child Health **Strategy:** Three of the four choices relate to antibiotics, so the correct response is likely to be one of them. Choose the time frame that is not immediate and not too lengthy. **Reference:** Ball, J., Bindler, R., & Cowen, K. (2010). *Child health nursing: Partnering with children and families* (2nd ed.). Upper Saddle River, NJ: Pearson Education, p. 1336.

6 **Answer: 4** **Rationale:** The child with meningitis will hyperextend the neck and head in an arching position referred to as *opisthotonos*. The child does this to relieve discomfort from the meningeal irritation. Decerebrate posturing is a symptom of dysfunction at the level of the midbrain and is characterized by rigid extension and pronation of arms and legs. Decorticate posturing is a symptom of a dysfunction of the cerebral cortex and is characterized by adduction of the arms at the shoulders, the arms flexed on the chest with hands in fists and wrists flexed, and lower extremities extended and adducted. Jacksonian seizure is a simple motor seizure characterized by clonic movements that begin in a foot, hand, or face and then spread to include sometimes the entire body. **Cognitive Level:** Applying **Client Need:** Physiological Adaptation **Integrated Process:** Nursing Process: Implementation **Content Area:** Child Health **Strategy:** Visualize and distinguish between the positioning seen in various neurological defects. **Reference:** Ball, J., Bindler, R., & Cowen, K. (2010). *Child health nursing: Partnering with children and families* (2nd ed.). Upper Saddle River, NJ: Pearson Education, p. 1335.

7 **Answer: 1, 2, 4** **Rationale:** Keeping the head of the bed slightly elevated promotes flow of cerebrospinal fluid. Oxygen can serve as a vasodilator, decreasing the ICP. Turning the head to one side can occlude the flow of CSF or impair venous drainage from the brain, increasing the ICP. Diuretics are often part of the medical treatment to decrease ICP. Promoting oral fluids would not be appropriate; fluid restriction may be ordered. **Cognitive Level:** Applying **Client Need:** Physiological Adaptation **Integrated Process:** Nursing Process: Implementation **Content Area:** Child Health **Strategy:** Eliminate any activities that would increase intracranial pressure such as incorrect positioning and increased fluid intake. **Reference:** Ball, J., Bindler, R., & Cowen, K. (2010). *Child health nursing: Partnering with children and families* (2nd ed.). Upper Saddle River, NJ: Pearson Education, p. 1335.

8 **Answer: 1** **Rationale:** Epidural hematomas are characterized by arterial bleeding. Arterial bleeding is rapid, and onset of symptoms occurs within minutes to hours. Injury that leads to venous bleeding generally has a slower onset of symptoms, which could occur over a few days, weeks, or months. **Cognitive Level:** Applying **Client Need:** Physiological Adaptation **Integrated Process:** Nursing Process: Assessment **Content Area:** Child Health **Strategy:** Recall that an epidural hematoma is characterized by bleeding that is arterial in origin, which would mean symptoms would appear quickly. **Reference:** Ball, J., Bindler, R., & Cowen, K. (2010). *Child health nursing: Partnering with children and families* (2nd ed.). Upper Saddle River, NJ: Pearson Education, p. 1371.

9 **Answer: 3** **Rationale:** Obtunded indicates a diminished level of consciousness with limited response to the environment. The child will fall asleep unless given verbal or tactile stimulation. Stupor is a diminished level of consciousness with response only to vigorous stimulation. Semicomatose is when a child only responds to painful stimuli. Lethargy is when a child sleeps if left undisturbed and has sluggish speech and movement. **Cognitive Level:** Analyzing **Client Need:** Physiological

Adaptation **Integrated Process:** Communication and Documentation **Content Area:** Child Health **Strategy:** Recognize that this child is not fully conscious. At the same time, he is not in a stupor or semicomatose. Then choose between lethargic and obtunded based on knowledge of levels of consciousness. **Reference:** Ball, J., Bindler, R., & Cowen, K. (2010). *Child health nursing: Partnering with children and families* (2nd ed.). Upper Saddle River, NJ: Pearson Education, pp. 1319–1320.

10 Answer: 2 Rationale: The most common form of cerebral palsy involves spasticity of muscles. Because of the excessive energy expended, these children often need more calories than other children their age and size (not fewer). Feeding difficulties are often a component of cerebral palsy, but whether a child needs assistance with feedings is dependent upon the muscle groups affected. Inactivity does not increase the risk of obesity because of the pathophysiology involved. **Cognitive Level:** Analyzing **Client Need:** Physiological Adaptation **Integrated Process:** Teaching and Learning **Content Area:** Child Health **Strategy:** The child with spasticity has hypertonic muscles, so consider the effect that this has on cellular nutritional needs. **Reference:** Ball, J., Bindler, R., & Cowen, K. (2010). *Child health nursing: Partnering with children and families* (2nd ed.). Upper Saddle River, NJ: Pearson Education, p. 1362.

Posttest

1 Answer: 3 Rationale: The priority in assessing any critically ill child follows the ABC rule: airway, breathing, and circulation. Neurological status (including pupillary reaction, level of consciousness, and response to verbal stimuli) is important to assess, but does not take priority over status of the airway and breathing. **Cognitive Level:** Analyzing **Client Need:** Physiological Adaptation **Integrated Process:** Nursing Process: Assessment **Content Area:** Child Health **Strategy:** Utilize the ABCs; airway is always the first physiological priority. **Reference:** Ball, J., Bindler, R., & Cowen, K. (2010). *Child health nursing: Partnering with children and families* (2nd ed.). Upper Saddle River, NJ: Pearson Education, p. 1340.

2 Answer: 3 Rationale: This position opens the intervertebral spaces and allows easier access to the spinal canal. The position does not decrease pain or help to restrain the child. All lumbar punctures are done below L4 (the level of the spinal nerves), so injury to the spinal cord is always avoided. **Cognitive Level:** Analyzing **Client Need:** Reduction of Risk Potential **Integrated Process:** Nursing Process: Implementation **Content Area:** Child Health **Strategy:** Visualize the procedure and positioning. Compare each option to the information in the stem, looking for an option that fits with the question. To choose correctly, recall that the spinal vertebrae need to be separated to allow easier access by the

spinal needle. **Reference:** Ball, J., Bindler, R., & Cowen, K. (2010). *Child health nursing: Partnering with children and families* (2nd ed.). Upper Saddle River, NJ: Pearson Education, p. 1591.

3 Answer: 4 Rationale: It is important to never forcibly restrain a child during a seizure or insert a padded tongue blade; both are more likely to add trauma than prevent it. Oxygen via mask is of little benefit. Overall, the child must be protected from injury from the environment. **Cognitive Level:** Applying **Client Need:** Reduction of Risk Potential **Integrated Process:** Nursing Process: Implementation **Content Area:** Child Health **Strategy:** First eliminate two items that are not used during a seizure, leaving two options. Consider the client's risk for injury with seizure activity to choose correctly. **Reference:** Ball, J., Bindler, R., & Cowen, K. (2010). *Child health nursing: Partnering with children and families* (2nd ed.). Upper Saddle River, NJ: Pearson Education, p. 1331.

4 Answer: 1, 3, 4 Rationale: Treatment for viral meningitis is aimed at reducing the symptoms. The child should be allowed to assume a position of comfort. The room should be kept dim and stimulation reduced. Acetaminophen may be given to treat pain. Seizures can occur, although the disease is usually self-limiting. Viral meningitis does not require antibiotics. **Cognitive Level:** Applying **Client Need:** Physiological Adaptation **Integrated Process:** Nursing Process: Implementation **Content Area:** Child Health **Strategy:** Differentiate between treatment of viral and bacterial meningitis. Consider measures that may increase comfort. Eliminate any options that would increase stimulation. **Reference:** Ball, J., Bindler, R., & Cowen, K. (2010). *Child health nursing: Partnering with children and families* (2nd ed.). Upper Saddle River, NJ: Pearson Education, pp. 1339–1340.

5 Answer: 3 Rationale: This therapy involves an implanted pump that must be accessed through the skin to refill the pump. Parents are not taught to refill the pump. Baclofen does inhibit the neurotransmitter GABA; however, this is not the essential data to be shared with the parents. Promising the parents that the child will be able to run with normal gait offers false hopes. The implanted pump's dosage cannot be changed without special equipment. **Cognitive Level:** Analyzing **Client Need:** Physiological Adaptation **Integrated Process:** Teaching and Learning **Content Area:** Child Health **Strategy:** To determine the correct answer, first determine which responses are accurate and then prioritize the information that the parents will need. **Reference:** Ball, J., Bindler, R., & Cowen, K. (2010). *Child health nursing: Partnering with children and families* (2nd ed.). Upper Saddle River, NJ: Pearson Education, pp. 1361–1362.

6 Answer: 3 Rationale: Guillain-Barré syndrome is an ascending paralysis. It is expected that the child will have increasingly less muscle tone in the extremities. Hoarseness could indicate involvement in the muscles of respiration. Serious concern is raised when the respiratory muscles are affected. Sometimes mechanical ventilation is indicated. Tingling is a common sign of Guillain-Barré and is not related to respiratory distress. **Cognitive Level:** Applying **Client Need:** Physiological Adaptation **Integrated Process:** Nursing Process: Assessment **Content Area:** Child Health **Strategy:** Consider which option can have serious implications. Knowledge of Guillain-Barré as an ascending paralysis would indicate which symptom is the gravest sign of impending difficulty. **Reference:** Ball, J., Bindler, R., & Cowen, K. (2010). *Child health nursing: Partnering with children and families* (2nd ed.). Upper Saddle River, NJ: Pearson Education, pp. 1342–1343.

7 **Answer: 3** **Rationale:** Discharge instructions will include the necessity of waking the child to check neurological status throughout the night. Vomiting could be a sign of increasing intracranial pressure and should be reported. Narcotics are not given after a head injury because they could mask deteriorating neurological signs. Amnesia for the events surrounding the injury may be permanent. It is not a sign of increasing intracranial pressure. **Cognitive Level:** Analyzing **Client Need:** Physiological Adaptation **Integrated Process:** Nursing Process: Evaluation **Content Area:** Child Health **Strategy:** Consider care of the client with a head injury and determine which response is not in line with the normal care. **Reference:** Ball, J., Bindler, R., & Cowen, K. (2010). *Child health nursing: Partnering with children and families* (2nd ed.). Upper Saddle River, NJ: Pearson Education, pp. 1322–1323.

8 **Answer: 4** **Rationale:** No eye opening, no verbal response, and no motor response are the lowest criteria on the scale. Confusion is a criterion applicable only for the older child and adult but is comparable to "irritable and cries" for the infant (which rates a four out of five on the verbal response subscale). "Eyes open only to pain" is the next to the lowest level on the eye-opening category.

Cognitive Level: Analyzing **Client Need:** Physiological Adaptation **Integrated Process:** Nursing Process: Diagnosis **Content Area:** Child Health **Strategy:** First eliminate two options that are normal findings. Determine which of the two remaining responses shows the least brain functioning. **Reference:** Ball, J., Bindler, R., & Cowen, K. (2010). *Child health nursing: Partnering with children and families* (2nd ed.). Upper Saddle River, NJ: Pearson Education, p. 1322.

9 **Answer: 3** **Rationale:** The Moro or startle, tongue extrusion, and tonic neck reflexes are all neonatal reflexes that should have disappeared by this child's age. A developmental delay and the presence of a neonatal reflex are some of the earliest clues to cerebral palsy. Lack of head lag indicates good motor development. **Cognitive Level:** Applying **Client Need:** Physiological Adaptation **Integrated Process:** Nursing Process: Diagnosis **Content Area:** Child Health **Strategy:** Differentiate normal from abnormal findings in a 7-month-old infant. **Reference:** Ball, J., Bindler, R., & Cowen, K. (2010). *Child health nursing: Partnering with children and families* (2nd ed.). Upper Saddle River, NJ: Pearson Education, p. 1360.

10 **Answer: 4, 5** **Rationale:** All of the symptoms indicate increased ICP or hydrocephalus. Head enlargement and bulging fontanels would not be seen in the child after closure of the sutures (12 to 18 months). A shrill, high-pitched cry is a late-stage symptom in children. Headache and vomiting on arising would be early symptoms in an older child. **Cognitive Level:** Analyzing **Client Need:** Physiological Adaptation **Integrated Process:** Nursing Process: Assessment **Content Area:** Child Health **Strategy:** The key concept here is the age of the child. At 4 years old, the sutures and fontanels have closed, eliminating two of the four options. **Reference:** Ball, J., Bindler, R., & Cowen, K. (2010). *Child health nursing: Partnering with children and families* (2nd ed.). Upper Saddle River, NJ: Pearson Education, pp. 1320–1321, 1335.

References

Ball, J., Bindler, R., & Cowen, K. (2012). *Principles of pediatric nursing: Caring for children* (5th ed.). Upper Saddle River, NJ: Pearson Education.

Ball, J., Bindler, R., & Cowen, K. (2010). *Child health nursing: Partnering with children and families* (2nd ed.). Upper Saddle River, NJ: Pearson Education.

Hockenberry, M., & Wilson, D. (2011). *Wong's essentials of pediatric nursing* (8th ed.). St. Louis, MO: Elsevier.

Hockenberry, M., & Wilson, D. (2011). *Wong's nursing care of infants and children* (9th ed.). St. Louis, MO: Elsevier.

Lefever Kee, J. (2009). *Prentice Hall handbook of laboratory & diagnostic tests with nursing implications* (6th ed.). Upper Saddle River, NJ: Pearson Education.

London, M., Ladewig, P., Ball, J., Bindler, R., & Cowen, K. (2011). *Maternal & child nursing care* (3rd ed.). Upper Saddle River, NJ: Pearson Education.

Perry, S., Hockenberry, M., Lowdermilk, D., & Wilson, D. (2010). *Maternal child nursing care* (4th ed.). St. Louis, MO: Elsevier.

Pillitteri, A. (2009). *Maternal and child health nursing: Care of the childbearing and childrearing family* (6th ed.). Philadelphia: Lippincott Williams & Wilkins.

ANSWERS & RATIONALES

7 Renal and Genitourinary Health Problems

Chapter Outline

Overview of Anatomy and
Physiology of Renal
System
Diagnostic Tests and
Assessments of Renal
System

Common Nursing Procedures
for Children with Renal
Health Problems
Surgical Interventions for
Children with Renal Health
Problems

Congenital Renal Health
Problems
Acquired Renal Health Problems
Infectious Renal Health
Problems: Urinary Tract
Infections

NCLEX-RN® Test Prep

Use the accompanying online resource,
NursingReviewsandRationales, to test
yourself with hundreds of NCLEX®-style
practice questions.

Objectives

➤ Identify data essential to the assessment of alterations in health
of the renal system of the child.
➤ Discuss the clinical manifestations and pathophysiology of
alterations in health of the renal system of a child.
➤ Discuss therapeutic management of a child with alterations in
health of the renal system.
➤ Describe nursing management of a child with alterations in health
of the renal system.

Review at a Glance

anuria complete or almost complete
cessation of urine production by
kidneys
azotemia retention of excess nitrogenous wastes in blood
chordee ventral curvature of penis
caused by a fibrous band of tissue
circumcision operation to remove
part or all of prepuce (foreskin) of penis
creatinine substance produced daily
in body; found in blood, muscle, and
urine; measurement of its excretion is
used to evaluate kidney function
cryptorchidism failure of one or
both testes to descend
cystitis inflammation of urinary
bladder
epispadias a malformation in
which urethra opens on dorsum of penis;

frequently associated with exstrophy of
bladder
exstrophy congenital eversion of a
hollow organ; a congenital gap in anterior
wall of bladder and abdominal wall in
front of it, with posterior wall of bladder
being exposed
glomerulonephritis inflammation
of glomerulus of nephron
glomerulus a tuft formed of capillary
loops at beginning of each nephric tubule in
kidney; this tuft with its capsule (Bowman's
capsule) constitutes the corpusculum renis
hemodialysis filtering of blood to
remove toxins (nitrogenous wastes)
hypospadias a malformation in
which urethra opens on ventral aspect of
penis; frequently associated with congenital chordee

micturition act of urinating
nephron a long, convoluted tubular
structure in kidney, consisting of renal corpuscle, proximal convoluted tubule, neph-
ronic loop, and distal convoluted tubule
oliguria a urine output of less than
0.5–1.0 mL/kg/hour
peritoneal dialysis filtering blood
to remove toxins via a catheter inserted
into peritoneal cavity
prepuce free fold of skin that covers
glans penis
pyelonephritis inflammation of
renal parenchyma, calyces, and pelvis,
particularly due to local bacterial infection
uremia excess of urea and other
nitrogenous waste products in blood
ureteritis inflammation of a ureter
urethritis inflammation of the urethra

PRETEST

1 A male newborn is found to have exstrophy of the bladder. The nurse should evaluate the infant for which of the following? Select all that apply.

1. Hypospadias
2. Epispadias
3. Cryptorchidism
4. Acute tubular necrosis
5. Bilateral inguinal hernias

2 A child has been admitted to the hospital with a diagnosis of "rule out nephrotic syndrome." The nurse would assess the child for which of the following symptoms?

1. Hematuria
2. Edema
3. Petechial rash
4. Dehydration

3 The nurse is caring for a toddler who is not toilet trained. The doctor has ordered intake and output measurement. The nurse will most accurately measure the urine using which method?

1. Estimating output as small, moderate, or large and recording on the child's chart
2. Weighing each wet diaper and recording the weight of the diaper as the amount of urine output
3. Subtracting the weight of a dry diaper from a wet diaper and recording this amount
4. Determining urine output by the number of diaper changes in each 24-hour period

4 The nurse has provided parents of a preschooler with information about urinary tract infections (UTIs) and how to reduce their recurrence. Which statements from the parents indicate they learned the information? Select all that apply.

1. "I should try to get her to drink a lot of water and juices."
2. "I will buy her underwear made with cotton."
3. "Soaking in a bubble bath will reduce irritation."
4. "If I notice her starting to wet the bed again, I need to have her checked for another urinary tract infection."
5. "I should avoid giving her cranberry juice as it has been shown to make the urine more acidic."

5 The nurse would include which of the following in the care of a child with acute glomerulonephritis? Select all that apply.

1. Carefully handling edematous extremities
2. Measuring the blood pressure to monitor for hypertension
3. Providing fun activities for the child on bedrest
4. Monitoring the urine for hematuria
5. Encouraging fluid intake

6 A urinalysis is ordered for a child with a throat culture positive for group-A beta-hemolytic streptococcus (strep throat). When the mother asks why this test is being ordered, what would the nurse include in a response?

1. The urinalysis will indicate whether an HIV infection is also present.
2. Urinary tract infections are common with streptococcal infections and need to receive prompt treatment.
3. Pyelonephritis is a potential complication of antibiotic therapy.
4. Group-A beta-hemolytic streptococcus infections can be followed by the complication of acute glomerulonephritis.

7 What would the nurse select as an appropriate nursing diagnosis for an infant with unrepaired exstrophy of the bladder?

1. Disorganized Infant Behavior
2. Impaired Parent–Infant Attachment
3. Urinary Retention
4. Risk for Infection

8 A child has been admitted to the unit with acute glomerulonephritis. What test does the nurse anticipate will be ordered to confirm this diagnosis?

1. Antistreptolysin-O (ASO) titer
2. Urinalysis
3. Blood cultures
4. White blood cell (WBC) count

9 The health care provider prescribes that a urine culture be obtained on an infant who is not toilet trained. The nurse implements which of the following as the best means of collecting this urine specimen?

1. Perform a straight catheterization.
2. Apply a urine collection bag.
3. Use diaper analysis.
4. Perform Foley catheterization.

10 A 14-year-old is being treated for chronic renal failure. The nurse would assist the child in making food selections that are part of which prescribed diet?

1. High-sodium
2. High-protein
3. Low-sodium
4. Low-fiber

➤ *See pages 160–162 for Answers and Rationales.*

I. OVERVIEW OF ANATOMY AND PHYSIOLOGY OF RENAL SYSTEM

A. Structures of the renal system

1. Kidney
   a. Internal structures: cortex, medulla, pyramids, papilla, and pelvis
   b. Microscopic structures: key functional unit is a **nephron** that consists of a renal corpuscle, loop of Henle, and renal tubules; renal corpuscle consists of **glomerulus** (a capillary tuft) enclosed within Bowman's capsule
2. Ureter: narrow, long tube with an expanded upper end that lies inside kidney pelvis; ureters are lined with mucous membrane and drain urine from kidney pelvis to urinary bladder
3. Bladder: elastic muscular organ that is capable of great expansion; lined with mucous membrane arranged in rugae, like stomal mucosa; bladder stores urine before voiding occurs and also initiates voiding
4. Urethra: narrow tube from urinary bladder to exterior of body lined with mucous membrane; urethral opening to exterior of body is the urinary meatus; urethra passes urine from bladder to outside the body and in the male, reproductive fluid (semen) from the body

B. Functions of the renal system

1. Forms and excretes urine
2. Regulates fluid and electrolyte balance within body
3. Regulates acid–base balance within body
4. Regulates blood pressure
5. Stimulates production of erythropoietin, which promotes production of red blood cells (RBCs) in bone marrow
6. Regulates calcium metabolism in body

!

Practice to Pass

For each of the six functions of the renal system, name at least two clinical symptoms the client might manifest if that function were impaired.

C. **Renal system differences between child and adult**

   1. Fluid is more important to body chemistry of infants and small children because it constitutes a larger fraction of their total body weight
   2. During first two years of life, kidneys are less efficient at regulating electrolyte and acid–base balance; infants are more prone to excess fluid volume and dehydration
   3. Bladder capacity increases from 20 to 50 mL at birth to 700 mL in adulthood
   4. Innervation of "stretch" receptors in bladder wall, which initiates urination and control of bladder sphincters, does not occur before the age of 2; most children under age 2 cannot maintain bladder control
   5. Urethra is shorter in children than in adults and may contribute to a higher frequency of urinary tract infections in children
   6. Kidneys are more susceptible to trauma in children because children do not have as much fat padding as adults

II. DIAGNOSTIC TESTS AND ASSESSMENTS OF RENAL SYSTEM

A. **Urine specimen**: urinalysis for dipstick results, microscopic examination, or for culture; refer to Table 7-1 for normal urinalysis results and to Table 7-2 for significance of color changes

   1. Clean-catch specimen: urine specimen is collected in a clean specimen container following cleansing of urinary meatus and surrounding tissue; in infants and toddlers who are not toilet trained, a straight catheterization is performed; parental assistance is needed for school-age, toilet-trained children, and specimens are obtained individually by adolescents after careful instruction
   2. Sterile urine specimen: obtained by urinary catheterization only

B. **IVP**: intravenous pyelogram; an x-ray or series of x-rays of renal pelvis and ureters following injection of a contrast medium; special preprocedure care may be necessary

C. **KUB**: an x-ray showing kidneys, ureters, and bladder

D. **Ultrasound**: used to obtain location, measurement, or delineation of deep structures that may not show up on x-ray; gives a two-dimensional image through transmission of high-frequency ultrasonic waves

E. **Retrograde/antegrade pyelogram**: a ureteral catheter is passed via a cystoscope; contrast dye is injected and a series of x-rays are taken

F. **Cystogram**: an x-ray of bladder only; dye is injected into bladder via a urethral catheter until bladder is full; several films are taken and dye is then drained via catheter; a final picture is taken when bladder is emptied

G. **Voiding cystourethrogram**: same process as a cystogram except when bladder is filled with contrast dye, urethral catheter is removed; when client feels urge to void, he or she is asked to do so; films are taken during bladder filling, during micturition (voiding) and after micturition

Table 7-1	Normal Urinalysis Results		
Macroscopic Exam		**Microscopic Exam**	
Color	Pale yellow	Red blood cells	0–5/HPF (high-power field)
Turbidity	Clear	White blood cells	0–5/HPF
Odor	Ammonia-like smell	Casts	1 per every 10–20/LPF (low power field)
Specific gravity	1.003–1.030		
pH	4.6–8.0	Crystals	None
Protein	Negative; <10–150 mg/24 hr	Bacteria	<1000 colonies/mL
Glucose	<250 mg/24 hr		
Ketones	Negative		
Bilirubin	Negative		

Table 7-2	Interpreting Changes in Urine Color
Color	**Possible Meaning**
Pale yellow	Normal
Yellow	Concentrated urine
Amber	Bile in urine
Orange	Alkaline or concentrated urine
Red orange	Acidic urine, medication effect
Red	Blood, menses
Pink	Dilute blood
Burgundy	Laxatives
Tea	Melanin, hematuria
Dark gray	Medications, dyes
Blue	Medications, dyes

H. **CT (computed tomography)**: visualization of urinary tract after an oral iodine-containing preparation is taken; provides a much more detailed picture than an x-ray

I. **MRI (magnetic resonance imaging)**: study based on reaction of protons and electrons in living tissues to a magnetic field; images are obtained by measuring energy utilized by protons and electrons during reaction to magnetic field

J. **Serum blood tests**
   1. Hemoglobin and hematocrit: clients with alterations in renal health are often anemic; hemoglobin and hematocrit levels are decreased
   2. BUN (blood urea nitrogen): measures amount of urea in blood; urea is end product of protein metabolism and is excreted by kidneys; clients with alterations in renal health will have an elevated BUN
   3. **Creatinine**: substance produced daily as an end product of metabolism; it is excreted entirely by kidneys and is therefore directly proportional to renal excretory function; serum creatinine level should remain normal and constant; clients who have renal impairment will have an elevated creatinine

   4. Serum electrolytes: measure sodium, potassium, chloride, magnesium, and calcium; the kidneys conserve water and necessary electrolytes; children under age 2 years have immaturely functioning glomeruli, tubules, and nephrons, resulting in more water loss in urine; because of this, infants and toddlers are at greater risk for dehydration and electrolyte imbalances

III. COMMON NURSING PROCEDURES FOR CHILDREN WITH RENAL HEALTH PROBLEMS

A. **Urine specimen collection**

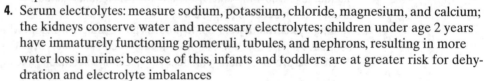

   1. Clean-catch specimen collection
      a. See Box 7-1 for directions for applying a urine collection bag for infant and toddler specimen collection; this procedure can be used also for urine culture
      b. See Box 7-2 for instructions for parent/client education for assisted specimen collection

B. **Assessment**
   1. Newborn assessment: newborn assessment often identifies anomalies of renal system, including the following:

Box 7-1	
Applying a Urine Collection Bag for Infants	

- Gather a urine collection bag, soap solution, sterile water, sterile cotton balls, and urine specimen container.
- Apply gloves and remove diaper. Cleanse and dry the infant's genital area and buttocks if soiled. Change gloves.
- Using one cotton ball at a time that is moistened in soapy water or agency approved cleanser, wipe the genital area three times.
- For males, clean from the tip of the penis towards the scrotum. For females, spread the labia and clean from front to back. Rinse with cotton balls moistened in sterile water. **Use each cotton ball only once and discard.** Dry skin with a sterile cotton ball.
- Remove the adhesive backing from the urine collection bag. Place the bag around the labia for females and gently press to skin. Place the bag around the scrotum for males and gently press to skin. Make sure the seal is tight to avoid urine leakage.
- Diaper the infant. Check frequently for urine. Approximately 20 mL of urine is needed.
- When specimen bag is adequately filled, gently pull the bag away from the skin. Fold the opening over and place the entire urine bag in the specimen container. Cap the container tightly and transport immediately to the lab.

Box 7-2	
Client/Parent Education for Obtaining a Clean-Catch Urine Specimen	

Females
- Do not touch the inside of the specimen cup or lid.
- Wash hands with soap and water.
- Spread the outer folds of the labia with one hand. Using separate antiseptic towelettes, wipe each side of the labia with a separate towelette. With a third towelette, wipe the urinary meatus in the center; **wipe front to back only**, keeping the labia separate.
- While keeping the labial folds spread apart **(do not let go)**, allow the first portion of the urine stream to fall into the toilet.
- **Catch the middle portion** of the urine stream in the specimen cup. **Do not allow specimen cup to touch skin.** Fill one-half full if possible.
- Replace lid (touching outside only) and place container where directed to by health care provider.

Males
- Do not touch the inside of the specimen cup or lid.
- Wash hands with soap and water.
- Clean the head of the penis (after pulling back foreskin if not circumcised) three times using a separate antiseptic towelette. Cleaning should move from the urinary meatus outward.
- Begin to urinate into the toilet and then **insert cup into urine stream** and fill approximately one-half full.
- Replace lid (touching the outside only) and place container where directed to by health care provider.

    a. Hypospadias: a malformation in which urethra opens on ventral aspect of penis; frequently associated with congenital chordee, a fibrous band of tissue that causes ventral curvature of penis

    b. Epispadias: a malformation in which urethra opens on dorsum of penis; frequently associated with exstrophy of bladder

    c. Exstrophy: congenital eversion of a hollow organ (the bladder); a congenital gap in anterior wall of bladder and abdominal wall in front of it, with posterior wall of bladder being exposed

  2. Observation and documentation of voiding patterns: frequent, wet diapers are normal for well-hydrated children; a decrease in voiding frequency can indicate dehydration and potential electrolyte imbalances; early identification of abnormal urinary excretion can help prevent serious urinary tract disease, including renal failure

C. Catheter care

1. Straight catheterization: most commonly utilized to obtain sterile urine samples; use strict aseptic technique to avoid introducing harmful pathogens into urinary tract
2. Indwelling urethral catheters: used postoperatively with children undergoing surgery of renal system; maintain a closed drainage system and perform frequent assessments for catheter patency; if a child is discharged with an indwelling catheter, document parent education and understanding of catheter care and maintenance
3. Suprapubic catheters: drain urine directly from bladder, bypassing urethra
   a. Suprapubic catheters are frequently used postoperatively when surgery is performed on urethra
   b. In addition to maintaining a closed drainage system and assessing for catheter patency, incision care at catheter insertion site is another important nursing responsibility
   c. Provide parent education regarding home care of suprapubic catheters for client who is discharged home with a suprapubic catheter
4. Nephrostomy tubes: inserted directly into renal pelvis of kidney; may be unilateral or bilateral
   a. Nursing interventions include maintaining a closed drainage system and frequently assessing for patency and incisional care of catheter insertion site
   b. Output from nephrostomy tubes must be calculated and documented individually; this helps to quickly identify sources of urinary flow changes
   c. Perform irrigation of nephrostomy tubes only with a health care provider order using sterile technique, which requires a minimum amount of fluid to be used (since renal pelvis is small, irrigating with too large of a fluid volume can cause serious renal damage)

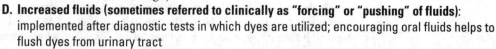

Practice to Pass

Describe the differences in methods used to collect urinalysis specimens from infants, toddlers, school-age children, and adolescents. For each age group, identify developmental factors that impact the method used.

D. Increased fluids (sometimes referred to clinically as "forcing" or "pushing" of fluids): implemented after diagnostic tests in which dyes are utilized; encouraging oral fluids helps to flush dyes from urinary tract

E. Fluid restriction: health care provider may order an oral fluid intake restriction in renal system disorders when edema is present or fluid volume excess is a potential complication

F. Intake and output

1. A measurement of fluid balance in body
   a. Intake: measurement of fluids (in mL) of what is delivered to child through parenteral or oral routes
   b. Output: measurement (in mL) of fluid expelled, drained, secreted, or suctioned from body; for infants, counting wet diapers per day (four to eight per day is normal) is one method of measuring urine output; weighing a dry diaper before it is placed on infant and then after infant has voided is another method of measuring urine output for an infant; each 1 gram of diaper weight is equal to 1 mL of urine output

G. Medication administration

1. Antimicrobial therapy: specific antibiotics are administered for specific pathogens
2. Pathogens causing urinary tract infections are identified by urine culture and sensitivity
3. Sensitivity describes what antimicrobials the identified pathogen will be eradicated by and which ones it is resistant to
4. Nursing management includes administering antibiotics when scheduled as well as parent/client education regarding importance of completing entire course of drug therapy even though symptoms may subside

IV. SURGICAL INTERVENTIONS FOR CHILDREN WITH RENAL HEALTH PROBLEMS

A. Urinary diversion procedures

1. Ureterostomy: surgical implantation of ureters to outside abdominal wall; allows urine to bypass bladder and drain directly into a collection device
2. Vesicostomy: surgical opening into bladder in which bladder wall is brought to surface of abdomen
3. Ileal or colon conduit: ureters are removed from bladder and attached to a segment of ileum or colon, which has been separated from bowel; this segment then acts as a bladder without voluntary control of voiding; client has a stoma on abdominal wall and must wear an appliance for urine collection

B. Issues in psychosocial support for children undergoing surgery of renal system

1. Implementation of psychological interventions in daily care to address the following concerns of the client or parents
   a. Increased physical care of client, especially if stomas or tubes are involved
   b. Hygiene concerns
   c. Skin problems, especially with urinary diversion procedures
2. Difficulty leaving client in the care of others
3. Frequent trips to clinic add stress to everyday life
4. Toddlers may be unable to achieve toilet training
5. School-age children are affected by being "different" and may develop a distorted perception of body image
6. Adolescents may experience low self-esteem and have concerns regarding body image and sexuality

C. Priority nursing diagnoses for children undergoing renal surgery

1. Anxiety related to the surgical experience
   a. Provide surgical tour, especially the "wake-up" room
   b. Determine client's words for genitalia, urination, etc.
   c. Encourage parents to remain with client as appropriate
   d. Provide support and reassurance
2. Risk for Ineffective Airway Clearance related to poor cough effort associated with postanesthesia state, postoperative immobility, or pain
   a. Assist client to turn, cough, and breathe deeply; reposition infants frequently
   b. Perform frequent vital signs monitoring
   c. Teach splinting of incision and incentive spirometry preoperatively and reinforce as needed postoperatively
3. Pain
   a. Assess and monitor for bladder spasms and incisional pain
   b. Provide analgesics as ordered
   c. If an older child is using a PCA (patient controlled analgesia), educate parents about importance of allowing only the client to push the button
4. Risk for Deficient Fluid Volume related to client's age, surgery, catheters, and refusal to drink
   a. Regulate IV fluids
   b. Keep accurate intake and output records
   c. Measure daily weights
   d. Record separate output for each drainage tube
   e. Promote oral intake, when allowed, by offering preferred liquids and using special enticements such as fancy straws

5. Health-Seeking Behaviors regarding ostomy care
   a. Teach need to keep skin dry and odor free
   b. Demonstrate ostomy care procedures to parents and to client as appropriate to age
   c. Provide written instructions to parents
   d. Provide contact number should problems occur

V. CONGENITAL RENAL HEALTH PROBLEMS

A. Hypospadias and epispadias

1. Description
   a. Hypospadias: congenital defect in which urinary meatus is not at end of penis but is located on lower or underside of shaft (see Figure 7-1a)
   b. Epispadias: congenital defect in which urinary meatus is not at end of penis but on upper side of penile shaft; less common than hypospadias (see Figure 7-1b)

2. Etiology and pathophysiology
   a. In hypospadias, opening can be anywhere on underside of penis to base of penis; in epispadias, meatal opening can be anywhere along upper shaft; most frequent anomalies are minor with openings off-center but still on glans
   b. Hypospadias is the more common anomaly, occurring in 1 in 500 newborns
   c. Hypospadias is often accompanied by **chordee**, a downward curvature of penis
   d. Epispadias is often associated with exstrophy of bladder
   e. Both males and females can be affected by hypospadias or epispadias; in most instances, the female anomaly does not require surgical correction

3. Assessment: noted on admission to newborn nursery; defect does not interfere with voiding but could interfere with reproduction if not repaired before adulthood

4. Priority nursing diagnoses
   a. Risk for Impaired Parent–Infant Attachment
   b. Risk for Ineffective Family Coping
   c. Anxiety (parental)
   d. Disturbed Body Image (in unrepaired school-age or adolescent client)

5. Planning and implementation
   a. Document findings carefully and report to physician
   b. **Circumcision** (operation to remove part or all of **prepuce**) is delayed as prepuce may be used in reconstruction
   c. If chordee present, curvature of penis may be released before hypospadias repair

Figure 7-1

A. Hypospadias,
   B. Epispadias.

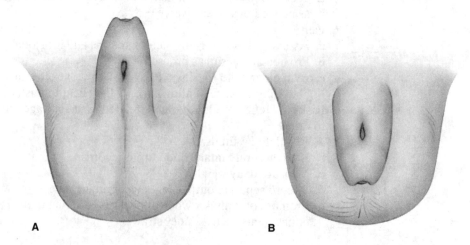

A   B

        d. Surgical correction is usually begun before 18 months of age

        e. Postoperative care

          1) Penis may have a urethral stent in place and be wrapped with a pressure dressing

          2) Arm and leg restraints may be needed to prevent accidental removal of the stent

          3) Encourage increased fluid intake to maintain urine output and stent patency

          4) Call health care provider if no urine output occurs for one hour; there may be kinks in the system or occlusion by sediment

          5) Medication therapy includes antibiotics until the stent falls out, acetaminophen (Tylenol) for pain, and anticholinergics such as oxybutynin (Ditropan) for bladder spasms

    6. Client and family education

        a. Parents need explanation of disorder and information about surgical repair

        b. Postsurgical discharge teaching includes double-diapering technique to protect stent, limiting activity for approximately two weeks, restricting activities that put pressure on site (riding toys, sitting on lap), medication administration, maintaining adequate fluid intake, monitoring for signs of infection, and calling health care provider if urine leaks from anywhere but penis (urine will also be blood-tinged for several days)

    7. Evaluation: parents show positive infant bonding; parents describe surgical plans

B. Exstrophy of bladder

    1. Description: lower portion of abdominal wall and anterior bladder wall are missing, resulting in bladder being open and exposed on abdomen

    2. Etiology and pathophysiology

        a. Occurs more frequently in boys than girls and is most frequently associated with epispadias

        b. Bladder appears as an angry red mass glistening with urine

        c. Continuous drainage of urine from ureters may lead to excoriation of skin surrounding bladder

        d. Exstrophy of bladder can be life threatening and therefore needs to be corrected as soon after birth as possible

    3. Assessment: immediately obvious at birth; evaluate infant for other anomalies

    4. Priority nursing diagnoses

        a. Risk for Infection

        b. Risk for Impaired Parent–Infant Attachment

        c. Risk for Ineffective Family Coping

        d. Impaired Skin Integrity

    5. Planning and implementation

        a. Bladder closure is corrected during first 48 to 72 hours of life

        b. Correction of exstrophy of bladder is usually a staged surgical correction, with epispadias repair at about 9 months of age (if present) and bladder neck reconstruction with ureteral reimplantation at 2 to 3 years of age

        c. Preoperative nursing care involves covering bladder with sterile plastic wrap and maintaining skin integrity of surrounding area using skin sealant to protect it from excoriating effects of urine

        d. Postoperative nursing care may involve Bryant's traction to facilitate healing, and avoiding abduction of legs (places stress on surgical area); changing dressings as ordered by surgeon; monitoring urinary output and characteristics and observing for signs of obstruction, bladder spasms, and urine or blood draining from meatus

        e. Emotional support of infant and parents is important; activities to support bonding as well as helping parents accept deformity are a major component of nurse's activities

6. Client and family education

   a. Parents will need an explanation of anomaly as well as instructions for care

   b. As soon as possible, parents should participate in care of infant and will need appropriate instructions

7. Evaluation: parents identify positive attributes of infant and visit baby often; skin surrounding bladder remains intact

C. Cryptorchidism

   1. Description: a failure of one or both testes to descend from inguinal canal into scrotum

   2. Etiology and pathophysiology

      a. Normal descent of testes occurs in late gestation

      b. More frequently seen in premature infants than in full-term infants

      c. Failure to descend exposes testes to heat of body, leading to low sperm counts at sexual maturity

      d. Undescended testes are also at greater risk for torsion (twisting of testis on its blood supply) and trauma; undescended testes have a higher incidence of cancer

      e. Undescended testes are frequently associated with an inguinal hernia

   3. Assessment: absence of one or both testes in scrotal sac may be noted at birth; if testes are not felt on examination, condition should be monitored as testes may descend later

   4. Priority nursing diagnoses

      a. Risk for Injury

      b. Risk for Disturbed Body Image (in older child with undescended testes)

   5. Planning and implementation

      a. Often testes descend on their own during first year of life

      b. If this does not occur, human chorionic gonadotropin (hCG) hormone is given to induce descent

      c. If testes remain undescended, an orchiopexy is performed before age 2; increased risk of testicular cancer if not performed; if testes are damaged or absent, a prosthesis may be placed in the scrotum

      d. Nursing care preoperatively is directed at preparing client and family for surgery

      e. Postoperative nursing care includes placing ice on surgical area, giving analgesics for pain, monitoring client for infection and maintaining bedrest

   6. Client and family education

      a. Educate parents about surgical process

      b. Since client will likely go home after recovering from anesthesia, parents will need instructions on how to care for client at home

      c. Symptoms of infection should be described

   7. Evaluation: client recovers without signs and symptoms of infection; parents describe appropriate home care for client

VI. ACQUIRED RENAL HEALTH PROBLEMS

A. Acute glomerulonephritis

   1. Description

      a. A disease process that affects primarily the glomerulus of kidney

      b. May be acute or chronic

      c. Most common form is post-streptococcal **glomerulonephritis**

   2. Etiology and pathophysiology

      a. Acute inflammation of glomeruli

      b. Acute post-infectious glomerulonephritis is preceded by a streptococcal infection, usually of skin or respiratory tract

      c. Damage is caused by an antigen-antibody complex that lodges in glomeruli

---

Practice to Pass

What discharge instructions/parent education should be included for the child being discharged after a urinary diversion procedure?

3. Assessment

   a. Diagnostic tests: elevated BUN indicates impaired renal function; elevated erythrocyte sedimentation rate (ESR) indicates inflammation in body; elevated antistreptolysin O (ASO) titer indicates a previous streptococcal infection; renal ultrasound shows enlarged kidneys, while urine exams demonstrate gross hematuria, proteinuria, and red blood cell casts; serum samples may also display **azotemia** (retention of excess nitrogenous wastes in blood), elevated creatinine, and electrolyte imbalance

   b. Nursing assessments include observing for edema, hematuria, lethargy, and anorexia; hypertension can lead to headache, decreased level of consciousness, and convulsions

4. Priority nursing diagnoses

   a. Risk for Excess Fluid Volume

   b. Imbalanced Nutrition

   c. Risk for Injury related to hypertension and CNS involvement

   d. Activity Intolerance

   e. Diversional Activity Deficit

5. Planning and implementation (see Table 7-3)

   a. Bedrest is required during acute period

   b. Monitor for fluid and electrolyte imbalances; measure intake and output; weigh daily to monitor fluid balance; maintain fluid restriction if ordered; sodium, potassium, and possibly protein intake will be limited; monitor dietary intake to optimize calories consumed

   c. Provide skin care to limit effects of edema and immobility

   d. Monitor vital signs including mental status; report increasing hypertension and deterioration of mental status immediately

6. Medication therapy: to treat hypertension and prevent CNS involvement

   a. Antihypertensives, such as hydralazine (Apresoline)

   b. Diuretics, such as furosemide (Lasix)

Table 7-3 **Comparison of Features of Acute Glomerulonephritis and Nephrotic Syndrome**

Assessment Factor	Acute Glomerulonephritis	Nephrotic Syndrome
Cause	Immune reaction to group A beta-hemolytic streptococcal infection	Idiopathic; possibly a hypersensitivity reaction
Onset	Abrupt	Insidious
Hematuria	Grossly bloody	Rare
Proteinuria	3+ or 4+, not massive	Massive
Edema	Mild	Massive
Hypertension	Marked	Mild
Hyperlipidemia	Rare or mild	Marked
Peak age frequency	5–10 years of age	2–3 years of age
Interventions	Limited activity; anti-hypertensives as needed; symptomatic therapy if CHF occurs	Bedrest during edema stage; corticosteroid administration
Diet	Normal for age; no added salt if child is hypertensive	Nutritious for age; no added salt; small, frequent meals may be desirable
Prevention	Prevention through treatment of group A beta-hemolytic streptococcal infections	None known
Course	Acute 2–3 weeks	Chronic—may have relapses

7. Client and family education

    a. Parents and client need information about disease, treatment, and prognosis

    b. Parents need information on safely administering medications

    c. Instructions may be needed on monitoring blood pressure and weight and how to test urine for protein

8. Evaluation: parents demonstrate safe administration of medications; parents and client describe necessary home monitoring

B. Nephrotic syndrome

1. Description: clinical state characterized by edema, massive proteinuria, and hyperlipidemia

2. Etiology and pathophysiology

    a. Cause is unknown

    b. Increased permeability of glomerular membrane allows albumin to pass into urine; kidneys reabsorb salt and water

    c. Protein deficiency leads to decreased osmotic pressure, allowing fluids to escape into tissues; massive edema results

    d. Loss of protein leads to decreased immunoglobulins and susceptibility to infection

    e. Hyperlipidemia occurs secondary to liver stimulation by decreased volume of albumin

    f. Relapses often occur but frequency of relapses diminishes with puberty

3. Assessments

    a. Gradual onset of massive edema, starting as periorbital then shifting to abdomen and extremities, resulting in dramatic weight gain and abdominal pain

    b. Secondary symptoms of irritability, general malaise, and anorexia occur

    c. Urinalysis reveals proteinuria

4. Priority nursing diagnoses

    a. Risk for Infection

    b. Excess Fluid Volume

    c. Risk for Impaired Skin Integrity

    d. Imbalanced Nutrition: Less Than Body Requirements

5. Planning and implementation

    a. Monitor weight and intake and output; measure abdominal girth

    b. Promote nutrition by allowing child's preferences; fluids are not usually restricted; diet may be "no added salt"

    c. Promote rest; provide diversional activities as necessary

    d. Prevent skin breakdown: turn and reposition on a regular basis; use special mattresses as needed to help prevent breakdown; keep skin dry and clean

    e. Prevent infection: use careful handwashing; restrict visitors with infectious diseases; children with nephrotic syndrome are often not kept in the hospital after initial diagnosis to reduce exposure to organisms; encourage diet to replace lost protein

    f. Refer again to Table 7-3 for comparison of acute glomerulonephritis and nephrotic syndrome according to manifestations, interventions, prevention, and course

6. Medication therapy

    a. Intravenous albumin and/or diuretics may be administered to reduce edema

    b. Corticosteroids reduce inflammatory process, which reduces proteinuria

    c. Alkylating agents may be used if steroid therapy is unsuccessful

C. Acute renal failure (ARF)

1. Description: sudden onset of diminished renal function

2. Etiology and pathophysiology

    a. Occurs suddenly and is often reversible; generally follows ischemic or toxic trauma to the kidney

---

Practice to Pass

What nursing measures are specific to caring for children with acute glomerulonephritis? What nursing measures are specific to caring for children with nephrotic syndrome? How do they differ?

       b. Three causes

          1) Prerenal causes include decreased glomerular filtration secondary to decreases in renal blood flow

          2) Intrarenal causes include direct kidney damage or changes caused by toxic substances or infection

          3) Postrenal causes include obstruction in urinary tract (from renal tubules to urethral meatus) caused by cancer, calculi, or trauma

  3. Assessment

       a. Laboratory findings include hyperkalemia, hyponatremia, and hypocalcemia; BUN and serum creatinine are elevated

       b. Clinically, client will be pale and lethargic with edema; hypertension occurs secondarily to fluid volume overload

       c. Nursing history may indicate possible causes of acute renal failure

       d. Prognosis depends upon cause as well as kidneys' response to therapy

  4. Priority nursing diagnoses

       a. Impaired Urinary Elimination

       b. Risk for Imbalanced Nutrition: Less Than Body Requirements

       c. Excess Fluid Volume

       d. Anxiety

       e. Risk for Ineffective Family Coping

       f. Disturbed Body Image

  5. Planning and implementation

       a. Medical management depends upon cause

       b. Clients with ARF are catabolic and at risk for calorie and protein malnutrition related to decreased appetite and fluid restriction; help client choose a diet that has necessary nutrients while restricting sodium, potassium, and phosphorus as needed; initially, parenteral or enteral nutrition may be needed

       c. Dialysis may be required during acute period to correct electrolyte and fluid balances while eliminating wastes

       d. Monitor intake and output and weigh client daily; maintain fluid restrictions, which are calculated to replace insensible losses (1/3 daily maintenance requirements); febrile children usually have a 12% increase in fluid intake for each 1° Celsius increase in temperature

       e. Monitor blood pressures and report changes to prevent complications

       f. Child will be susceptible to infection so wash hands carefully, protect from infectious visitors, and promote nutrition

       g. Provide emotional support for client and parental anxiety, possible parental feelings of guilt; assist parents and older siblings to participate in care to increase their sense of control

  6. Medication therapy

       a. Antibiotic therapy may be ordered

       b. Avoid nephrotoxic drugs (such as aminoglycosides, cephalosporins, sulfonamides, tetracycline, contrast dye with iodine, indomethacin, aspirin, and heavy metals)

  7. Client and family education

       a. Teach dietary management, including protein, water, and sodium restrictions

       b. Teach parents symptoms of progressive renal failure and how to monitor weight, intake and output, and blood pressure

       c. Discuss with parents principles of safe and effective drug administration

  8. Evaluation: parents describe symptoms of renal failure and discuss monitoring that will be done in the home; dietary restrictions are followed

D. Chronic renal failure (CRF)

  1. Description: progressive deterioration of renal function

2. Etiology and pathophysiology
   a. Etiology of CRF includes congenital abnormalities, damage from disease such as glomerulonephritis, hemolytic-uremic syndrome, infections, and exposure to toxins
   b. Gradual loss of functioning nephrons
   c. End-stage renal disease refers to a disease where kidneys can no longer maintain body homeostasis and would lead to death without dialysis
3. Assessment
   a. Laboratory test results (rising BUN, creatinine) indicate a failure of kidneys to cleanse blood, with resulting **uremia** (excess of urea and other nitrogenous waste products in blood)
   b. Renal biopsy determines diagnosis and provides a basis for determining treatment
   c. Assessment findings will include **oliguria** (urine output less than 0.5–1 mL/kg/hour) or **anuria** (complete/almost complete cessation of urine production by kidneys); sudden weight gain indicates fluid retention; assess for signs and symptoms of fluid overload; monitor for manifestations of fluid and electrolyte imbalances (see Table 7-4)
   d. Assess cardiac, hematological, gastrointestinal, neurological, dermatological, urinary, and skeletal systems for changes secondary to renal failure (see Table 7-5)
4. Priority nursing diagnoses
   a. Risk for Infection
   b. Excess Fluid Volume
   c. Caregiver Role Strain
   d. Impaired Growth and Development
   e. Disturbed Body Image
5. Planning and implementation
   a. Medical management is aimed at maintaining fluid and electrolyte balance as close to normal as possible
   b. Dialysis will be used to maintain client's fluid and electrolyte balance when renal function is no longer able to maintain homeostasis
   c. Chronic renal failure is permanent; kidney transplant may be indicated
   d. Renal replacement therapy

Table 7-4 **Symptoms of Electrolyte Imbalance**

Electrolyte Imbalance	Manifestations
Hyponatremia (decreased sodium)	Headache, muscle weakness, fatigue, apathy, confusion, coma, postural hypotension, anorexia, nausea, vomiting, abdominal cramping, weight loss
Hypernatremia (increased sodium)	Dry mucous membranes, decreased urine output, rubbery skin turgor, excitement, tachycardia
Hypokalemia (decreased potassium)	Anorexia, nausea, vomiting, abdominal distention, lethargy, confusion, depression, weakness, decreased BP while standing, arrhythmias, thirst, increased urine output
Hyperkalemia (increased potassium)	Nausea, vomiting, diarrhea, irritability, weakness, oliguria, numbness, tingling, arrhythmias, sudden death
Hypocalcemia (decreased calcium)	Osteoporosis, fractures, tingling, convulsions, muscle spasms, tetany, calcium deposits in tissue, nausea, vomiting, diarrhea, arrhythmias
Hypercalcemia (increased calcium)	Renal calculi, coma, decreased reflexes, lethargy, arrhythmias, muscle fatigue, bone pain, osteoporosis, fractures
Acidosis (decreased bicarbonate)	Headache, malaise, rapid deep respirations, disorientation, stupor, coma, hyperkalemia

Table 7-5	Clinical Manifestations of Renal Failure	
Body System	**Clinical Manifestations**	**Cause of Manifestations**
Cardiovascular	Hypervolemia, hypertension, tachcardia, arrhythmias, congestive heart failure, pericarditis	Increased fluid volume, build-up of metabolic wastes, chronic hypetension, change in renin-angiotensin mechanism
Hematologic	Anemia, leukocytosis, decreased platelet function, thrombocytopenia	Decreased production of erythropoietin and RBCs, decreased survival of RBCs, decreased platelet activity; blood loss through dialysis and bleeding
Gastrointestinal	Anorexia, nausea, vomiting, abdominal distention, diarrhea, constipation, bleeding	Build-up of uremic toxins, electrolyte imbalances, changes in platelet activity, conversion of urea to ammonia by saliva
Neurologic	Lethargy, confusion, convulsions, stupor, coma, sleep disturbances, behavioral changes, muscle irritability	Uremic toxins, electrolyte imbalances, cerebral swelling caused by fluid shifts
Dermatologic	Pallor, pigmentation, pruritus, ecchymosis, excoriation, uremic frost	Anemia, decreased activity of sweat glands, dry skin, phosphate deposits on skin
Urinary	Decreased urine output, decreased specific gravity, proteinuria, casts and cells in the urine	Damage to the nephron
Skeletal	Osteoporosis, renal rickets, joint pain	Decreased calcium absorption, decreased phosphate excretion

1) **Hemodialysis**: filtering of blood with a dialyzer to remove toxins (nitrogenous wastes) using a special machine; requires vascular access site with frequent monitoring for potential infection; involves a 4- to 6-hour treatment approximately three times a week and is the most effective dialysis treatment in clearing nitrogenous wastes from blood

2) **Peritoneal dialysis**: filtering of blood to remove toxins via a catheter inserted into peritoneal cavity (see Figure 7-2); peritoneal dialysis is relatively easy to learn for home dialysis treatment; it is the most widely used renal replacement therapy in children; however, clients are at increased risk for peritonitis

3) Renal transplantation: kidney transplantation from a cadaver (organ donor) or a living relative donor; donation of a kidney from a histocompatible family-related donor (has human leukocyte antigen [HLA] system match) improves survival rate of graft; transplantation is considered to be optimal renal replacement therapy because it provides for normal homeostasis and offers optimal chance for normal growth and development; disadvantages include rejection episodes and complications of immunosuppression

e. General nursing care involves monitoring intake and output, weight, and vital signs; assess for signs of electrolyte imbalances; support good nutrition while maintaining dietary and fluid restrictions

f. Nursing care of client receiving peritoneal dialysis includes carrying out dialysis procedure and using aseptic technique to prevent *peritonitis* (fever, vomiting, diarrhea, abdominal pain, tenderness, and cloudy dialysate)

g. Nursing care of client receiving hemodialysis includes monitoring for complications that can suddenly occur, including hypotension (nausea and vomiting, abdominal cramping, tachycardia, and dizziness), rapid fluid and electrolyte shifts (muscle cramps, nausea and vomiting, and dizziness), and disequilibrium syndrome

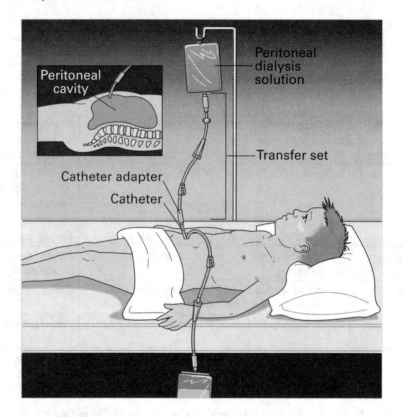

Figure 7-2

Peritoneal dialysis

(restlessness, headache, blurred vision, altered level of consciousness, nausea and vomiting, muscle twitching)

h. Both client and parents will have emotional needs related to chronic nature of disease, ongoing life-sustaining treatment, and possibility of death; assist with physical and emotional preparation for dialysis and renal transplant

6. Medication therapy

   a. Sodium bicarbonate may be needed for severe metabolic acidosis

   b. Diuretics are given to promote fluid elimination

   c. Vitamins are necessary because of dietary deficiencies; vitamin D and calcium supplements may be ordered

   d. Erythropoietin (epoetin alfa, Epogen) may be given to stimulate red blood cell production

   e. Antihypertensives may be necessary

7. Client and family education

   a. Teach parents and client to manage client's disease at home, including dietary restrictions and needs

   b. Teach parents safe and effective administration of medications and potential side effects

   c. Provide parents with information about symptoms of electrolyte imbalances

   d. Provide individualized instruction to client and parents about dialysis and possible renal transplant

8. Evaluation: parents describe safe medication administration; client maintains dietary and fluid restrictions; parents and client describe preparation for dialysis and/or renal transplant; parents demonstrate adequate coping mechanisms; client's growth and development is maintained at an optimal level

Practice to Pass

What are the three types of renal replacement therapy? For each type, describe one advantage and disadvantage for the child with renal failure.

VII. INFECTIOUS RENAL HEALTH PROBLEMS: URINARY TRACT INFECTIONS

A. Description: urinary tract infection (UTI) is an infection caused by bacteria, virus, or fungus that occurs in the urinary tract

B. Etiology and pathophysiology

1. Site of infection within urinary tract determines consequences of infection within it

   a. Infections of upper urinary tract, which include **pyelonephritis** (inflammation of renal parenchyma, calyces, and pelvis, particularly due to local bacterial infection) or **ureteritis** (inflammation of a ureter), are associated with or may result in permanent renal damage or scarring

   b. Infections confined to lower urinary tract, such as **cystitis** (inflammation of urinary bladder) and **urethritis** (inflammation of urethra), may be followed by recurrent episodes, but have not been associated with long-term sequelae

2. Acute pyelonephritis is the most commonly occurring bacterial infection documented in young children, with *Escherichia coli* being responsible for approximately 85% of UTIs in infants and young children, followed by *Klebsiella* and *Proteus* organisms

3. UTI is second most common infection in children; it is more common in girls than boys (girls have a shorter urethra); approximately 7% of girls and 2% of boys will have a UTI by age 6

C. Assessment

1. Urinalysis: microscopic urinalysis shows large numbers of white blood cells (greater than 10 WBC/mm^3) as well as large numbers of bacteria

   a. Obtain catheter specimens in infants and young children without urinary control

   b. Obtain clean-catch specimens from toilet-trained children (refer back to Box 7-2)

2. Urine culture: *Escherichia coli* is the most frequently found organism after 48 hours of growth

3. Signs and symptoms

   a. Infants: fever, weight loss, failure to thrive, vomiting, increased voiding, foul-smelling urine, and persistent diaper rash

   b. Older children: urinary frequency, pain during micturition, onset of bedwetting in a previously "dry" child, abdominal pain, hematuria, fever, chills, and flank pain

D. Priority nursing diagnoses

1. Pain

2. Impaired Urinary Elimination

3. Risk for Injury

E. Planning and implementation

1. Monitor intake and output; renal function should be 1 mL/kg/hr; obtain daily weights

2. Encourage frequent voiding in toilet-trained child

3. Encourage increased fluid intake

4. Acidify the urine with ascorbic acid or cranberry juice (adjunct measure)

5. All clients under age 5 at time of first UTI are evaluated by ultrasound and voiding cystourethrogram (VCUG)

F. Medication therapy

1. Give antibiotic therapy

   a. Must continue to give/take doses for full course of therapy to prevent recurrent infection

   b. Untreated lower UTIs can ascend further into the urinary system and lead to acute pyelonephritis

2. Give antipyretic therapy as needed for temperature control

Box 7-3

Client and Family Education for Preventing Urinary Tract Infections in Children

- Encourage complete bladder emptying and explain the need for this as age permits. "Standing urine" in the bladder is susceptible to the growth of pathogens.
- Remind client to void frequently. The bladder flushes away organisms by ridding itself of urine; this prevents organisms from accumulating and invading nearby structures. The convalescent bladder is less resistant to invasion than is a healthy bladder.
- Suggest avoidance of hot tubs, whirlpool baths, water softeners, or bubble baths. Oils in these products are known to irritate the urethra and can be potential sources of infection.
- Teach girls the importance of wiping themselves after toileting from front to back to avoid contamination of the urethra with *Escherichia coli*, which is found in stool. Have girls demonstrate this technique on a doll.
- Encourage the use of showers rather than tub baths to help prevent infection.
- Explain the need for cotton underwear, which is more absorbent than nylon or other synthetic materials.
- Suggest apple or cranberry juices to maintain acidity of urine; acidifying the urine may decrease rate of bacterial multiplication; an acid-ash diet consisting of meats, cheese, prunes, cranberries, plums, and whole grains is also beneficial.
- Recommend frequent pad change for menstruating girls and proper genital cleansing during menses. Old, pooled blood fosters growth of organisms.

G. Client and family education

1. Teach parents ways to reduce UTIs (see Box 7-3): avoid bubble baths, tight underwear
2. Encourage client to void frequently and to drink plenty of liquids
3. Teach parents to administer medications and to complete therapy

H. Evaluation: parents describe ways to reduce UTIs; parents describe safe administration of antibiotics

Case Study

A school-age child with end-stage renal disease (ESRD) is evaluated for renal replacement therapy. Please answer the following questions regarding the child's nursing management in terms of the type of replacement therapy prescribed, as well as general management principles.

1. What type of diet (including fluids) is prescribed for the child with ESRD? Why?

2. What type of renal replacement is considered to be the most effective for a child with ESRD? Why?

3. What are the potential complications of hemodialysis? What are the advantages of hemodialysis over peritoneal dialysis?

4. Why is peritoneal dialysis more widely used in the treatment of children with ESRD?

5. What psychosocial concerns need to be addressed with the child with ESRD?

For suggested responses, see page 353.

POSTTEST

1 The nurse would place highest priority on which nursing activity in managing a young child diagnosed with urinary tract infection (UTI)?

1. Provide adequate nutrition to prevent dehydration.
2. Prevent enuresis.
3. Administer ordered antibiotics on schedule.
4. Restrict fluids to provide kidney rest.

2 When reviewing a urinalysis report of a client with acute glomerulonephritis, the nurse expects to note which of the following?

1. Decreased creatinine clearance
2. Decreased specific gravity
3. Proteinuria
4. Decreased erythrocyte sedimentation rate (ESR)

3 While a child is receiving prednisone (Deltasone) for treatment of nephrotic syndrome, the nurse determines that it is important to assess the child for which of the following?

1. Infection
2. Urinary retention
3. Easy bruising
4. Hypoglycemia

4 The nurse is admitting a 12-year-old girl to the hospital prior to surgery. The physician has ordered a urinalysis. What should the nurse do to ensure that proper procedure is followed for obtaining the specimen?

1. Encourage fluids to 1000 mL prior to specimen collection.
2. Cleanse the specimen container with antiseptic prior to collecting the specimen.
3. Allow the urine to cool to room temperature before taking it to the lab.
4. Provide information about specimen collection before it is obtained.

5 The parents of a child diagnosed with glomerulonephritis ask the nurse why the child needs a daily weight. In formulating a response, the nurse includes which benefit of measuring daily weight?

1. Determine if the child's caloric intake is adequate.
2. Indicate the need for dietary restrictions of sodium and potassium.
3. Keep track of possible loss or gain of fluid retained in body tissues.
4. Track the amount of fluid ingested orally each day.

6 A child has been diagnosed with acute renal failure secondary to an infectious organism. The nurse would question a prescription for which medication?

1. Aqueous penicillin
2. Gentamicin (Garamycin)
3. Hydralazine (Apresoline)
4. Prednisone (Deltasone)

7 The newborn has been diagnosed with cryptorchidism and the health care provider has explained treatment options to the parents. The nurse reinforces which point about the treatment plan when questioned by the parents?

1. Surgery will be done before age six months.
2. Drugs to stimulate peristalsis may be given to indirectly exert a downward pushing effect on undescended testes.
3. There will be heightened monitoring for testicular cancer until 10 years of age.
4. The infant will be observed at this time because the testes may descend spontaneously.

8 The nurse admits children with the following diseases to the unit. The nurse determines that the children with which diseases are at risk for the development of acute renal failure (ARF)? Select all that apply.

1. Leukemia
2. Cryptorchidism
3. Acute tubular necrosis
4. Phenylketonuria
5. Urinary tract infection

POSTTEST

9 A child has recurrent nephrotic syndrome. The mother reports to the nurse that she is overwhelmed with the care of her child. After the nurse discusses options with the mother, which statement by the mother indicates continued coping difficulties?

1. "I joined a support group like you suggested. I hope it does some good."
2. "I'm going to ask my mother-in-law to come on a regular basis to allow me an afternoon out."
3. "My husband has agreed to help me manage my son's medication."
4. "We're going to skip his dietary restrictions one day a week to allow us both some relaxation."

10 A child returning to the unit after an intravenous pyelogram (IVP) has an order to drink extra fluids. When the mother asks the purpose of these fluids, what should the nurse include in a response?

1. "The fluids are needed to overhydrate your child."
2. "Increased fluids will help to raise serum creatinine levels."
3. "This will make up for fluid losses from the NPO status before tests."
4. "The fluids will help to flush any remaining dye from the urinary tract."

➤ *See pages 162–163 for Answers and Rationales.*

ANSWERS & RATIONALES

Pretest

1 **Answer: 2, 5 Rationale:** Epispadias and bilateral inguinal hernias are frequent anomalies associated with exstrophy of the bladder. Hypospadias, cryptorchidism, and acute tubular necrosis are not. **Cognitive Level:** Analyzing **Client Need:** Physiological Adaptation **Integrated Process:** Nursing Process: Assessment **Content Area:** Child Health **Strategy:** Analyze each of the options and recall commonly associated defects with exstrophy of the bladder to choose correctly. **Reference:** Ball, J., Bindler, R., & Cowen, K. (2010). *Child health nursing: Partnering with children and families* (2nd ed.). Upper Saddle River, NJ: Pearson Education, p. 1203.

2 **Answer: 2 Rationale:** Edema is the major clinical symptom of nephrotic syndrome. The child may gain twice his or her normal weight in severe cases. Hematuria and petechial rash are not associated with nephrotic syndrome. Dehydration is the opposite problem of what the client is experiencing. **Cognitive Level:** Applying **Client Need:** Physiological Adaptation **Integrated Process:** Nursing Process: Assessment **Content Area:** Child Health **Strategy:** Nephrotic syndrome is a renal/urinary condition, so look first for the options related to urinary function. Recall that body fluid is involved in dehydration and edema, which are opposites. If the kidneys are not working effectively, there will be problems eliminating fluid. **Reference:** Ball,

J., Bindler, R., & Cowen, K. (2010). *Child health nursing: Partnering with children and families* (2nd ed.). Upper Saddle River, NJ: Pearson Education, p. 1215.

3 **Answer: 3 Rationale:** Diapers are weighed on a gram scale before using them and after removal (1 gram = 1 mL). The weight of the dry diaper is then subtracted from the weight of the wet diaper to determine urine output. Estimating output does not provide valid, objective data. Recording the weight of the wet diaper does not account for the weight of the dry diaper as baseline. Counting the number of diaper changes has no value when there is a need to measure the actual output. **Cognitive Level:** Applying **Client Need:** Physiological Adaptation **Integrated Process:** Nursing Process: Implementation **Content Area:** Child Health **Strategy:** Notice that two options are very similar. Determine which of the two would provide the most accurate information. **Reference:** Ball, J., Bindler, R., & Cowen, K. (2010). *Child health nursing: Partnering with children and families* (2nd ed.). Upper Saddle River, NJ: Pearson Education, p. 751.

4 **Answer: 1, 2, 4 Rationale:** Drinking an increased amount of fluids helps flush microbes from the bladder. Cotton is a fabric that does not trap moisture, and is preferred to nylon or other fabrics that retain moisture. Bed-wetting may be a sign of urinary tract infection, and the parents should have the child seen by the health care provider. Bubble baths are irritating to the meatus and increase the incidence of urinary tract infections. Cranberry juice may acidify urine or may prevent bacteria from sticking to bladder wall, which is desirable. **Cognitive Level:** Applying **Client Need:** Physiological Adaptation **Integrated Process:** Nursing Process: Evaluation **Content Area:** Child Health **Strategy:** The core concept being tested in the question is factors that influence UTI or are signs of UTI. The wording of the question indicates that more than option will be correct. **Reference:** Ball, J., Bindler, R., & Cowen, K. (2010). *Child health nursing: Partnering with children and families* (2nd ed.). Upper Saddle River, NJ: Pearson Education, pp. 1202–1203.

5 **Answer: 2, 3, 4** **Rationale:** Glomerulonephritis can be associated with hypertension, so regular blood pressure monitoring is important. Although children with acute glomerulonephritis may feel well, they are confined to bed until hematuria resolves. This can lead to boredom, making diversional activities helpful. Hematuria accompanies glomerulonephritis, and the nurse needs to monitor for this as part of routine care. Severe edema of the extremities that would require careful handling is not generally seen in glomerulonephritis. Fluid intake should not be encouraged or increased because the kidneys have difficulty handling the fluid load in glomerulonephritis. **Cognitive Level:** Applying **Client Need:** Physiological Adaptation **Integrated Process:** Nursing Process: Implementation **Content Area:** Child Health **Strategy:** With glomerulonephritis, there is damage to the glomerular capillary causing the loss of red blood cells through the urine, decreased urine output, and hypertension. Consider any interventions related to these symptoms. **Reference:** Ball, J., Bindler, R., & Cowen, K. (2010). *Child health nursing: Partnering with children and families* (2nd ed.). Upper Saddle River, NJ: Pearson Education, p. 1221.

6 **Answer: 4** **Rationale:** Urinalysis allows for early diagnosis and treatment of acute glomerulonephritis, which is a serious complication that can follow group-A beta-hemolytic streptococcal infection. HIV screening is done initially by enzyme-linked immunosorbent assay (ELISA). Urinary tract infections are not commonly associated with streptococcal infections, although they would require prompt treatment if they were present. Pyelonephritis is an infection of the pelvis of the kidney, and is often a complication of ascending infection from the urinary bladder. **Cognitive Level:** Analyzing **Client Need:** Physiological Adaptation **Integrated Process:** Nursing Process: Implementation **Content Area:** Child Health **Strategy:** Remember to associate strep infections with the common complications of rheumatic fever and glomerulonephritis. **Reference:** Ball, J., Bindler, R., & Cowen, K. (2010). *Child health nursing: Partnering with children and families* (2nd ed.). Upper Saddle River, NJ: Pearson Education, p. 1219.

7 **Answer: 4** **Rationale:** The open bladder allows bacteria to enter the urinary system, and urinary tract infections are common. Disorganized behavior does not apply. Although there is a risk for Impaired Parent–Infant Attachment at the time of birth, this diagnosis is written as an actual nursing diagnosis, and there is no evidence to support this with the information given. The unformed bladder does not hold urine, so urinary retention would not be an appropriate diagnosis. **Cognitive Level:** Analyzing **Client Need:** Physiological Adaptation **Integrated Process:** Nursing Process: Diagnosis **Content Area:** Child Health **Strategy:** Recall the pathophysiology of exstrophy of the bladder, which is a congenital defect where the bladder does not have an anterior wall so cannot collect urine. Consider the risks of an open bladder to choose correctly. **Reference:** Ball, J., Bindler, R., & Cowen, K. (2010). *Child health nursing: Partnering with children and families* (2nd ed.). Upper Saddle River, NJ: Pearson Education, p. 1204.

8 **Answer: 1** **Rationale:** The ASO titer indicates a preceding infection with group A beta-hemolytic streptococcus, which can lead to glomerulonephritis as a complication. The urinalysis would show hematuria, but this alone would not be diagnostic of acute glomerulonephritis. Blood cultures may be negative as the infection preceded the illness by one to three weeks. A WBC count could be elevated with any inflammatory or infectious process in the body, and thus, is not diagnostic for glomerulonephritis. **Cognitive Level:** Applying **Client Need:** Physiological Adaptation **Integrated Process:** Nursing Process: Planning **Content Area:** Child Health **Strategy:** Recall the nature of the disorder, and then select the method that will be most specific to the etiology of the disorder. **Reference:** Ball, J., Bindler, R., & Cowen, K. (2010). *Child health nursing: Partnering with children and families* (2nd ed.). Upper Saddle River, NJ: Pearson Education, p. 1220.

9 **Answer: 1** **Rationale:** Catheterization is necessary as this will provide a specimen that is not contaminated by microorganisms outside the urinary bladder. The urine does need to be obtained at the time of voiding. Clean-catch urine specimens, such as those obtained using a urine collection bag, are less reliable urine samples; therefore, catheterization is preferred. Diaper analysis is not valid for performing a culture, although weighing dry and wet diapers may be used to calculate urine output. A Foley catheter is an indwelling urinary catheter and is unnecessary for obtaining a urine culture. **Cognitive Level:** Applying **Client Need:** Basic Care and Comfort **Integrated Process:** Nursing Process: Implementation **Content Area:** Child Health **Strategy:** Determine whether the specimen should be sterile or clean, then select the option that would provide an uncontaminated specimen. **Reference:** Ball, J., Bindler, R., & Cowen, K. (2010). *Child health nursing:*

Partnering with children and families (2nd ed.).Upper Saddle River, NJ: Pearson Education, p. 1201.

10 **Answer: 3** **Rationale:** With the inability to secrete urine, electrolytes will build up in the blood, including sodium and potassium. The child should be on a low-sodium, low-potassium diet with restricted fluids and proteins. Fiber is necessary for GI function and this client has a renal disorder. **Cognitive Level:** Analyzing **Client Need:** Physiological Adaptation **Integrated Process:** Nursing Process: Implementation **Content Area:** Child Health **Strategy:** In renal failure, the kidneys have difficulty excreting waste products. Therefore, the diet will reduce the amount of substances that are hard to clear. **Reference:** Ball, J., Bindler, R., & Cowen, K. (2010). *Child health nursing: Partnering with children and families* (2nd ed.). Upper Saddle River, NJ: Pearson Education, p. 1230.

Posttest

1 **Answer: 3** **Rationale:** Urinary tract infections are ascending in nature; an untreated UTI can lead to acute pyelonephritis with resulting kidney scarring and damage. Early diagnosis and prompt antimicrobial therapy will prevent or minimize permanent renal damage. Dehydration is not a primary concern, although increased fluid intake will help flush the urinary system. Enuresis or bedwetting can occur as a symptom of urinary tract infection in a young child, but this should resolve as the infection is treated. Fluids should be increased rather than decreased to help eliminate microorganisms from the urinary bladder. **Cognitive Level:** Analyzing **Client Need:** Physiological Adaptation **Integrated Process:** Nursing Process: Evaluation **Content Area:** Child Health **Strategy:** With any infectious disease, recall that it is important that antibiotics be administered on schedule. **Reference:** Ball, J., Bindler, R., & Cowen, K. (2010). *Child health nursing: Partnering with children and families* (2nd ed.). Upper Saddle River, NJ: Pearson Education, p. 1203.

2 **Answer: 3** **Rationale:** The presence of protein in the urine is a prime manifestation of acute glomerulonephritis. Decreased creatinine clearance would be found with renal failure. A decreased urine specific gravity would be found with dilute urine, but this is not an associated finding with glomerulonephritis. The ESR is a blood test that is a non-specific indicator of inflammation in the body. **Cognitive Level:** Analyzing **Client Need:** Reduction of Risk Potential **Integrated Process:** Nursing Process: Assessment **Content Area:** Child Health **Strategy:** Eliminate those tests that are blood exams. That leaves proteinuria and specific gravity. Both findings would be abnormal, but specific gravity would not be specific for glomerulonephritis. **Reference:** Ball, J., Bindler, R., & Cowen, K. (2010). *Child health nursing: Partnering with children and families* (2nd ed.). Upper Saddle River, NJ: Pearson Education, pp. 1220–1221.

3 **Answer: 1** **Rationale:** Prednisone is a synthetic corticosteroid that depresses the immune response and increases susceptibility to infection. Steroids mask infection;

therefore, the child must be assessed for subtle signs and symptoms of infection. Urinary retention is not a concern with administration of a corticosteroid such as prednisone. Easy bruising would be of concern if the client were taking an anticoagulant or antiplatelet medication. Hyperglycemia, rather than hypoglycemia, would be a possible concern in the client taking corticosteroids. **Cognitive Level:** Applying **Client Need:** Pharmacological and Parenteral Therapies **Integrated Process:** Nursing Process: Implementation **Content Area:** Child Health **Strategy:** The core concept is side effects of the drug. Recall the side effects of corticosteroids to choose correctly. **Reference:** Ball, J., Bindler, R., & Cowen, K. (2010). *Child health nursing: Partnering with children and families* (2nd ed.). Upper Saddle River, NJ: Pearson Education, p. 1218.

4 **Answer: 4** **Rationale:** Education about proper specimen collection technique will minimize contamination of the urine sample and help ensure accurate results. It is unnecessary to increase fluid intake prior to specimen collection. The specimen container is not cleansed, although the urinary meatus will be cleansed. The specimen should be sent to the lab immediately after collection to prevent urine degradation. **Cognitive Level:** Applying **Client Need:** Reduction of Risk Potential **Integrated Process:** Nursing Process: Implementation **Content Area:** Child Health **Strategy:** Eliminate any response that would adversely affect the results, including technique and timing. **Reference:** Ball, J., Bindler, R., & Cowen, K. (2010). *Child health nursing: Partnering with children and families* (2nd ed.). Upper Saddle River, NJ: Pearson Education, p. 1203.

5 **Answer: 3** **Rationale:** With glomerulonephritis, the kidneys' ability to filter and reabsorb salt and water is altered, resulting in edema. Weight can be an easy and effective measure to determine the current fluid load. Adequacy of caloric intake can be determined by weight gain, but a daily weight would not be required. Fluid gain or loss is best detected using daily weight measurements. Serum levels of sodium and potassium would be monitored to detect need for their restriction in the diet, and this would be of concern with renal failure. Monitoring of ingested fluids is done by documenting oral liquid intake. **Cognitive Level:** Applying **Client Need:** Physiological Adaptation **Integrated Process:** Nursing Process: Implementation **Content Area:** Child Health **Strategy:** Two of the options deal with fluids. Determine if one of these is the right response. Then review the other options to ensure the right response. **Reference:** Ball, J., Bindler, R., & Cowen, K. (2010). *Child health nursing: Partnering with children and families* (2nd ed.). Upper Saddle River, NJ: Pearson Education, p. 1222.

6 **Answer: 2** **Rationale:** Gentamicin is an aminoglycoside antibiotic that is nephrotoxic. Nephrotoxic drugs should be avoided in a child with acute renal failure. Penicillin, propranolol, and prednisone do not belong to drug groups that are particularly nephrotoxic. **Cognitive Level:** Applying **Client Need:** Pharmacological and

Parenteral Therapies **Integrated Process:** Nursing Process: Implementation **Content Area:** Child Health **Strategy:** The core concept is which medication has side effects that would be detrimental to kidney function. **Reference:** Ball, J., Bindler, R., & Cowen, K. (2010). *Child health nursing: Partnering with children and families* (2nd ed.). Upper Saddle River, NJ: Pearson Education, p. 1221.

7 **Answer: 4** **Rationale:** In most cases, the testes descend spontaneously by three months of age. Surgery is done near one year of age, to allow time for testes to descend spontaneously while preventing further damage and avoiding psychological consequences for the child. Drugs that increase gastrointestinal motility will not be effective in treating undescended testes. The risk of testicular cancer is higher in clients who have undescended testes, but the occurrence is after puberty, necessitating diligent testicular self-examination at that time and onward. **Cognitive Level:** Applying **Client Need:** Pharmacological and Parenteral Therapies **Integrated Process:** Teaching and Learning **Content Area:** Child Health **Strategy:** Consider the pathophysiology of cryptorchidism and the usual course of treatment to choose correctly. **Reference:** Ball, J., Bindler, R., & Cowen, K. (2010). *Child health nursing: Partnering with children and families* (2nd ed.). Upper Saddle River, NJ: Pearson Education, pp. 1242–1243.

8 **Answer: 3, 5** **Rationale:** Injury to the renal tubules in the kidneys is the most common cause of intrinsic renal failure in children. Urinary tract infections and obstructions can lead to acute renal failure if untreated or inadequately treated. Leukemia is a malignant disorder of white blood cells that does not cause acute renal failure as a complication. Cryptorchidism is the term for undescended testes and is not related to acute renal failure. Phenylketonuria is a genetic disorder in which the infant cannot properly metabolize phenylalanine. **Cognitive Level:** Analyzing **Client Need:** Physiological Adaptation **Integrated Process:** Nursing Process: Assessment **Content Area:** Child Health **Strategy:** Eliminate those conditions that are not associated with kidney disease. **Reference:** Ball, J.,

Bindler, R., & Cowen, K. (2010). *Child health nursing: Partnering with children and families* (2nd ed.). Upper Saddle River, NJ: Pearson Education, p. 1226.

9 **Answer: 4** **Rationale:** The parents must understand the need for compliance with medical orders to promote the child's health. Relaxation should be accomplished without harming the child. Joining a support group is a positive coping strategy. Getting help from others is helpful so that the parent is able to get short periods of respite from child care. Assistance from a family member in managing an aspect of the client's care helps relieve part of the workload of raising a child with chronic illness. **Cognitive Level:** Analyzing **Client Need:** Psychosocial Integrity **Integrated Process:** Nursing Process: Evaluation **Content Area:** Child Health **Strategy:** Consider which response would have inappropriate consequences for the child. **Reference:** Ball, J., Bindler, R., & Cowen, K. (2010). *Child health nursing: Partnering with children and families* (2nd ed.). Upper Saddle River, NJ: Pearson Education, p. 1219.

10 **Answer: 4** **Rationale:** The additional fluids will increase urinary output, causing greater urine volume and more frequent voiding, thus flushing the dye from the urinary system. The goal of the therapy is not to overhydrate the child, which could have other adverse consequences. Increased fluids should not affect the serum creatinine level, although it could reduce the blood urea nitrogen (BUN) level. Although this is a plausible explanation, fluids are not encouraged for the purpose of replacing fluids missed while on NPO status. **Cognitive Level:** Analyzing **Client Need:** Reduction of Risk Potential **Integrated Process:** Teaching and Learning **Content Area:** Child Health **Strategy:** Consider the testing methods to determine the correct response. Knowledge that the test uses a dye to visualize the kidney's collection system and that the dye needs to be excreted will help to choose the correct answer. **Reference:** Ball, J., Bindler, R., & Cowen, K. (2010). *Child health nursing: Partnering with children and families* (2nd ed.). Upper Saddle River, NJ: Pearson Education, p. 1591.

References

Ball, J., Bindler, R., & Cowen, K. (2012). *Principles of pediatric nursing: Caring for children* (5th ed.). Upper Saddle River, NJ: Pearson Education.

Ball, J., Bindler, R., & Cowen, K. (2010). *Child health nursing: Partnering with children and families* (2nd ed.). Upper Saddle River, NJ: Pearson Education.

Hockenberry, M., & Wilson, D. (2011). *Wong's essentials of pediatric nursing* (8th ed.). St. Louis, MO: Elsevier.

Hockenberry, M., & Wilson, D. (2011). *Wong's nursing care of infants and children* (9th ed.). St. Louis, MO: Elsevier.

Lefever Kee, J. (2009). *Prentice Hall handbook of laboratory & diagnostic tests with nursing implications* (6th ed.). Upper Saddle River, NJ: Pearson Education.

London, M., Ladewig, P., Ball, J., Bindler, R., & Cowen, K. (2011). *Maternal & child nursing care* (3rd ed.). Upper Saddle River, NJ: Pearson Education.

Perry, S., Hockenberry, M., Lowdermilk, D., & Wilson, D. (2010). *Maternal child nursing care* (4th ed.). St. Louis, MO: Elsevier.

Pillitteri, A. (2009). *Maternal and child health nursing: Care of the childbearing and childrearing family* (6th ed.). Philadelphia: Lippincott Williams & Wilkins.

Smith, S., Duell, D., & Martin, B. (2012). *Clinical nursing skills: Basic to advanced skills* (8th ed.). Upper Saddle River, NJ: Pearson Education, Inc.

ANSWERS & RATIONALES

Endocrine Health Problems

Chapter Outline

Overview of Anatomy and
Physiology of Endocrine
System

Congenital Endocrine Health
Problems

Acquired Endocrine Health
Problems

 NCLEX-RN® Test Prep

Use the accompanying online resource,
NursingReviewsandRationales, to test
yourself with hundreds of NCLEX®-style
practice questions.

Objectives

➤ Identify data essential to the assessment of endocrine health
problems in a child.
➤ Discuss the clinical manifestations and pathophysiology of
endocrine health problems of a child.
➤ Discuss therapeutic management of a child with alterations in
health of the endocrine system.
➤ Describe nursing management of a child with alterations in health
of the endocrine system.

Review at a Glance

constitutional delay delayed
growth in which serum gonadotropins
are normal, but bone age is mildly
delayed and there is history of small
stature in client's family
epiphyseal growth plate
cartilaginous end of long bones allowing
bone growth
estrogen female hormone that is
secreted by ovaries and promotes
secondary sexual characteristics
exophthalmos protrusion of the
eyeballs
**follicle stimulating hormone
(FSH)** secreted by anterior pituitary
gland and stimulates secretion
of estrogen
glucagon a hormone produced by
pancreas that helps release stored
glucose from liver
hypothalamus an endocrine gland
located in brain that secretes
gonadotropin-releasing hormone

hypotonia lack of muscle tone that
may be seen in infants who have
congenital hypothyroidism
insulin a hormone released from beta
cells of pancreas that aids in energy
metabolism
islets of Langerhans cells of
pancreas involved in energy metabolism
karyotype a picture of the cell during
division allowing identification of
chromosomes
ketoacidosis a state when glucose
is unavailable to cells for energy and that
source of energy is provided by free fatty
acids; is a serious complication of
diabetes mellitus
Kussmaul respirations deep,
pauseless respirations that are
characteristic of metabolic acidosis
luteinizing hormone (LH) a hormone secreted by anterior lobe of pituitary
gland that stimulates secretion of andro-
gens in males and progesterone in females

phenylalanine an essential amino
acid found in most natural protein foods
polydipsia excessive thirst—a
symptom of diabetes mellitus
polyphagia excessive hunger—a
symptom of diabetes mellitus
polyuria passage of a large amount
of urine—a symptom of diabetes mellitus
testosterone hormone responsible
for production of sperm and development
of male sex characteristics
**thyroid-stimulating hormone
(TSH)** a hormone produced by anterior
pituitary gland that stimulates thyroid
hormone secretion
thyroxine (T4) secreted by thyroid
gland; stimulates cellular growth rate
thyrotoxicosis excessive amount of
thyroid hormone in blood causing rapid
heart rate, tremors, and elevated basal
body temperature

PRETEST

1 A mother of a 4-month-old tells the nurse that her child has been diagnosed with hypothyroidism. The mother asks the nurse what symptoms led to the diagnosis. The nurse explains that which symptoms are consistent with this diagnosis? Select all that apply.

1. High-pitched, shrill cry
2. Prolonged jaundice at birth
3. Less than expected motor activity
4. Constipation
5. Tall for gestation age at birth

2 An infant was born 24 hours ago. The nurse has been instructed to collect blood by heel stick for neonatal screening for congenital hypothyroidism before the baby is discharged. The nurse explains to the mother that a follow-up test will likely be needed for which reason?

1. At 24 hours, the T4 level will be extremely low
2. There is an immediate rise in the TSH after birth
3. The baby needs to digest formula before a blood sample can be taken
4. A thyroid scan should be done first

3 The nurse is administering propylthiouracil (PTU) to a 12-year-old recently diagnosed with Graves' disease. The child has been receiving the drug three times a day for three weeks. She suddenly reports onset of a severe sore throat. What would be the appropriate nursing action?

1. Continue to give the medication or she will continue to exhibit signs of Graves' disease.
2. Offer lozenges for the relief of the sore throat.
3. Withhold the dose and report this to the physician.
4. Question whether she is trying to avoid doing assigned schoolwork while in the hospital.

4 A 10-year-old diabetic client visits the school nurse after recess and reports feeling sweaty and jittery. What should be the nurse's recommendation to the child?

1. Take an extra injection of regular insulin.
2. Drink six ounces of orange juice.
3. Skip the next dose of insulin.
4. Sit quietly in class after exercising.

5 The nurse is teaching a 15-year-old client about the different types of insulin. The client takes NPH insulin at 8:00 a.m. The nurse interprets that the adolescent understands this type of insulin when the child states that which of the following would be the most likely time for a hypoglycemic reaction? Select all that apply.

1. While in gym class at 9:00 a.m
2. While taking a test at 10:00 a.m
3. While eating lunch at noon
4. While golfing after school at 2:15 p.m
5. While waiting for an early supper at 4:00 p.m

6 A teenage mother arrives at the clinic with her new baby who was recently diagnosed with congenital hypothyroidism. When instructing the mother about administering levothyroxine medication, what information should the nurse include?

1. Crush the medication and place it in a full bottle of formula or juice to disguise the taste.
2. Administer the medication every third day.
3. Give the crushed medication in a syringe or in the nipple mixed with a small amount of formula.
4. Understand that the medication will not be needed after age 5.

7 A mother attends the pediatric clinic with her 10-year-old daughter who has diabetes mellitus (DM). After completing a diabetic teaching session, the nurse evaluates learning. Which statement by the mother indicates a satisfactory understanding of DM?

1. "I worry about my daughter maintaining control since children with diabetes have more complications that adults do."
2. "My daughter should drink vanilla milkshakes to maintain a high caloric intake."
3. "Complications from diabetes could include cataracts and kidney stones."
4. "My child won't need a mid-afternoon snack since she takes a gym class in the afternoon."

8 A 4-month-old infant who has been diagnosed with phenylketonuria (PKU) has eczema and sensitivity to sunlight. The mother asks the nurse why her child's skin is so sensitive. What is an appropriate explanation by the nurse?

1. "Some children just have sensitive skin. There is no reason to be excessively concerned."
2. "Your child will outgrow his sensitivity when he is 5 years old. Just use sunscreen for now."
3. "Your child has a deficiency in melanin because of decreased tyrosine. You will always have to take special care of his skin."
4. "The phenylketones in your baby's blood concentrate the sun's rays, making burning more likely. Children with PKU can never be in the sun."

9 The nurse has completed family teaching on dietary restrictions necessary for a child with phenylketonuria. The parents are given sample menus to choose a meal for their child. Which menu choice best indicates understanding of the dietary instructions?

1. A hamburger and a diet soda sweetened with aspartame
2. Steak and mashed potatoes with orange juice
3. A large bowl of dry cereal with strawberries and apple juice
4. Milkshakes and grilled cheese sandwich

10 Mothers in the waiting room of the endocrine clinic are discussing their children's illnesses. The nurse determines that the mothers of children with phenylketonuria (PKU) and congenital hypothyroidism recognize a common goal in the early treatment of their children when they state they are hoping to avoid which complication?

1. Mental retardation
2. Secondary liver disease
3. Obesity
4. Premature cataract development

➤ *See pages 185–186 for Answers and Rationales.*

I. OVERVIEW OF ANATOMY AND PHYSIOLOGY OF ENDOCRINE SYSTEM

A. Thyroid gland

1. Structure
   a. Reddish-brown soft mass with right and left pear-shaped lobes that extend from sides of thyroid and cricoid cartilage to sixth tracheal cartilage just below larynx
   b. A narrow isthmus connecting right and left lobes
2. Thyroid gland functions
   a. Regulates and accelerates cellular functions of all cells including protein, fat, and carbohydrate catabolism; has a major role in controlling basal metabolic rate
   b. Helps maintain cardiac output, respiratory rate, and utilization of oxygen and carbon dioxide
   c. Regulates body heat production and mechanisms of control
   d. Aids in growth hormone secretion and skeletal maturation
   e. Metabolizes substances as nutrients
      1) Maintains appetite
      2) Regulates calcium utilization by decreasing calcium concentration
      3) Aids in utilization of glucose and cholesterol; promotes sensitivity to insulin
3. Thyroid hormones
   a. Thyroid hormones include **thyroxine (T4)**, triiodothyronine (T3), and thyrocalcitonin

    b. The secretion of thyroid hormones is controlled by **thyroid-stimulating hormone (TSH)**, which is secreted by anterior pituitary gland; TSH is regulated by thyrotropin-releasing factor (TRF)

    c. Hypothyroidism may occur because of deficient levels of thyroid hormone and either hypothyroidism or hyperthyroidism may occur because of malfunction in secretion of TSH or TRF

B. Pituitary gland

  1. Structure

    a. A round, pea-sized gland that is ½-inch in diameter; it is supported by sella turcica, a bony depression of sphenoid bone and is attached to **hypothalamus** (an endocrine gland located in the brain)

    b. Is composed of an anterior lobe and a posterior lobe; anterior pituitary is considered to be the "master gland"

  2. Anterior pituitary hormones and functions

    a. Somatotropin or growth hormone (GH) promotes somatic growth and maintains blood glucose levels; it promotes growth of bone and soft tissues

    b. **Follicle stimulating hormone (FSH)** stimulates secretion of **estrogen** (a female hormone secreted by ovary) and progesterone in females; stimulates seminiferous tubules to produce sperm in males

    c. **Luteinizing hormone (LH)** stimulates ovulation in females; stimulates secretion of **testosterone** (reproductive or sex hormone) in males

    d. Luteinizing-releasing hormone stimulates release of FSH and LH by pituitary gland

    e. Gonadotropins stimulate gonads to mature and produce sex hormones and germ cells

    f. Adrenocorticotropic hormone (ACTH) stimulates adrenal cortex to convert cholesterol into adrenal steroids

    g. Prolactin maintains milk production after childbirth

    h. Thyroid-stimulating hormone (TSH) stimulates thyroid gland to synthesize and release thyroxine

    i. Melanocyte-stimulating hormone promotes pigmentation of skin

  3. Posterior pituitary hormones and functions

    a. Antidiuretic hormone (ADH or vasopressin) stimulates distal loop of kidney to reabsorb water and sodium

    b. Oxytocin stimulates uterine contractions and let-down reflex in breastfeeding women

C. Ovary

  1. Structure

    a. Female gonads are located in pelvis behind and below fallopian tubes

    b. Size and shape of large almonds

  2. Ovarian hormones and functions

    a. Estrogen stimulates overall cellular RNA and protein synthesis, breast development during puberty and pregnancy, growth of pubic and axillary hair, pelvic enlargement, and growth of mammary glands; promotes epiphyseal closure of bones and stimulates water and sodium retention in renal tubules

    b. Progesterone prepares uterus for fertilized ovum; promotes growth of breasts; during pregnancy, progesterone keeps uterine smooth muscle calm; it also promotes salt and water retention

D. Testes

  1. Structure

    a. Lobular male gonads that are composed of tiny tubules called seminiferous tubules, implanted in tissue containing interstitial cells

    b. Two testes are located in scrotum; each is located in a compartment with ducts emerging from top of gland to join head of epididymis

    2. Testes hormones and function

        a. Testosterone stimulates testes to produce spermatozoa

        b. Promotes secondary sex characteristics and closure of bone epiphyses

        c. Accelerates protein synthesis for growth of long bones, muscle development, external genitalia enlargement, and growth of body hair

E. Islets of Langerhans/pancreas

    1. Structure: pancreas is a fish-shaped organ that extends from duodenal curve to spleen

    2. Islets of Langerhans hormones and function

        a. Islets of Langerhans are ductless clusters of cells located in pancreas, consisting of alpha, beta, and delta cells

        b. Alpha cells secrete **glucagon**, which increases blood glucose by accelerating liver glycogenolysis; glucagon acts as an antagonist to insulin

        c. Beta cells produce **insulin**, a hormone that promotes glucose, protein, and fatty acid transport into cells; it accelerates movement of potassium and phosphate ions through cell membranes with glucose, thereby decreasing blood glucose and increasing glucose utilization

        d. Delta cells produce somatostatin, which inhibits secretion of both insulin and glycogen

II. CONGENITAL ENDOCRINE HEALTH PROBLEMS

A. Hypothyroidism

    1. Description

        a. A condition present from birth in which thyroid gland does not produce enough thyroid hormone to meet metabolic needs of body; it occurs in 1 in 4000 live births and is twice as common in girls as in boys; it is less prevalent in African Americans

        b. Untreated congenital hypothyroidism leads to mental retardation

    2. Etiology and pathophysiology

        a. Usually caused by a spontaneous gene mutation, an autosomal recessive genetic transmission of an enzyme deficiency, iodine deficiency, or a failure of central nervous system–thyroid feedback system mechanism to develop

        b. When these hormones are not available to stimulate specific target cells, growth delay and mental retardation usually develop

    3. Assessment

        a. Routine neonatal screening by state mandate is done prior to hospital discharge to evaluate levels of thyroid hormones, although optimal testing occurs at two to six days after birth since an early test may show TSH as falsely high

            1) Neonatal screening for congenital hypothyroidism: a filter-paper blood-spot thyroxine (T4) evaluation is taken by a heel-stick blood sample on a newborn between 2 and 6 days of age; some specimens are taken within first 24 to 48 hours along with other metabolic screenings; if specimen is obtained too early, it may result in a false interpretation caused by an immediate rise in TSH shortly after birth; if T4 values are low, a sample of TSH is measured; an increased TSH level indicates that hypothyroidism originates in thyroid gland (not pituitary); this test is mandatory in all 50 states

            2) Serum measurement of T4, triiodothyronine (T3), resin uptake, free T4, and thyroid-bound globulin may be needed for further testing for potential causes of congenital hypothyroidism

3) If client is discharged prior to 24 hours of life, a home health nurse may make a home visit to assess neonate and perform neonatal screening at that time; screening may also be done at a health care facility

b. An infant who has a T4 level under 3 mcg/100mL and a TSH level greater than 40 mcg/mL is considered to have primary hypothyroidism

c. If diagnosed with congenital hypothyroidism, serial measurements of height, weight, and head circumference are performed at each follow-up visit to assess for inadequate growth; screening should also be done to assess developmental milestones

d. Signs and symptoms include lethargy, prolonged jaundice, constipation, feeding problems, being cold to touch, excessive sleeping, hoarse cry, large tongue, **hypotonia** (lack of muscle tone), and distended abdomen; infant is often described as "a good baby" because crying is infrequent; baby may appear puffy and pale

4. Priority nursing diagnoses: Risk for Injury; Imbalanced Nutrition: Less Than Body Requirements; Hypothermia; Constipation; Fatigue; Risk for Ineffective Health Maintenance

5. Planning and implementation

a. Teach family about disorder and its treatment; genetic counseling may be indicated if condition is suspected to be genetic in origin

b. Monitor growth and development of infant

c. Provide ongoing client/family education including ongoing medication administration

d. Provide information to family regarding infant stimulation programs or special education centers if client has cognitive delays; assess for delayed physical growth; if mental retardation has already occurred, provide support to parents and family

6. Medication therapy: thyroid hormone replacement (Synthroid or Levothroid) therapy to eliminate signs of hypothyroidism; this will establish normal physical and mental growth and development; it is imperative to evaluate blood levels of thyroxine periodically to ensure appropriate dosage and optimal outcome

7. Client and family education

a. Instruct client and family regarding importance of daily administration of medication; drug therapy is needed for life; noncompliance can lead to mental retardation and slow growth and development

b. Medication can be crushed and added to a small amount of formula, food, or water; it can be offered through a syringe or a nipple mixed with formula

c. Medication should never be put in a whole bottle of formula in case infant does not finish the formula

d. Signs of overdose include irritability, rapid pulse, dyspnea, sweating, and fever; include instructions on taking a pulse in teaching plan

e. Signs of ineffective treatment are fatigue, constipation, and decreased appetite

8. Evaluation: client is free of signs of hypothyroidism (disease) or hyperthyroidism (excesive medication); physical and developmental growth is within normal parameters; parents/caregivers verbalize importance of daily administration of thyroid hormone and administer as ordered

B. Hyperthyroidism

1. Description

a. Occurs when thyroid hormone levels are increased (**thyrotoxicosis**), with an accompanying enlarged thyroid gland and exophthalmos

b. Graves' disease is one cause; incidence is highest in adolescent girls, but may be present at birth when mother has Graves' disease

2. Etiology and pathophysiology

Practice to Pass

An infant client was discharged from the newborn nursery prior to having the newborn screening done for congenital hypothyroidism. How should the public health nurse respond if the mother of the client refuses to have the blood drawn on the first home visit?

    a. Graves' disease is an autoimmune disorder; body produces an autoantibody, thyroid-stimulating immunoglobulin (TSI), which attacks thyroid gland cells; serum TSI causes oversecretion of thyroid hormones

    b. There is evidence of familial association and female to male ratio is 4:1

3. Assessment

    a. Serum measurement of T4 and T3 levels: if elevated may indicate diagnosis of hyperthyroidism; if elevated, a TSH level may need to be obtained

    b. Graves' disease is diagnosed by serum blood test results of elevated T3 and T4 levels and a decreased TSH level; autoantibodies are noted as positive also

    c. Signs and symptoms include: tachycardia, tremor, excessive perspiration, irritability, weight loss, diarrhea, increased appetite, muscle weakness, and fatigue; **exophthalmos** (protrusion of eyeballs) may occur

    d. Findings will include a non-tender, enlarged thyroid gland (goiter); exophthalmos may be present in children, with accompanying blurred vision

    e. Subtle signs may go undetected for one to two years prior to diagnosis

    f. School work may be affected as changes in behavior will be exhibited

    g. Pulse and blood pressure may be elevated

4. Priority nursing diagnoses: Risk for Injury; Imbalanced Nutrition: Less Than Body Requirements; Ineffective Thermoregulation (elevated); Fatigue; Disturbed Body Image; Ineffective Therapeutic Regimen Management

5. Planning and implementation

    a. Be aware of signs of disorder such as weight loss, inability to sit still in school, academic problems, short attention span, fatigue, fine motor problems, and exophthalmos

    b. Once diagnosed, give instruction to parents/family members and school personnel as appropriate regarding signs and symptoms, dietary requirements, medication therapy, and pre- and postoperative care, since management may include antithyroid drug therapy, radioactive iodine therapy, or surgery

    c. Offer ongoing support to client and family

    d. A rare complication of hyperthyrodism is thyrotoxicosis or thyroid storm; thyroid storm is characterized by sudden onset of tachycardia, restlessness, and severe irritability, caused by sudden release and subsequent high level of thyroid hormones; it can be fatal; monitor client for this condition following surgical treatment or during periods of stress and infection

6. Medication therapy: goal is to decrease secretion of thyroid hormone; the following medications may be used:

    a. Propylthiouracil (PTU) or methimazole (MTZ, Tapazole) may interfere with biosynthesis of thyroid hormone by preventing incorporation of iodine into tyrosine

       1) These medications are usually given three times per day and may take six to twelve weeks to produce full effect

       2) They must be taken as directed and doses should not be skipped

       3) Severe leukopenia may occur; report sore throat, cervical lymph node enlargement, GI disturbances, fever, skin rashes, itching, and jaundice to physician immediately

       4) Medication may alter taste of foods, so extra seasoning may be needed; sources of iodine (iodized salt, shellfish, turnips, cabbage, and kale) should be omitted from diet

    b. Ablation with radioiodine (131I-iodine) is usually not recommended for children because of potential for carcinoma or genetic damage

    c. A beta-adrenergic blocking agent (propranolol [Inderal]) may be indicated for two to three weeks after thyrotoxicosis or thyroid storm to reduce symptoms of adrenergic hyperresponsiveness

Practice to Pass

An adolescent client has recently been diagnosed with Graves' disease. She continues to have periods of fatigue, especially during school hours. She has decided that she does not want to go to school. As a school nurse, how would you approach this issue to meet her health and school needs?

7. Client and family education
   a. If drug therapy is needed, instruct client to take medication as directed; missed doses may cause signs of hyperthyroidism to occur
   b. Teach parents to offer frequent rest periods for client; school attendance may be possible, but physical education classes should be discontinued until thyroid hormone levels have returned to normal
   c. Explain importance of eating healthy foods versus "junk" or "fast" foods
   d. Parents should be aware of signs of hypothyroidism caused by excessive dose of drug regimen
   e. Instruct parents to provide ventilation and a cool environment for client until symptoms subside
   f. Provide preoperative education if a thyroidectomy is indicated; emotional support is essential for client and family because of distress caused by diagnosis, client's emotional lability, and/or surgical intervention
   g. Prepare client for surgical dressing and a possible endotracheal tube after surgery; teach child how to support neck (maintaining midline position) when sitting up
8. Evaluation: client is free of symptoms of hyperthyroidism; client grows at an age-appropriate rate; bowel movements are normal; family demonstrates compliance with medication regimen as ordered; family and client describe side effects of medication

C. Phenylketonuria (PKU)

1. Description
   a. An inherited disorder that affects body's protein utilization caused by abnormal metabolism of amino acid **phenylalanine**
   b. Inherited as an autosomal recessive trait or a mutation affecting 1 in 10,000 to 25,000 live births; it affects mostly Caucasian children; PKU is rare in African Americans, Japanese, and the Jewish population
2. Etiology and pathophysiology
   a. Phenylalanine is an essential amino acid found in most natural protein foods
   b. In PKU, there is a deficiency in liver enzyme phenylalanine hydroxylase, which normally breaks down the amino acid phenylalanine into tyrosine; as a result, phenylalanine metabolite levels increase in blood, leading to musty body and urine odor (caused by excretion of phenol acids), seizures, hyperactivity, irritability, vomiting, and an eczema-type rash
   c. Decreased levels of tyrosine cause a deficiency of the pigment melanin, causing most children with PKU to have blond hair, blue eyes, and fair skin that is prone to eczema
   d. Decreased levels of dopamine (neurotransmitter) and tryptophan (amino acid), which affect protein synthesis and myelinization, cause degeneration of gray and white matter in brain; mental retardation and seizures occur if high levels of phenylalanine are not decreased
3. Assessment
   a. Many infants with PKU appear normal at birth; if treatment is not started to lower phenylalanine levels immediately, infant's IQ can drop as many as 10 points within first month and will continue to decline
   b. Compulsory newborn screening is done by use of Guthrie blood test in all 50 states at 48 hours after birth
      1) The Guthrie blood test is a bacterial inhibition assay for serum phenylalanine; *Bacillus subtilis* is present in blood if increased levels of phenylalanine are present
      2) Infant should ingest adequate protein (usually 24 hours of normal feedings of breast milk or formula) prior to test being performed

3) Heel blood should be used for specimen; heel stick sample should be collected after first 24 hours but no later than seven days after birth

4) A normal level is <2 mg/dL; Guthrie test will detect levels greater than 4 mg/dL; if level is elevated, a repeat test is performed to validate original results

5) If infant is discharged prior to 48 hours, Guthrie test should be performed within one week after discharge from hospital or birthing center by a public health nurse, pediatrician, or pediatric nurse practitioner

c. Although client will appear normal at birth, symptoms will develop as levels of phenylalanine metabolites rise; symptoms include failure to thrive, vomiting, irritability, and unpredictable behavior in infant; urine will have a musty odor; client may experience myoclonic or tonic-clonic seizures

4. Priority nursing diagnoses: Risk for Injury; Impaired Growth and Development; Risk for Imbalanced Nutrition; Ineffective Family Processes; Ineffective Role Performance (client)

5. Planning and implementation

a. Mental retardation can occur if condition is left untreated; ensure that Guthrie blood test has been done correctly and results have been received; repeat blood test if phenylalanine levels are elevated on first test

b. Phenylalanine is maintained at a level that allows for normal growth but does not allow buildup of phenylalanine metabolites; monitor phenylalanine levels closely; phenylalanine is allowed in diet based on client's weight (usually at a level of 20 to 30 mg of phenylalanine per kilogram of body weight); consult with registered nutritionist to aid in food calculations

c. Client is placed on a protein-restricted diet; some protein is allowed to provide phenylalanine essential to life; careful control of dietary protein levels is essential; encourage use of mature breast milk or modified protein hydrolysate formula with phenylalanine removed to keep phenylalanine level at 2 to 6 mg/dL; special protein foods are used that are free of phenylalanine; dietary restrictions used to be lifted after maximum brain growth has occurred (around age 8) or end of adolescence, but current recommendation is to maintain lifelong restriction

d. Serum phenylalanine levels should be measured periodically throughout client's life; children of women with PKU may be born with congenital defects including mental retardation unless mother resumes or maintains a low phenylalanine diet before conception

e. In young children who were not adequately screened after birth and who develop PKU, dietary modification at time of diagnosis will usually provide benefits in terms of behavior and other symptoms; retardation that has occurred will not be reversed, but further damage may be prevented

f. At first, parents may be overwhelmed by diagnosis and dietary restrictions; emotional support is essential; genetic counseling is suggested because each child born to a mother and father who are both carriers has a 1 in 4 chance of having the disease

6. Medication therapy: anti-epileptic medications may be needed if client is having seizures; a modified protein hydrolysate formula with phenylalanine removed is used for infant nutrition and as a supplement in childhood

7. Client and family education

a. Support parents and teach them about disease and its management

b. Instruct parents that Guthrie test may need to be repeated if initial test was done before 24 to 48 hours of age or if the test was positive initially

c. Review low phenylalanine diet with parents and offer written instructions to validate teaching; specifically review preparation of low phenylalanine formula; teach family to avoid giving client high-protein foods (meats and dairy products) and

Practice to Pass

An infant client with phenylketonuria (PKU) arrives in the pediatric clinic with a severe sunburn. Her mother informs you that they attended a baseball game the day before and the baby got a little too much sun. What advice would you give to this mother to avoid future sunburns?

products containing aspartame as they contain large amounts of phenylalanine; teach parents to read food labels for contents

d. If teaching an adolescent with PKU, encourage resumption of low phenylalanine diet, especially if client is having difficulty with attention span, concentration, and school tasks

e. Offer emotional support and refer older children and parents to a support group dealing with issues and problems related to chronic illness

8. Evaluation: parents identify dietary restrictions and requirements for client; client's growth and development remains within normal limits; family complies with follow-up blood testing of phenylalanine levels

III. ACQUIRED ENDOCRINE HEALTH PROBLEMS

A. Diabetes mellitus (DM)

1. Description

a. A metabolic disease causing a malfunction of carbohydrate (CHO), protein, and fat metabolism

b. Most children have type 1 DM, formerly called insulin-dependent diabetes mellitus

c. Some children may have type 2 DM, formerly called non-insulin-dependent diabetes mellitus; this disease is usually acquired as an adult, but may develop in overweight adolescents

d. Incidence of type 1 DM is 15 per 100,000 people in North America; peak ages of onset are between 10 to 12 years in girls and 12 to 14 years in boys; the risk increases if child or adolescent has a first-degree relative or identical twin with the disease

2. Etiology and pathophysiology

a. Type 1 DM does not show any specific pattern of inheritance but may show a familial tendency; it may be caused by a genetic component, an autoimmune response, or environmental influences such as viruses; an autoimmune response causes destruction of insulin-secreting cells (beta cells) of pancreas in islets of Langerhans

b. Because over 90% of pancreatic insulin-secreting cells are destroyed, there is an absence of insulin available to metabolize CHOs for energy; this in turn causes fats and proteins to be burned for energy; excess amount of unused CHOs causes hyperglycemia when blood glucose levels exceed normal level of 70 to 110 mg/dL

c. As blood glucose level exceeds renal threshold of 160 mg/dL, kidneys are unable to reabsorb all glucose, allowing excess glucose to enter urine (called glucosuria or glycosuria); large amounts of electrolytes and water are lost with glucose, leading to increased urination (**polyuria**) and dehydration; the resulting dehydration leads to excessive thirst (**polydipsia**); additional manifestations of hunger (**polyphagia**), fatigue, and weight loss may occur because of cellular starvation, since insulin cannot enter cells (see Figure 8-1)

d. During fat metabolism for cellular use, the liver produces ketones (acidic waste products of fat metabolism); ketones cannot be utilized by cells in absence of insulin; therefore, ketones accumulate in blood (causing metabolic acidosis or **ketoacidosis**) and in urine, called ketonuria (presence of ketones in urine); the respiratory system attempts to rid body of excess carbon dioxide by increasing depth and rate of respirations, called **Kussmaul respirations**; if acidosis is not corrected, acute renal failure, severe dehydration, coma, and subsequent death may occur

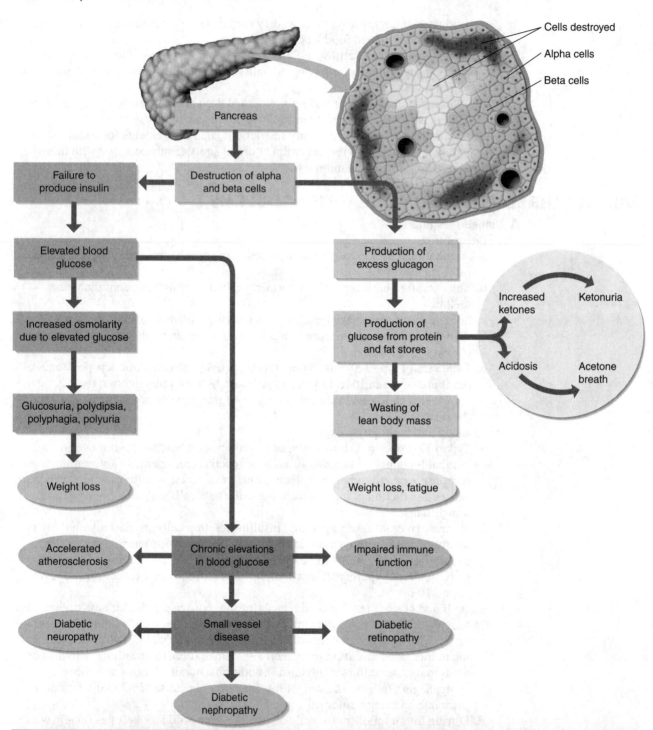

Figure 8-1

Pathophysiology of diabetes mellitus

Source: Ball, Jane W.; Bindler, Ruth C., *Child health nursing: Partnering with children and families*, 1st Ed., ©2006. Reprinted and Electronically reproduced by permission of Pearson Education, Inc. Upper Saddle River, NJ.

    e. About 5% of teens who develop diabetes have type 2 DM, especially those who are overweight; they may be prescribed an oral hypoglycemic with or without accompanying insulin

    f. Acute complications of DM are hyperglycemia (that can lead to diabetic ketoacidosis in clients with type 1 DM) and hypoglycemia

    g. Chronic complications of DM include retinopathy, nephropathy, neuropathy, and vascular complications such as peripheral vascular disease (from accelerated atherosclerosis); these occur more frequently with poor diabetic control; goal of treatment is to prevent such complications

    h. Complications related to growth and development include delays in growth and puberty, menstrual disturbances, and emotional disturbances

3. Assessment

    a. Elevated serum glucose level (>126 mg/dL for a fasting sample and >200 mg/dL for a random sample) on two separate samples, accompanied by classic signs of diabetes: lethargy, confusion, dry skin, thirst, weakness, abdominal pain, fruity breath, and diminished reflexes; ketonuria and glycosuria possible

    b. Polyuria (enuresis in a toilet-trained child), polyphagia, and polydipsia with accompanying weight loss and fatigue

    c. Dehydration, as indicated by poor skin turgor (tenting), dry mucous membranes, and low urine output

    d. A complete physical examination, including dietary and caloric intake and long-term/short-term history is indicated; history rules out presence of other illnesses, causing elevated blood glucose (stress-related illness, corticosteroid use, fracture, acute infection, cystic fibrosis, pancreatitis, and liver disease)

    e. Diagnosis is based on the following:

        1) Eight-hour fasting blood glucose (BG) level (>126 mg/dL)

        2) Ensure that the client has fasted completely for eight hours or more prior to collection of blood

        3) Label blood collection tube as a "fasting sample"

        4) Serum electrolytes, pH, PO_2, PCO_2, blood urea nitrogen are used to evaluate state of diabetic ketoacidosis

4. Priority nursing diagnoses: Risk for Injury; Risk for Deficient Fluid Volume; Risk for Imbalanced Nutrition; Impaired Skin Integrity; Ineffective Breathing Pattern; Deficient Knowledge; Powerlessness; Ineffective Therapeutic Regimen Management

5. Planning and implementation

    a. Provide emotional support to both the client and family, especially if this is a new diagnosis

    b. Continuously monitor vital signs, respiratory status, and level of consciousness; monitor hydration status by checking skin turgor, urine output, and mucous membranes

    c. Administer intravenous fluids (IV) as ordered that may include electrolytes to regulate acidosis and continuous insulin infusion

    d. Keep strict intake and output records

    e. Monitor glucose levels with blood testing as indicated; monitor urine for ketones during illness

        1) Test BG level using blood chemstrip or blood glucose meter method; report results immediately, especially if BG is >240 mg/dL; it is usually recommended that BG levels be checked before each meal and at bedtime daily

        2) Test urine for ketones using fresh urine and follow directions on package insert; report elevated levels as ordered

    f. When a continuous IV insulin infusion is discontinued, administer insulin subcutaneously as ordered to maintain normal BG levels

    g. Diet and exercise work together with insulin to allow normal growth and development

        1) Dietary plan includes providing sufficient calories for normal growth and development; diet is usually low in saturated fat and avoids concentrated CHOs (simple sugars)

        2) Three meals per day and mid-afternoon and bedtime snacks are usually recommended

        3) Exercise assists body to become more sensitive to insulin and reduces insulin requirement; if child exercises without decreasing insulin or without increasing intake, child may develop hypoglycemia; exercise is encouraged

        4) Importance of exercise must be considered during initial hospitalization while child is being stabilized on insulin but may not be as active as normal; after discharge when regular activities are resumed, hypoglycemia may occur

    h. A glycosylated hemoglobin (usually HgbA1c) is usually performed every three months to evaluate long term control; a non-diabetic person will have HBA1c levels of 4 to 7%, whereas client with DM will have higher levels; the higher the value, the poorer the control over the last three months

6. Medication therapy

    a. For type 2 DM, oral agents may be used to increase insulin production in pancreas; included are sulfonylureas and meglitinides; biguanides reduce glucose production from liver, thus they rarely cause hypoglycemia; insulin sensitizers improve body's ability to use insulin in liver and skeletal tissues; these medications also decrease production and release of glucose by liver; side effects from all oral agents may include headache, dizziness, and edema; liver enzyme levels may increase and must be monitored

    b. For type 1 DM, basal-bolus insulin therapy consists of basal insulin once daily (Lantos or glargine) or twice daily (Humulin or Ultralente), plus bolus of rapid-acting insulin with each meal and snack; the different types of insulin are: rapid-acting, short-acting, intermediate-acting, long-acting, and fixed combinations; the vials of insulin can be kept safely at room temperature (above freezing and below 86°F) but should be discarded in one month after opening, even if refrigerated (see Table 8-1)

Table 8-1 **Insulin Action (Subcutaneous Route)**

Type	Onset	Peak	Duration
Rapid-Acting			
Lispro, glulisine, aspart	5–10 minutes	½–2 hours	3–4 hours
Short-Acting			
Regular	½ to 1 hour	2–5 hours	6–8 hours
Intermediate-Acting			
NPH	1–3 hours	5–8 hours	12–18 hours
Lente	1–2 hours	6–12 hours	24–26 hours
Long Acting			
Ultralente	4–8 hours	10–20 hours	28–36 hours
Very Long Acting			
Glargine, detemir	1½–4 hours	None	20–24 hours

Source: Ball, Jane W.; Bindler, Ruth C., *Child health nursing: Partnering with children and families,* 1st Ed., ©2006. Reprinted and Electronically reproduced by permission of Pearson Education, Inc. Upper Saddle River, NJ.

1) Most insulin is administered subcutaneously (subQ)

2) Only regular insulin may be administered intravenously (IV)

3) Glucagon (pancreatic hormone that helps release stored glucose from liver) may be given subQ or intramuscularly (IM) to a hypoglycemic client; usually children under 7 years of age will receive 0.5 mg while children over 7 receive 1 mg subQ

4) Insulin pumps are also available and may be used as early as age 2 years

c. Glucose paste or glucose tablets should be available to all clients with DM, especially those that have documented hypoglycemic events

7. Client and family education

a. Assess family's ability to learn concepts and adjust teaching to level assessed; optimally, offer teaching at least three to four days after initial diagnosis because of time needed for psychological adjustment of client and family

b. Offer psychological support and provide education and reinforcement of information

c. Keep information sessions limited to 15 to 20 minutes for client and 45 to 60 minutes for parents or adults involved; utilize audio-visual methods, books, pictures, and actual diabetic equipment for sensory stimulation to encourage learning

d. Review pathophysiology of type 1 or type 2 DM as indicated; answer all questions and anticipate unvoiced questions; encourage parent to purchase a MedicAlert identification bracelet for client

e. Review meal and snack planning; refer to a nutritionist with expertise in diabetes education; familiarize family with CHO, protein, and fat exchange lists; consider periods of rapid growth and levels of growth and development during teaching; discuss events such as travel, school parties, and holidays; these and other events often represent times when compliance is difficult for clients

f. Provide an overview of insulin and specifically instruct client and family on administration, absorption rates, dosage, storage, injection sites, side effects, and alternatives to syringe and needle with syringe-loaded injector (Injectease); if client is receiving short-acting and intermediate-acting insulin at same time, ensure appropriate mixing technique; teach appropriate disposal of equipment (see Box 8-1 and Figure 8-2)

Figure 8-2

Insulin injection sites. Rotation of sites is important to promote absorption and prevent tissue damage. Injections should be spaced 0.5 inch apart.

Source: Hogan, MaryAnn; Brancato, Vera; White, Judy; Falkenstein, Kathleen, *Prentice Hall Reviews & rationales: Child health nursing*, 2nd Ed., ©2007. Reprinted and Electronically reproduced by permission of Pearson Education, Inc. Upper Saddle River, NJ.

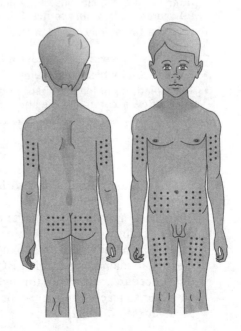

Box 8-1

Administration of Insulin

Insulin Storage

- Store insulin in a cool room. Do not expose to extreme heat or cold (freezer).
- Do not use an opened bottle of insulin for longer than one month due to loss of potency.

Insulin Administration

If mixing two types: Fast-acting (Regular) and intermediate-acting (such as NPH) insulin, follow this procedure:

- Place the two bottles of insulin on a table and read the labels.
- Clean the tops of both vials with alcohol.
- Open the U-100 syringe and draw up air that would equal the amount of intermediate-acting insulin (20 units of air = 20 units of insulin). Inject the air into the intermediate-acting insulin vial without allowing the needle to touch the liquid insulin. (Keep the vial upright on the table; do not invert.)
- Remove the syringe. Draw up the amount of air that would equal the amount of fast-acting insulin and inject that air into the fast-acting insulin vial.
- Slowly invert the bottle of fast-acting insulin and withdraw the ordered amount of insulin.
- Invert the immediate-acting insulin vial, puncture the rubber cap with the needle and slowly withdraw the ordered amount of immediate-acting insulin without injecting any fast-acting insulin into the intermediate-acting insulin vial. Some clients may choose to use a syringe-loaded injector (Injectease) or a preloaded pen (Novapen).

Subcutaneous Injection

- Cleanse the site for injection by wiping with an alcohol wipe or washing with soap and water and allowing skin to dry.
- Plan to rotate injection sites to enhance absorption of the insulin. Hypertrophy or atrophy of the area can occur with repeated injections into the same area, slowing insulin absorption by the fat pads that develop in overused areas of injection. Choose an anatomical area and administer insulin in that area six to eight times, with each injection about 1 inch apart. Move to another anatomical area and repeat the process. This aids in more consistent absorption of the insulin since the different sites absorb it at a different rate.
- With one of the client's hand, or with help from the parent, gently pinch or bunch up the skin at the site, insert the needle quickly, and inject the insulin at a 90-degree angle. Count to five, release the skin, and withdraw the needle.
- Wipe the site of injection with alcohol.

Continuous Subcutaneous Insulin Infusion

- Requires a portable insulin pump.
- Teach methods of loading the syringe, inserting the catheter, and adjusting the insulin flow according to metabolic needs.

g. Teach and supervise BG monitoring using manual and mechanical BG meter; competence in manual technique is necessary if BG meter malfunctions; reinforce teaching with client if he or she will be performing testing at home; instruct family to call health care provider if BG result is above or below expected parameters; explain that this procedure must be done as recommended to maintain control of BG levels; many clients may need to perform this procedure many times throughout day; if testing is necessary during school day, offer to teach school nurse or personnel appropriate procedure to ensure accuracy (see Box 8-2)

Box 8-2	**Blood Monitoring**
Glucose Monitoring Techniques	• Use a manual or spring-loaded puncturing device. • Hold finger under warm water for a few seconds to encourage blood flow to that area. • Use the side of the finger to avoid repeated discomfort to obtain blood samples and release the puncturing device. Squeeze the finger and apply a droplet of blood to the glucose measuring strip. • Read blood glucose level displayed on the meter, record on appropriate document, and report as needed. **Urine Testing** • Read instructions on reagent strip bottle. • Immerse strip into a urine sample and compare strip color with graph on bottle. • Record results and report as needed.

h. Demonstrate procedure for testing urine for ketones; if BG level is elevated or if there is a sudden onset of infection or illness, urine testing is indicated; daily urine testing for ketones may not be necessary (see Box 8-2 again)

i. Ensure that client and family know signs and symptoms of hyperglycemia and hypoglycemia to avoid complications (see Table 8-2); prior to exercise, less insulin or more food may be needed to avoid hypoglycemia; acute illness, such as gastroenteritis, may cause hyperglycemia and may change needs for insulin also

j. Stress importance of a regular exercise program and review alternate insulin needs during times of increased activity; exercise is equally important with type 2 DM and may aid in weight loss for overweight and obese clients (and thus aid in BG control)

Table 8-2   A Comparison of Hypoglycemia and Hyperglycemia with Ketoacidosis

	Causes	Symptoms	Treatment
Hypoglycemia	Too much insulin, inadequate intake or missed meals, strenuous exercise without increased intake.	1. Blood glucose levels drop below normal. 2. Diaphoresis, tremors, hunger, weakness, pallor, dizziness, somnolence, coma and convulsions, death.	Depends on severity of symptoms but involves replacement of glucose. Mild or moderate: juice, or regular soda, glucose tablets or gel. Severe: cake frosting available in tube form or glucose paste, parents may be taught to administer glucagon subQ.
Hyperglycemia with ketoacidosis	Insufficient insulin. Infection or other illness may contribute to development.	1. Blood glucose >250 mg/dL. 2. Blood pH of <7.2; bicarbonate <15 mEq/L. 3. Glycosuria and ketonuria, elevated serum potassium and chloride levels. Serum levels of sodium, phosphate, calcium, and magnesium are decreased. 4. Kussmaul respirations, acetone breath, dehydration, weight loss, tachycardia, flushed facial skin, hypotension, and decreased level of consciousness, death. 5. Reports of stomach ache or chest pain are common, vomiting may occur.	Intravenous insulin. Fluid and electrolytes are replaced as needed in a timely fashion. Normal saline is given by IV until glucose decreases to 250–300 mg/dL; then solution is changed to $D_5\frac{1}{2}$ NS to prevent rebound hypoglycemia. Potassium levels are monitored; initial hyperkalemia may change to hypokalemia following fluid and insulin therapy.

k. Teach appropriate record-keeping for BG levels and insulin dosage

l. Consider developmental level when formulating a teaching plan for a child or adolescent client (see Table 8-3); encourage client to assume responsibility for own care with parental supervision

m. Teach sick day guidelines: notify health care provider for fever or other signs of an infection; monitor blood glucose every one to four hours (instead of routine); monitor urine for ketones when BG exceeds 200 mg/dL; do not skip insulin doses (prescriber may even increase dose because stress of illness increases BG); ensure large fluid intake (more than 8 ounces hourly) of a beverage containing CHOs and notify health care provider if this cannot be done or maintained

8. Evaluation: client and/or family exhibit specific knowledge of type 1 or type 2 DM; they demonstrate ability to inject appropriate insulin dosage, perform home BG monitoring, and identify signs and symptoms of hyperglycemia and hypoglycemia

B. Delayed puberty

1. Description

   a. A condition noted in girls if breast development has not occurred by age 13, pubic hair has not appeared by age 14, or if menarche has not resulted within four years after onset of breast development, usually by age of 16

   b. In boys, delayed puberty is a concern if there is no testicular enlargement or scrotal changes by 13½ or 14 years of age, pubic hair has not appeared by age 15, or if genital growth is not complete by four to five years after testicular enlargement

2. Etiology

   a. Delayed puberty can be hereditary; family members may have **constitutional delay** (delay of overall growth and puberty)

   b. Delayed puberty may be caused by hypogonadism, where ovaries and testicles are not secreting their homones—estrogen or testosterone

      1) Hypogonadism may be caused by decreased stimulation of gonads secondary to abnormality of pituitary gland or hypothalamus

      2) Pituitary gland may malfunction as a result of brain tumors, hypothyroidism, anorexia, and other chronic illnesses

Practice to Pass

A client's parent informs you that sometimes the parent and child draw up the regular insulin first and other times they draw up the NPH first when combining insulins. They do not understand why the order is important. What would be your response and plan for teaching?

Table 8-3 Developmental Care Ideas for the Child with Type 1 Diabetes Mellitus

Infants and Toddlers	Preschoolers	School-Age	Teen
Allow the toddler to make choices in food selection while monitoring carbohydrate levels.	Allow the preschooler to make food choices while monitoring carbohydrate levels. Be prepared to substitute snacks at birthday parties and at daycare.	Encourage independence of the school-age child in food selection and glucose monitoring and insulin injections. Assess level of knowledge.	Assess the teen's body image and sense of identity. Assess compliance with other tasks.
The toddler may wish to help with the finger stick by cleaning his or her finger.	Encourage guided independence during the blood glucose/fingerstick procedure.	Assure that the school personnel will be available and knowledgeable if a hypoglycemic complication should occur during school hours.	Encourage independence with food selection, blood glucose monitoring, and insulin injections. Supervise diabetic tasks if teen is noncompliant.
Monitor temper tantrums as a possible sign of hypoglycemia.	Have appropriate snacks available if needed during sports activities that require a high expenditure of energy.	Encourage exercise but have snacks available for the child. Discourage fast food or snack machine selections.	Discuss future plans with the teen. Include diabetic issues, but promote a normal lifestyle.

    3) There may also be a problem with testicle itself as exhibited in Klinefelter's syndrome, or with the ovary as in Turner's syndrome; these syndromes are secondary to chromosomal abnormalities and can be evaluated by studying client's **karyotype** (number and types of chromosomes)

        a) Klinefelter's syndrome is manifested by IQ scores below normal range, tall stature, and overly long arms and legs; boys have one or more extra X chromosomes, commonly 47 chromosomes with an XXY karyotype; are usually sterile

        b) Girls who have Turner's syndrome exhibit delayed puberty, short stature, webbed neck, and cubitus valgus (where forearm deviates laterally); karyotype demonstrates a female with a missing X chromosome (45XO); are usually infertile

3. Assessment

  a. Assessment of family growth history is extremely important in diagnosis of delayed puberty; growth patterns of parents are of interest to pediatrician or pediatric endocrinologist; a complete examination includes measurements of arm span and (in males) testicular size and penile length; client may need a bone age test (an x-ray of left hand and wrist that indicates acceleration of skeletal growth and determines status of the **epiphyseal growth plate** closure); the beginning of puberty better correlates with bone age than with client's chronological age; an MRI or CT scan may be needed to determine a CNS lesion if a brain tumor is suspected

  b. Other tests may include blood levels of FSH (follicle stimulating hormone), LH (leutinizing hormone), and sex hormones; a complete blood count, thyroid function tests, and a chemistry panel may also be helpful for diagnosis; a karyotype should be done if Turner's or Klinefelter's syndromes are suspected; the gonadotropin-releasing hormone stimulation test may be used for diagnosis also

  c. Many clients with delayed puberty have short stature and may be treated as a child by teachers, coaches, and community members; during adolescent years, these children and teens may have difficulty in social situations

4. Priority nursing diagnoses: Disturbed Body Image; Impaired Social Interaction; Anxiety; Deficient Knowledge

5. Planning and implementation

  a. Assure clients with a constitutional delay and delayed bone age that they usually do not require any treatment as they will eventually begin puberty and go through those stages; medical intervention of low-dose injections of testosterone may be initiated if the adolescent client is over the age of 14

  b. If a client has hypogonadism and other conditions have been ruled out, client may receive hormone therapy to stimulate development of secondary sexual characteristics (see below)

  c. Provide psychological support to client, especially if he or she has social concerns

6. Medication therapy: males receive testosterone enanthate injections; females receive oral ethinyl estradiol with a combination of medroxyprogesterone

7. Client and family education

  a. Provide information regarding different stages of puberty and causes of delayed puberty; gear discussion to client's chronological age (if a client had a cognitive delay, then discussion is geared toward developmental age)

  b. Instruct client and family on administration of hormones if ordered; arrange for home nursing care to provide injections if needed

8. Evaluation: client and family exhibit knowledge and causes of delayed puberty; adolescent client exhibits evidence of good self-esteem

C. Precocious puberty

1. Description
   a. A condition characterized by early onset of puberty, usually occurring before age 8 in females and age 9 in males
   b. Is accompanied by appearance of secondary sexual characteristics and an advanced growth rate and bone maturation; this rapid bone growth will cause early fusion of epiphyseal plates and eventual short stature as an adult
2. Etiology and pathophysiology
   a. Most cases of precocious puberty in both males and females are idiopathic; some cases are caused by benign hypothalamic tumors, other brain tumors, infection, cranial radiation, and head trauma
   b. In normal puberty, hypothalamus secretes gonadotropin-releasing hormone (GnRH), which stimulates pituitary gland to secrete LH and FSH in males and females
      1) In females, FSH causes ovaries to produce estrogen that leads to development of secondary sexual characteristics
      2) In males, FSH causes testes to develop sperm and LH stimulates production of testosterone, leading to development of secondary sexual characteristics
      3) During this time, both males and females have accelerated linear and skeletal growth
   c. In precocious puberty, premature hormone secretion causes early onset of sexual characteristics; linear and skeletal growth is apparent as these children appear very tall early on, but because of early epiphyseal closure, short stature results as an adult
3. Assessment
   a. Signs of precocious puberty in females include breast development, pubic hair, axillary hair, acne, adult body odor, and onset of menstrual periods
   b. Signs of precocious puberty in males include testicular enlargement, pubic hair, penile enlargement, axillary and chest hair, facial hair, acne, adult body odor, and deepening voice
   c. GnRH stimulation test aids in diagnosis; synthetic GnRH is given IV, which stimulates secretion of FSH and LH in child; blood samples of LH and FSH are obtained every two hours to determine levels; if LH level is higher than FSH level, puberty has occurred
   d. Bone age x-rays will aid in determining epiphyseal maturation and closure; if bone age is more advanced than chronological age, skeletal growth acceleration is apparent
4. Priority nursing diagnoses: Disturbed Body Image; Impaired Social Interaction; Anxiety
5. Planning and implementation
   a. Support clients with precocious puberty by discussing their concerns and issues about body image and sexuality
   b. Offer support as family deals with sensitive issues dealing with premature appearance of secondary sexual characteristics and sexuality
   c. Encourage clients to express their feelings about their body changes; role-playing may help with coping with issues of peer teasing
   d. Assure children that their friends will go through same body changes
   e. If synthetic LH-releasing factor is used to slow down or arrest progression of puberty and skeletal growth to preserve adult height, plan for monthly or daily injections with family
   f. Allow client an opportunity to speak without parents present in room to encourage discussion of embarrassing topics
6. Medication therapy: a synthetic form of LH-releasing factor (Lupron Depot and other preparations)

7. Client and family education
   a. Teach client and parents about condition and answer all questions or refer to a pediatric endocrinologist
   b. If client is receiving synthetic LH, instruct family on medication administration including technique of either subcutaneous or intramuscular injections; provide client and family with information about drug side effects as per product literature
8. Evaluation: client and family describe pathophysiology of precocious puberty and their treatment options; client and parents identify purpose of medications, describe safe administration, and identify potential side effects

Case Study

A 14-year-old female with type 1 diabetes mellitus has the flu and stayed home from school today. Her mother reports that she does not have much of an appetite and can only get her to eat toast and drink a little tea. You are the nurse in the pediatric office when the mother calls.

1. What questions will you ask the mother to assure a complete assessment?

2. What instructions would you give regarding insulin dosage?

3. What are your priorities when offering dietary instructions?

4. If urine ketones are present, what advice would you offer the client?

5. What complications of type I diabetes mellitus would warrant emergency care for this client?

For suggested responses, see page 353–354.

POSTTEST

POSTTEST

❶ A 12-year-old boy was just diagnosed with type 1 diabetes mellitus (DM). As the nurse teaches him about insulin injections, he asks why he can't take the diabetic pills that his aunt takes. What would be the best response by the nurse?

1. "You will be able to take the pills once you reach adult height."
2. "You have a different type of diabetes where the pill won't work."
3. "We have to test you to see if you can take the diabetic pills."
4. "You might be able to switch between taking the pills and insulin."

❷ An adolescent with diabetes mellitus (DM) has had several episodes demonstrating lack of diabetic control. Which statement would the nurse include when reviewing information about how to self-monitor control of DM?

1. "Check your urine glucose three times a week."
2. "Check the glycosolated hemoglobin every three months and then every six months when stable."
3. "Check the blood glucose twice a day and the glycosolated hemoglobin every three months."
4. "Do not check anything as long as you feel well."

3 A new mother of an infant diagnosed with phenylketonuria (PKU) has been informed that PKU follows autosomal recessive inheritance. The mother states that this is a relief since she now knows her next baby will not have the disease. What additional information should the nurse provide?

1. With autosomal recessive inheritance, each baby has a 25% chance of having the disease.
2. Only female babies will have PKU.
3. The mother passes the gene only to male offspring.
4. Since this baby has the disease, the next baby will probably be a carrier for the disease.

4 Considering a child's developmental level in diabetic care is essential. The nurse should include which information in teaching the parents of a recently diagnosed toddler with diabetes? Select all that apply.

1. Allow the toddler to assist with the daily insulin injections.
2. Prepare meat, vegetables, and potatoes for each dinner. The toddler should not be allowed many choices in food selection.
3. Test the toddler's blood glucose each time he or she goes outside to play.
4. Allow the toddler to assist with cleaning off a finger before blood glucose monitoring.
5. Allow the toddler to choose food selections from options offered.

5 A 2-month-old infant arrives at the pediatric clinic. Upon assessment, the baby exhibits the following characteristics. Which characteristic does the nurse relate to a diagnosis of congenital hypothyroidism? Select all that apply.

1. Open fontanels
2. Protruding tongue
3. Tachycardia
4. Hypertonia
5. Hypotonia

6 A 10-year-old girl visits the school nurse after recess. This is the child's first day back in school after hospitalization, where she was diagnosed with diabetes mellitus (DM). The child reports she took the dose of insulin as instructed at the hospital, but feels sweaty and sleepy. After noting pallor and hand tremors as additional signs, the nurse suspects which problem?

1. Exercise-induced hypoglycemia
2. Hyperglycemia caused by increased intake at lunch
3. Ketoacidosis caused by an infection
4. The child is embarrassed about having DM upon return to school

7 After being diagnosed with Graves' disease, a teenager begins taking methimazole (Tapazole) for treatment of the disease. What symptom would indicate to the nurse that the dose may be too high?

1. Weight loss
2. Polyphagia
3. Lethargy
4. Difficulty attending to schoolwork

8 A 13-year-old boy is being evaluated for delayed puberty. He has had an examination with a pediatric endocrinologist who states that the child has a constitutional delay. How would the nurse best reinforce the health care provider's explanation of the diagnosis?

1. "Your hormone levels are normal, so no medication is needed at this time. If you want to talk about it, I am happy to discuss it with you."
2. "I am worried about your stature. I think you should get another opinion."
3. "Your father's stature doesn't matter. We just look at your height."
4. "If you want testosterone shots, I will speak to others so we can arrange for them to be given."

9 A child has demonstrated a sudden onset of thyrotoxicosis. The nurse anticipates that, besides anti-thyroid therapy, the child is likely also to receive which type of drug?

1. Antacid
2. Beta-adrenergic blocker
3. Muscle relaxant
4. Cardiac glycoside

10 Four newborns have blood drawn for the Guthrie test for phenylketonuria (PKU). The nurse would question the results for which infant?

1. An infant whose test is performed at 48 hours of age
2. An infant who was breastfed for the 24 hours before the test
3. An infant who was fed glucose water followed by formula for 30 hours
4. An infant who was tested immediately after birth

➤ *See pages 187–188 for Answers and Rationales.*

ANSWERS & RATIONALES

Pretest

1 **Answer: 2, 3, 4** **Rationale:** Prolonged jaundice at birth is associated with hypothyroidism. Congenital hypothyroidism in infants is often diagnosed because of hypotonicity and hypoactivity. A gastrointestinal effect of hypothyroidism is constipation because of the slowed metabolic rate. An infant with hypothyroidism does not have a high-pitched shrill cry. Instead, the infant is often described as a "good baby" because the infant rarely cries. Hypothyroidism is characterized by a slowed metabolic rate and so the infant would not be tall for gestational age at birth. **Cognitive Level:** Applying **Client Need:** Physiological Adaptation **Integrated Process:** Nursing Process: Diagnosis **Content Area:** Child Health **Strategy:** Think of the baby with hypothyroidism as lethargic and consider which symptoms might be seen in a lethargic baby. **Reference:** Ball, J., Bindler, R., & Cowen, K. (2010). *Child health nursing: Partnering with children and families* (2nd ed.). Upper Saddle River, NJ: Pearson Education, pp. 1238–1239.

2 **Answer: 2** **Rationale:** Tests done 24 to 48 hours after delivery may be interpreted as high because of the rise in TSH that occurs immediately after birth. The follow-up testing may be done at the first health visit at 1–2 weeks of age. The T4 level is not extremely low 24 hours after birth. There is no requirement for formula intake before a blood sample can be obtained. There is no indication to perform a thyroid scan when this is a screening test. **Cognitive Level:** Analyzing **Client Need:** Health Promotion and Maintenance **Integrated Process:** Nursing Process: Implementation **Content Area:** Child Health **Strategy:** The learner should be familiar with common screening blood tests. With that knowledge, two options can be eliminated. Then determine whether the test response would be high or low after birth. **Reference:** Ball, J., Bindler, R., & Cowen, K. (2010). *Child health nursing: Partnering with children*

and families (2nd ed.). Upper Saddle River, NJ: Pearson Education, p. 1269.

3 **Answer: 3** **Rationale:** A sore throat can be a manifestation of leukopenia, which is a drug side effect. The dose should be withheld and the prescriber notified because a dosage decrease may be indicated. The medication dose should not be given as scheduled. Offering lozenges does not address the concern about the drug side effect. There is no basis for assuming the client is trying to avoid school work by reporting a sore throat. This is an inappropriate and nontherapeutic communication. **Cognitive Level:** Analyzing **Client Need:** Pharmacological and Parenteral Therapies **Integrated Process:** Nursing Process: Implementation **Content Area:** Child Health **Strategy:** Knowledge of the side effects of this drug is the core concept of this item. **Reference:** Ball, J., Bindler, R., & Cowen, K. (2010). *Child health nursing: Partnering with children and families* (2nd ed.). Upper Saddle River, NJ: Pearson Education, p. 1273.

4 **Answer: 2** **Rationale:** If a child exhibits signs of hypoglycemia, a source of sugar such as orange juice can elevate glucose levels and prevent further signs of hypoglycemia. A 10-year-old must remember to only take one serving and wait ten minutes for symptoms to be alleviated. Additional insulin will drop the blood glucose level even further and is a dangerous action. Skipping the next dose of insulin does not alleviate the current symptoms of hypoglycemia. Sitting quietly in class fails to treat the symptoms of hypoglycemia and puts the client at further risk. **Cognitive Level:** Analyzing **Client Need:** Physiological Adaptation **Integrated Process:** Nursing Process: Implementation **Content Area:** Child Health **Strategy:** Recognize that the child is showing signs of hypoglycemia and consider an action that will increase the blood glucose level. **Reference:** Ball, J., Bindler, R., & Cowen, K. (2010). *Child health nursing: Partnering with children and families* (2nd ed.). Upper Saddle River, NJ: Pearson Education, p. 1299.

5 **Answer: 4, 5** **Rationale:** The peak action of NPH insulin is five to eight hours after administration subcutaneously. During peak times, the client may need a snack to offset potential hypoglycemia. Because NPH insulin peaks at five to eight hours, the client is at risk for hypoglycemia during these times, especially before a meal. Although exercising does help utilize blood glucose, the NPH insulin does not peak this early. Sitting quietly for a test does not raise utilization of blood glucose, and the NPH insulin has not reached a peak action at this time. Eating raises blood glucose levels and so the client is not at risk for hypoglycemia during this time. **Cognitive Level:** Analyzing **Client Need:** Pharmacological and Parenteral Therapies **Integrated Process:** Nursing Process: Evaluation **Content Area:** Child Health **Strategy:** Recall that the peak action time for NPH insulin is 6–12 hours and use this information to calculate times when the client is most at risk. The wording of the question indicates that more than one option is correct. **Reference:** Ball, J., Bindler, R., & Cowen, K. (2010). *Child health nursing: Partnering with children and families* (2nd ed.). Upper Saddle River, NJ: Pearson Education, p. 1285.

6 **Answer: 3** **Rationale:** It is important that the infant takes the medication in a small amount of food or liquid to ensure the infant receives the full dose. It is important that the medication is not placed in the bottle since the infant may not receive the full dose if the entire bottle is not consumed. The medication is administered daily. Since hypothyroidism is a lifelong condition, the levothyroxine will need to be taken indefinitely. **Cognitive Level:** Applying **Client Need:** Pharmacological and Parenteral Therapies **Integrated Process:** Nursing Process: Implementation **Content Area:** Child Health **Strategy:** Consider that since two options discuss how to administer the medication in relation to the amount of formula, one of them is more likely to be correct. **Reference:** Ball, J., Bindler, R., & Cowen, K. (2010). *Child health nursing: Partnering with children and families* (2nd ed.). Upper Saddle River, NJ: Pearson Education, pp. 1269–1270.

7 **Answer: 1** **Rationale:** Long-term complications of type 1 DM can affect children and adults. The longer the child lives with diabetes, the greater the likelihood of complications. Milkshakes would be a source of concentrated carbohydrates, which should be avoided. Long-term complications of type 1 DM include retinopathy, nephropathy, neuropathy, and accelerated atherosclerosis, but not cataracts or kidney stones. Exercise increases the utilization of glucose, thus an afternoon snack would be very important. **Cognitive Level:** Analyzing **Client Need:** Physiological Adaptation **Integrated Process:** Nursing Process: Evaluation **Content Area:** Child Health **Strategy:** Recall that DM is a problem with carbohydrate metabolism, and that exercise affects this metabolism, to eliminate two options. **Reference:** Ball, J., Bindler, R., & Cowen, K. (2010). *Child health nursing: Partnering with children and families* (2nd ed.). Upper Saddle River, NJ: Pearson Education, p. 1290.

8 **Answer: 3** **Rationale:** Decreased levels of tyrosine cause a deficiency of the pigment melanin, causing most children with PKU to have blond hair, blue eyes, and fair skin that is prone to eczema. Dismissing the concern and implying that sensitive skin is a random occurrence fails to provide the mother with accurate information. The child will not outgrow the skin changes. Phenylketones do not concentrate the ultraviolet sun rays. **Cognitive Level:** Applying **Client Need:** Physiological Adaptation **Integrated Process:** Teaching and Learning **Content Area:** Child Health **Strategy:** Recall common symptoms of PKU to link the symptoms to the disease process. **Reference:** Ball, J., Bindler, R., & Cowen, K. (2010). *Child health nursing: Partnering with children and families* (2nd ed.). Upper Saddle River, NJ: Pearson Education, pp. 1307–1308.

9 **Answer: 3** **Rationale:** Foods with low phenylalanine levels include vegetables, fruits, juices, and some cereals and breads. Aspartame is not allowed on the diet as it contains large amounts of phenylalanine. The hamburger may or may not be allowed depending on current serum phenylalanine levels. Steak is a meat that is rich in phenylalanine and is, therefore, not the best choice. Mashed potatoes (if fresh potatoes and mashed by hand) and orange juice are acceptable. Dairy products (milkshake and cheese) are high in phenylalanine and should be limited in the diet. **Cognitive Level:** Applying **Client Need:** Physiological Adaptation **Integrated Process:** Nursing Process: Evaluation **Content Area:** Child Health **Strategy:** Eliminate any meal choice that has a lot of protein, especially meat and dairy products. **Reference:** Ball, J., Bindler, R., & Cowen, K. (2010). *Child health nursing: Partnering with children and families* (2nd ed.). Upper Saddle River, NJ: Pearson Education, pp. 1307–1308.

10 **Answer: 1** **Rationale:** Keeping the levels of phenylalanine at a low level in children with PKU and daily administration of levothyroxine in children with congenital hypothyroidism will decrease the incidence of mental retardation by allowing normal brain growth. Secondary liver disease is not a concern for the child with PKU or with congenital hypothyroidism. Obesity is not a complication of PKU although hypothyroidism can lead to weight gain if sufficient medication is not prescribed. Premature cataract development is not a complication of either PKU or congenital hypothyroidism. **Cognitive Level:** Analyzing **Client Need:** Physiological Adaptation **Integrated Process:** Nursing Process: Evaluation **Content Area:** Child Health **Strategy:** Review the disease process of PKU and hypothyroidism. Combine this knowledge with concerns regarding growth and development to make a selection. **Reference:** Ball, J., Bindler, R., & Cowen, K. (2010). *Child health nursing: Partnering with children and families* (2nd ed.). Upper Saddle River, NJ: Pearson Education, pp. 1269–1270, 1307–1308.

Posttest

1 **Answer: 2** **Rationale:** Children with type 1 DM must take insulin because they have a total absence of secretion of insulin from the pancreas. Type 2 DM may be associated with some insulin production so the client can take oral antidiabetic agents. Reaching adult height has nothing to do with the type of medication required to treat DM. Because of the pathophysiology involved with type 1 DM, testing has no place in determining the route of medication therapy. Alternating between oral medication and insulin injections is not an option. **Cognitive Level:** Applying **Client Need:** Physiological Adaptation **Integrated Process:** Nursing Process: Implementation **Content Area:** Child Health **Strategy:** The core concept in this question is the difference between type 1 and type 2 DM. The wording of the question indicates there is only once correct response. **Reference:** Ball, J., Bindler, R., & Cowen, K. (2010). *Child health nursing: Partnering with children and families* (2nd ed.). Upper Saddle River, NJ: Pearson Education, p. 1285.

2 **Answer: 3** **Rationale:** Checking the blood glucose at least twice a day prevents sustained levels of either high or low glucose readings. The glycosolated hemoglobin measures long-term control and is a very important value. Urine glucose is not checked because it is not reliable for current serum glucose. Urine would be tested for ketones during periods of illness or when blood glucose levels exceed 240 or 250 mg/dL, depending on health care provider's specific recommendation. A six-month interval between glycosylated hemoglobin evaluations would be insufficient. To refrain from checking anything while feeling well is dangerous advice and does not reflect any attempt at diabetic self-management. **Cognitive Level:** Analyzing **Client Need:** Physiological Adaptation **Integrated Process:** Teaching and Learning **Content Area:** Child Health **Strategy:** Recall that the more frequently blood glucose is checked, the better the control of diabetes. **Reference:** Ball, J., Bindler, R., & Cowen, K. (2010). *Child health nursing: Partnering with children and families* (2nd ed.). Upper Saddle River, NJ: Pearson Education, pp. 1290–1291.

3 **Answer: 1** **Rationale:** In each pregnancy, there is a 25% chance of the child having the disease, a 50% chance that the child will be a carrier of the gene, and a 25% chance that the child will be unaffected. PKU affects both sexes equally. The gene can be passed to asn infant of either gender. The disease follows patterns of probability for autosomal recessive inheritance. **Cognitive Level:** Applying **Client Need:** Health Promotion and Maintenance **Integrated Process:** Nursing Process: Evaluation **Content Area:** Child Health **Strategy:** The key concept is autosomal recessive inheritance. **Reference:** Ball, J., Bindler, R., & Cowen, K. (2010). *Child health nursing: Partnering with children and families* (2nd ed.). Upper Saddle River, NJ: Pearson Education, p. 1307.

4 **Answer: 4, 5** **Rationale:** The toddler needs to feel some control. Cleaning off his finger with alcohol, with supervision, will allow some control. One way to promote control would be for the toddler to choose food selections from options offered. It is inappropriate to allow the toddler to assist with injections. Prohibiting the toddler from having some choices in food selection does not support developmentally appropriate care. It is unnecessary to test glucose every time the toddler goes out to play. **Cognitive Level:** Applying **Client Need:** Physiological Adaptation **Integrated Process:** Nursing Process: Planning **Content Area:** Child Health **Strategy:** Consider the growth and development of the toddler to determine which activity can safely be assumed by a toddler. **Reference:** Ball, J., Bindler, R., & Cowen, K. (2010). *Child health nursing: Partnering with children and families* (2nd ed.). Upper Saddle River, NJ: Pearson Education, p. 1291.

5 **Answer: 2, 5** **Rationale:** Most babies with congenital hypothyroidism exhibit a protruding tongue. Hypotonia is a common feature of congenital hypothyroidism in an infant. Open fontanels are normal for a 2-month-old infant. Hypothyroidism would be more likely to result in bradycardia than tachycardia. Hypertonia is a finding that would be expected in hyperthyroidism. **Cognitive Level:** Analyzing **Client Need:** Physiological Adaptation **Integrated Process:** Nursing Process: Assessment **Content Area:** Child Health **Strategy:** First eliminate a finding that is normal in a 2-month-old infant. Next, differentiate between signs of hypothyroidism and hyperthyroidism to choose correctly. **Reference:** Ball, J., Bindler, R., & Cowen, K. (2010). *Child health nursing: Partnering with children and families* (2nd ed.). Upper Saddle River, NJ: Pearson Education, pp. 1268–1269.

6 **Answer: 1** **Rationale:** Exercise makes the body more sensitive to insulin, thus metabolizing the glucose faster. While hospitalized, the child was less active. Now that the child has returned to normal activity, it is possible that the insulin dose is too high or more glucose is required in the diet. The client's symptoms are consistent with hypoglycemia, not hyperglycemia. There is no evidence of either ketoacidosis or infection. There is no information to support any conclusion about how the child is feeling about returning to school. **Cognitive Level:** Analyzing **Client Need:** Physiological Adaptation **Integrated Process:** Nursing Process: Diagnosis **Content Area:** Child Health **Strategy:** First decide if the symptoms the child is displaying are hypo- or hyperglycemia. Recall the effect of exercise on glucose metabolism to aid in choosing correctly. **Reference:** Ball, J., Bindler, R., & Cowen, K. (2010). *Child health nursing: Partnering with children and families* (2nd ed.). Upper Saddle River, NJ: Pearson Education, p. 1300.

7 **Answer: 3** **Rationale:** Lethargy may indicate an overdose of the drug, causing the child to exhibit signs of hypothyroidism. Weight loss, polyphagia, and difficulty with schoolwork are consistent with a diagnosis of hyperthyroidism. **Cognitive Level:** Analyzing **Client Need:** Pharmacological and Parenteral Therapies **Integrated Process:** Nursing Process: Diagnosis **Content Area:** Child Health **Strategy:** Recall that Graves' disease is hyperthyroidism and drug therapy should suppress the thyroid gland. Consider that oversuppression could result in a hypothyroid state to choose correctly. **Reference:** Ball, J., Bindler, R., & Cowen, K. (2010). *Child health nursing: Partnering with children and families* (2nd ed.). Upper Saddle River, NJ: Pearson Education, pp. 1269–1270.

8 **Answer: 1 Rationale:** An adolescent client with delayed puberty may need to talk about issues of low self-esteem. If he has a constitutional delay, puberty will usually follow with time. There is no need for a second opinion. The assessment of the client is multifaceted. Hormone therapy is not given until after the age of 14. **Cognitive Level:** Applying **Client Need:** Physiological Adaptation **Integrated Process:** Teaching and Learning **Content Area:** Child Health **Strategy:** Consider which response would be therapeutic to determine the correct answer. **Reference:** Ball, J., Bindler, R., & Cowen, K. (2010). *Child health nursing: Partnering with children and families* (2nd ed.). Upper Saddle River, NJ: Pearson Education, p. 1260.

9 **Answer: 2 Rationale:** Propranolol, a beta-adrenergic blocking agent, provides relief from adrenergic hyperresponsiveness. It is usually needed for two to three weeks along with anti-thyroid hormone therapy. An antacid has no specific benefit for a client with thyrotoxicosis.

The use of muscle relaxants is not needed during thyrotoxicosis because the muscle tremors would be effectively treated with beta-adrenergic blockade. A cardiac glycoside improves cardiac contractility, and this is not needed by a client with thyrotoxicosis. **Cognitive Level:** Applying **Client Need:** Pharmacological and Parenteral Therapies **Integrated Process:** Nursing Process: Implementation **Content Area:** Child Health **Strategy:** Consider which drug would counteract the symptoms caused by excessive thyroid hormone. **Reference:** Ball, J., Bindler, R., & Cowen, K. (2010). *Child health nursing: Partnering with children and families* (2nd ed.). Upper Saddle River, NJ: Pearson Education, p. 1272.

10 **Answer: 4 Rationale:** The screening is done only after an adequate amount of protein has been ingested. The testing is usually done at 48 hours of age. Breast milk provides the protein needed before PKU screening. Formula meets the requirements for protein needed for PKU screening even though glucose water has no benefit. **Cognitive Level:** Analyzing **Client Need:** Health Promotion and Maintenance **Integrated Process:** Nursing Process: Implementation **Content Area:** Child Health **Strategy:** Knowing that 24 hours of formula/breast milk are required to provide adequate test results, eliminate any choice that would not provide this. **Reference:** Ball, J., Bindler, R., & Cowen, K. (2010). *Child health nursing: Partnering with children and families* (2nd ed.). Upper Saddle River, NJ: Pearson Education, p. 1308.

References

Adams, M., Holland, L., & Urban, C. (2011). *Pharmacology for nurses: A pathophysiological approach* (3rd ed.). Upper Saddle River, NJ: Pearson Education.

Ball, J., Bindler, R., & Cowen, K. (2012). *Principles of pediatric nursing: Caring for children* (5th ed.). Upper Saddle River, NJ: Pearson Education.

Ball, J., Bindler, R., & Cowen, K. (2010). *Child health nursing: Partnering with children and families* (2nd ed.). Upper Saddle River, NJ: Pearson Education.

Hockenberry, M., & Wilson, D. (2011). *Wong's essentials of pediatric nursing* (8th ed.). St. Louis, MO: Elsevier.

Hockenberry, M., & Wilson, D. (2011). *Wong's nursing care of infants and children* (9th ed.). St. Louis, MO: Elsevier.

Lefever Kee, J. (2009). *Prentice Hall handbook of laboratory & diagnostic tests with nursing implications* (6th ed.). Upper Saddle River, NJ: Pearson Education.

London, M., Ladewig, P., Ball, J., Bindler, R., & Cowen, K. (2011). *Maternal &*

child nursing care (3rd ed.). Upper Saddle River, NJ: Pearson Education.

Perry, S., Hockenberry, M., Lowdermilk, D., & Wilson, D. (2010). *Maternal child nursing care* (4th ed.). St. Louis, MO: Elsevier.

Pillitteri, A. (2009). *Maternal and child health nursing: Care of the childbearing and childrearing family* (6th ed.). Philadelphia: Lippincott Williams & Wilkins.

Smith, S., Duell, D., & Martin, B. (2012). *Clinical nursing skills: Basic to advanced skills* (8th ed.). Upper Saddle River, NJ: Pearson Education, Inc.

Musculoskeletal Health Problems

9

Chapter Outline

Overview of Anatomy and Physiology of Musculoskeletal System

Congenital Musculoskeletal Health Problems

Acquired Musculoskeletal Health Problems

Infectious Musculoskeletal Health Problems: Osteomyelitis

Accidents and Injuries Causing Musculoskeletal Health Problems: Fractures

Objectives

➤ Identify data essential to the assessment of alterations in health of the musculoskeletal system in a child.

➤ Discuss the clinical manifestations and pathophysiology of alterations in health of the musculoskeletal system of a child.

➤ Discuss therapeutic management of a child with alterations in health of the musculoskeletal system.

➤ Describe nursing management of a child with alterations in health of the musculoskeletal system.

NCLEX-RN® Test Prep

Use the accompanying online resource, NursingReviewsandRationales, to test yourself with hundreds of NCLEX®-style practice questions.

Review at a Glance

cartilage connective tissue that composes most of skeleton of an embryo and changes to bone through process of ossification

clubfoot congenital malposition of foot involving bone and soft tissue

developmental dysplasia of the hip (DDH) congenital condition leading to improper formation and function of hip socket

diaphysis long central shaft in long bones that constitutes major portion of bone

epiphysis rounded end portion of long bones that consist of layers of cartilage, subcondral bone, and spongelike cancellous bone

epiphyseal plate situated between diaphysis and epiphysis and plays major role in longitudinal growth in children

fracture discontinuity in bone caused by force to the bone

Legg-Calve-Perthes disease condition in which there is avascular necrosis of femoral epiphysis in school-age children

metaphysis columns of spongy tissue that unite diaphysis with epiphyseal plate

muscular dystrophy inherited condition where there is progressive weakness and wasting of symmetrical groups of skeletal muscle, with increasing disability and deformity

ossification process of gradual conversion of cartilage to bony structures, which begins in embryo and continues until 18 to 21 years of age

osteoblasts immature bone cells that replace cartilage cells as bones grow

osteogenesis imperfecta (OI) inherited disorder characterized by connective tissue and bone defects leading to bones that are fractured by the slightest trauma

osteomyelitis infection of bone that may be caused by any microorganism, but usually caused by bacteria

periosteum thin, tough membrane covering central shafts of all bones, containing blood vessels that nourish the bone

pseudohypertrophy enlargement of muscles as a result of infiltration by fatty tissue that occurs in Duchenne's muscular dystrophy

scoliosis lateral curvature of spine, which may be idiopathic or caused by neuromuscular disease

slipped capitol femoral epiphysis a condition where proximal femoral head displaces posteriorly and inferiorly in relation to neck of the femur during rapid adolescent growth spurt

traction involves pulling on a body part in one direction against a counter-pull exerted in opposite direction; used to reduce dislocations and immobilize fractures

PRETEST

1 A 6-year-old child has a cast applied for a fractured radius. The nurse completes an orthopedic assessment on this child. Which manifestation requires immediate attention and should be reported to the physician? Select all that apply.

1. Capillary refill of five seconds in the affected hand
2. Edema in the affected fingers that resolves with elevation
3. Child describes feeling of the affected hand being "asleep"
4. Skin surrounding the cast is warm
5. Pain that increases with elevation of the hand

2 Which of the following nursing care measures takes highest priority in caring for a child in skeletal traction?

1. Assessing bowel sounds every shift
2. Assessing temperature every four hours
3. Providing adequate nutrition
4. Providing age-appropriate activities

3 A nurse performs triage in a pediatric orthopedic clinic. Which of the following should the nurse recognize as a symptom of slipped capitol femoral epiphysis?

1. Pain in the hip of a preadolescent child
2. Acute onset of knee pain
3. Presence of a limp in a preschool-age child
4. Painful external rotation of the affected leg

4 Which statement made by the parent of a child being discharged with osteomyelitis requires further teaching by the nurse?

1. "I can stop the antibiotics when I see that my child is afebrile for one week."
2. "We will make sure that our child's diet has plenty of calcium and protein."
3. "I will look at the intravenous site for signs of infection a couple of times a day."
4. "My child won't take physical education at school until allowed by the doctor."

5 A 5-month-old infant is being evaluated for developmental dysplasia of the hip. The nurse assesses for which signs and symptoms that are exhibited with this disorder? Select all that apply.

1. Ortolani sign
2. A limp
3. Allis sign
4. Trendelenburg sign
5. Asymmetric thigh and gluteal folds

6 A nurse who is admitting a newborn to the newborn nursery is assessing for congenital defects. In addition to the abnormal position of the foot, the nurse would note which of the following if clubfoot is present?

1. Affected foot is larger and longer.
2. Affected limb is longer.
3. There is calf muscle atrophy of the affected limb.
4. Affected foot is cooler.

7 A child is admitted with osteogenesis imperfecta (OI). In reviewing laboratory findings, the nurse would expect to find abnormal levels of which of the following?

1. Calcium
2. Phosphorus
3. Precollagen type I
4. Vitamin D

8 Which statement made by a parent of a child with osteogenesis imperfecta (OI) needs clarification by the nurse?

1. "My child may be able to participate in sports."
2. "There are no medications available to help this disease process."
3. "Surgery may be needed to place rods in the bone for stability."
4. "My child will need to be home schooled to protect him from injury."

9 The physician has written the following orders for a child with Duchene muscular dystrophy hospitalized for a respiratory infection. The nurse should question the order for which of the following?

1. Physical therapy
2. Antibiotic therapy
3. Passive range of motion exercises
4. Strict bedrest

10 A 14-year-old adolescent has just been fitted for a Milwaukee brace. Which of the following should the nurse include in teaching about this brace?

1. The brace should be worn only when the adolescent is sleeping or in the recumbent position
2. The brace should be worn next to the skin
3. Exercises to increase pelvic tilt should be done several times per day while in the brace
4. The adolescent should experience no pain as a result of wearing this brace

➤ *See pages 208–210 for Answers and Rationales.*

I. OVERVIEW OF ANATOMY AND PHYSIOLOGY OF MUSCULOSKELETAL SYSTEM

A. *Ossification*: conversion of **cartilage** (embryonic connective tissue) to bony structures; begins in embryo and continues until child is 18 to 21 years old, when skeletal maturation is complete; **osteoblasts** are immature bone cells that replace cartilage cells as bones grow

1. Children's bones are less dense and more porous than adult bones; therefore, they are not as strong and fracture more easily

2. A **fracture** or break in contour of bone can result from minor falls or twists

3. Ossification progresses outwardly from **diaphysis** (hard shaftlike portion that constitutes a major portion of bone)

B. *Epiphysis*: located at end of long bones; consists of layers of cartilage, subchondral bone, and spongelike cancellous bone

C. *Epiphyseal plate*: plays a major role in longitudinal bone growth

1. Situated between diaphysis and epiphysis

2. Columns of spongy tissue, or **metaphysis**, unite diaphysis with epiphyseal plate

3. This is weakest point of long bones, thus a frequent site of damage

D. *Periosteum*: a thin, tough membrane that covers all bones and contains blood vessels that nourish bone

E. **Tendons and ligaments**: stronger than bone until puberty; as a child grows, muscles increase in length and circumference

 F. **Calcium intake**: during childhood and adolescence it is essential to provide sufficient calcium to promote adequate bone density and prevent osteoporosis later in life

II. CONGENITAL MUSCULOSKELETAL HEALTH PROBLEMS

A. Clubfoot

1. Description

a. In **clubfoot**, foot is twisted and fixed in an abnormal position; may be one or a combination of four deformities

1) Plantar flexion: foot is lower than heel

2) Dorsiflexion: heel is lower than foot

3) Varus deviation: foot turns in

4) Valgus deviation: foot turns out

b. Involves bone deformity and malposition with soft tissue contracture

c. One to two of every 1000 live-born children have clubfoot, with males affected twice as often as females

d. May be unilateral or bilateral

2. Etiology and pathophysiology
   a. Exact cause is unknown
   b. Abnormal intrauterine position may cause deformity
   c. Neuromuscular or vascular problems may cause deformity
   d. Strong familial tendency, with a 1 in 10 chance that a parent with clubfoot will have an affected offspring
3. Assessment
   a. Foot is twisted in a fixed abnormal position, which is easily recognized at birth; may be recognized on prenatal ultrasound
   b. Affected foot is usually smaller and shorter, with an empty heel pad and transverse plantar crease
   c. When defect is unilateral, affected limb is usually shorter with possible calf atrophy
4. Priority nursing diagnoses
   a. Impaired Physical Mobility related to cast wear
   b. Impaired Parenting related to emotional reaction following birth of infant with a physical defect
   c. Risk for Impaired Skin Integrity related to cast wear
   d. Deficient Knowledge: Deformity, Treatment and Home care
5. Planning and implementation
   a. Correction is achieved best if begun in newborn period, because small bones in foot begin to ossify shortly after birth
   b. Manipulation and serial casting begins immediately and continues for 8 to 12 weeks, with foot placed in a cast in an overcorrected position; casts are changed every 1 to 2 weeks because of rapid growth
   c. Parents need to perform passive range of motion (ROM) exercises to foot and ankle several times a day for several months once cast is off
   d. Infant may need to sleep in Denis Browne splints (shoes attached to a metal bar to maintain position) or wear corrective shoes for up to one year
   e. Surgery is performed when not able to achieve full correction with casting; most children have surgery between 4 to 12 months of age, which involves realigning bones in foot, held by steel pins, then foot is casted for 6 to 12 weeks
   f. Nursing care for client after casting and after surgical repair of clubfoot
      1) Neurovascular checks, at least every two hours
      2) Observe for any swelling around cast edges
      3) Elevate ankle and foot on pillows
      4) Monitor drainage on cast
      5) Pain management
      6) Appropriate distraction
6. Client and family education (see Box 9-1)
   a. Change diapers frequently to prevent soiled diapers from touching cast and causing cast to be soiled
   b. Sponge-bathe infant to keep cast dry
   c. Teach parents to evaluate crying episodes carefully, as they may be caused by tingling sensation of circulatory compression
   d. Reinforce need for passive ROM exercises several times a day for several months
   e. Reinforce use of Denis Browne splints or corrective shoes to maintain correction
   f. Discuss options for clothing that accommodates casts
7. Evaluation: client has corrected position of affected foot; parents demonstrate knowledge of care of a client with clubfoot

Box 9-1

Client and Family Education for a Client in a Brace or a Cast

Perform neurovascular checks

- Observe the fingers or toes for swelling, discoloration, and temperature.
- Check movement and sensation.
- Notify health care professional with any changes in neurovascular status.
- Teach the parents how to blanch the nail bed and watch for capillary refill.

Observe for infection

- Monitor for temperature increase.
- Assess for drainage through the cast/brace.
- Assess for odors coming from beneath the cast/brace.
- Notify health care professional for any of the above.

Assess and maintain skin around cast or brace edges

- Perform frequent assessment of the skin around the cast or brace edge for irritation, rubbing, or blistering.
- Keep edges clean and dry, avoiding the use of lotions, powders, or oils near the cast or brace.
- Petal the cast edges as needed.
- Do not allow the client to put anything down the cast.
- If the client is incontinent, protect the cast edges with waterproof tape and plastic.
- Keep the cast or brace clean and dry.

Activity

- Follow the health professional's orders for activity level, restriction of activity.
- Avoid allowing the affected extremity to hang in a dependent position for more than 30 minutes.
- Encourage frequent rest for the first few days following brace or cast application, keeping the injured extremity elevated while resting.
- Keep a clear path for ambulation, removing toys, hazardous floor rugs, pets, or other items over which the client might stumble.
- If in a body cast or brace, assist the client to be mobile with the use of a wagon, cart, or large skateboard.

Comfort

- Assess for discomfort and medicate according to health professional's orders.
- Contact the health care provider if pain is not relieved by any comfort measures.

Follow-up

- Encourage compliance with follow-up.
- Take the client to the health care professional if the cast becomes too loose, or becomes soft or cracked.

B. *Developmental dysplasia of hip (DDH) or congenital hip dysplasia*
   1. Description
      a. Refers to a variety of conditions in which femoral head and acetabulum are improperly aligned; DDH has been referred to as congenital hip dysplasia in the past
      b. Occurs in one to two per 1000 births, and condition affects females four to six times more often than males
      c. Unilateral in 80% of affected children
   2. Etiology and pathophysiology
      a. Cause is unknown; though certain factors are known to increase risk
      b. Family history increases risk tenfold

      c. Prenatal conditions may affect development of DDH
         1) Frank breech position
         2) Maternal hormones of relaxin and estrogen may cause laxity of hip joint and capsule, leading to joint instability
         3) Twinning
         4) Large infant size
      d. Sociocultural methods of childrearing, such as how infants are carried, may promote or decrease extent of involvement; infants held with hips abducted have decreased involvement

3. Assessment
      a. Diagnosis should be made in newborn period; treatment that is initiated before 2 months of age achieves highest rate of success
      b. All breech births now have ultrasound of hips before 6 months or hip x-ray after 6 months
      c. Assessment findings of DDH during newborn and infant period
         1) Shortening of affected limb
         2) Allis sign: client in supine position, thighs flexed to a 90-degree angle toward abdomen, unequal knee height
         3) Uneven number and placement of skin folds on posterior thighs
         4) Restricted abduction of hips after 6 to 10 weeks of age
         5) Wide perineum in bilateral dislocation
         6) Positive Ortolani or Barlow signs up to 2 to 3 months of age; to assess for this, lie infant supine and flex knees and hips to 90 degrees; place your middle fingers over greater trochanter and your thumb in internal side of thigh over lesser trochanter; abduct hips while applying pressure over greater trochanter and listen for a clicking sound, which would indicate a positive Ortolani's sign; no sound will be heard with a normal hip; with fingers in same position and holding knees and hips at 90 degrees, apply a backward pressure, and adduct hips; positive Barlow's sign is present if able to feel hips dislocate; hips should not be able to be dislocated
      d. Assessment findings in an older child
         1) Affected leg shorter than the other
         2) Telescoping or piston mobility of affected leg
         3) History of delay in walking
         4) Limp and toe walking
         5) Trendelenburg sign: when child bears weight on affected side, pelvis tilts downward on normal side instead of upward as it would with normal stability
         6) Waddling gait with bilateral dislocation
         7) Lordosis with bilateral dislocation

4. Priority nursing diagnoses
      a. Deficient Knowledge: Care of Client in Corrective Device
      b. Impaired Physical Mobility related to restriction of braces and casts
      c. Risk for Impaired Skin Integrity related to pressure from casts and braces
      d. Risk for Impaired Tissue Perfusion (peripheral) related to pressure from casts and braces
      e. Risk for Impaired Growth and Development related to limited mobility and potential decreased exposure to stimulation

5. Planning and implementation
      a. Correction involves positioning hip into a flexed, abducted (externally rotated) position to press femur head against acetabulum and deepen its contour

Figure 9-1

Pavlik harness

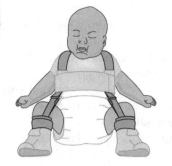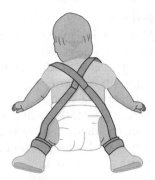

   b. For infants less than 3 months, most common treatment is a Pavlik harness, an adjustable chest halter that abducts legs; soft plastic stirrups hold hips flexed, abducted and externally rotated; may or may not be removed for bathing; usually worn for three to six months (see Figure 9-1)

   c. For infants older than 3 months of age, skin traction followed by spica cast application may be required

   d. Correction in child older than 18 months requires traction, operative reduction, and rehabilitation

6. Client and family education

   a. Pavlik harness: proper application, sponge bath, assess skin under straps daily for irritation or redness; t-shirt and knee socks should be worn under brace to prevent skin irritation; diaper should be placed under straps and changed without taking harness off

   b. For all abduction devices: modification of car seat, modification of positioning for nursing and eating

   c. Parents need to ensure client has adequate stimulation with toys and activities at appropriate eye level; encourage activities that stimulate upper extremities

   d. Client will catch up with developmental milestones once abduction splint is off

   e. Refer back to Box 9-1 for further information

7. Evaluation: client has normal growth and development; parent demonstrates care of a client with DDH

C. *Osteogenesis imperfecta (OI)*

1. Description

   a. Characterized by occurrence of pathologic fractures resulting from connective tissue and bone defects

   b. Occurs in several forms with variable degree of severity

   c. Bones are so fragile that fractures result from trauma, but also from simple walking or pressure of birth

   d. Occurs in 1 in 30,000 live births and affects boys and girls equally

   e. A client with this diagnosis should not be confused with client with fractures because of abuse

2. Etiology and pathophysiology

   a. Underlying pathology is a biochemical defect in collagen production

   b. There are normal calcium and phosphorus levels but abnormal precollagen type I, which prevents formation of collagen, the major component of connective tissue

   c. Bones consist of large areas of osseous tissue and increased numbers of osteoblasts

   d. Genetically transmitted, generally in an autosomal dominant inheritance pattern, although some types are transmitted in a recessive pattern

3. Assessment

   a. Major clinical manifestations include multiple and frequent fractures, some of which may be present at birth
   b. As client grows older, multiple breaks tend to cause limb and spinal column deformities, interfering with alignment or growth
   c. Other clinical manifestations include blue sclera; thin, soft skin with easy bruising; increased joint flexibility; weak muscles; short stature; conductive hearing loss often by adolescence or young adulthood
   d. May have dentinogenesis imperfecta: hypoplastic teeth with opalescent blue or brown discoloration
4. Priority nursing diagnoses
   a. Risk for Injury related to disease process
   b. Risk for Impaired Growth and Development
   c. Deficient Knowledge: Disease Process and Care of Child
5. Planning and implementation
   a. Keep floors dry; remove objects that could cause falls
   b. Handle client gently: avoid lifting by a single arm or leg; use a blanket for extra support when lifting and moving
   c. Never hold by ankles when being diapered, but lift gently by slipping a hand under buttocks
   d. Lightweight leg braces, splints, casting, and physical therapy may be helpful
   e. Intermedullary rods may be effective in strengthening bones
6. Medication therapy
   a. Calcitonin, which aids bone healing, may be used
   b. Bisphosphonates may be prescribed to increase bone mass
   c. Growth hormone may be given to stimulate growth
7. Client and family education
   a. Encourage a lifestyle that fosters growth and development, yet minimizes risk of trauma
   b. Teach how to support when bathing, dressing, and moving
   c. Encourage exercise, such as swimming, to improve muscle tone and prevent obesity
   d. Encourage realistic occupational planning
   e. Suggest genetic counseling
   f. Educational materials and information can be obtained from the Osteogenesis Imperfecta Foundation (http://oio.8k.com)
8. Evaluation: client has adequate growth and development with minimal fractures

III. ACQUIRED MUSCULOSKELETAL HEALTH PROBLEMS

A. *Legg-Calve-Perthes disease*

1. Description
   a. A self-limiting disorder in which there is aseptic necrosis of femoral head
   b. Affects clients between ages of 2 and 12 years, but is most common in those 5 to 7 years of age
   c. Occurs in about 1 in 12,000 children
   d. Male children are affected 4 to 5 times more often than females; Caucasian children are affected 10 times more often than African-American children
   e. The disease is bilateral in 10–15% of cases
2. Etiology and pathophysiology
   a. Cause is unknown, though research has shown a familial predisposition with incidence 20% higher in families with a history of this disease; in one-quarter of cases, disease is preceded by a mild traumatic injury

    b. There is a disturbance of circulation to femoral capitol epiphysis that produces an ischemic aseptic necrosis of femoral head

    c. Middle childhood is the time when blood supply to femoral head is most tenuous, being supplied almost entirely by lateral retinacular vessels; these vessels can become obstructed by trauma, inflammation, coagulation defects, among other causes

    d. Affected clients may have delayed skeletal maturation and abnormal thyroid levels

    e. Pathological events take place in four stages, which can last from one to four years

        1) Stage I: avascular stage; aseptic necrosis of femoral capitol epiphysis with degenerative changes producing flattening of femoral head

        2) Stage II: fragmentation or revascularization stage; old bone absorption and revascularization

        3) Stage III: reparative stage; new bone formation

        4) Stage IV: regeneration stage; gradual reformation of femoral head

    f. Undiagnosed or late-diagnosed Legg-Calve-Perthes disease can lead to osteoarthritis and hip dysfunction in later life

3. Assessment

    a. Mild pain in hip or anterior thigh and limp that are aggravated by increased activity and relieved by rest; referred pain to knee may occur

    b. Stiffness in morning or after rest

    c. As disease progresses there is limited range of motion, weakness, muscle wasting, possible shortening of affected limb, and positive Trendelenburg sign

4. Priority nursing diagnoses

    a. Impaired Physical Mobility related to brace or cast

    b. Deficient Knowledge: Disease Process, Potential Complications

    c. Pain related to disease process

    d. Diversional Activity Deficit related to brace or cast

5. Planning and implementation

    a. Prepare client for an x-ray (usual diagnostic test); there may be no radiological findings early in disease, but bone scans and MRIs are helpful to diagnose early disease

    b. Initial treatment includes rest to reduce inflammation and restore motion

    c. Goal is to keep head of femur in contact with acetabulum, which serves as a mold of spherical shape of femur head

    d. Treatment may be conservative, with rest and avoiding weight bearing on lower extremities, traction and containment with abduction braces, leg casts or leather harness slings

    e. Conservative therapy may be needed for two to four years

    f. Surgical correction may be done, which returns client to normal activities in three to four months

    g. Assist in selection of suitable activities for a client unable to maintain usual level of physical activity

    h. Ensure compliance with conservative devices

    i. Postoperative care following surgical treatment includes frequent neurovascular checks, pain management, and activity based on surgeon's orders

    j. Assist family with appropriate activities for client during treatment

6. Client and family education

    a. Teach purpose, function, application, and care of corrective device

    b. Stress importance of compliance to achieve desired outcome

    c. Stress importance of continuing school activities

    d. Promote normal growth and development with appropriate diversional activities

7. Evaluation: client has normal reformation of the femoral head; family is able to state the appropriate care for client

B. *Slipped capitol femoral epiphysis*

1. Description
   a. A condition in which upper femoral epiphysis gradually slips from its functional position
   b. Incidence is greatest during rapid growth spurt during adolescence; 13 to 16 years of age for males, and 11 to 14 years of age for females
   c. Is twice as frequent in African Americans as other races, and twice as frequent in males

2. Etiology and pathophysiology
   a. Etiology is unknown and thought to be multifactorial
   b. Is more common in obese or rapidly growing clients, suggesting that growth hormone or trauma from excessive weight may have an influence on the etiology
   c. There may be a genetic predisposition to development of this disorder
   d. Slippage of the femoral head occurs at proximal epiphyseal plate, and femur displaces from epiphysis; this is usually a gradual process, but may result from trauma
   e. If untreated, hip deformity with limited range of motion (ROM) will result

3. Assessment
   a. Onset of symptoms may be gradual, with persistent hip pain that is aching or mild, and can be referred to thigh and/or knee, along with limp and decreased ROM and internal rotation of hip; client may hold leg in an externally rotated position to relieve stress and pain in hip joint
   b. The client with an acute slip presents with sudden, severe pain and cannot bear weight
   c. Prepare client for an x-ray, which will confirm diagnosis

4. Priority nursing diagnoses
   a. Pain related to disease process
   b. Impaired Physical Mobility related to non-weight-bearing treatment
   c. Impaired Tissue Perfusion (peripheral) related to treatment
   d. Impaired Growth and Development related to mobility restrictions of treatment
   e. Deficient Knowledge: Disease Process and Treatment

5. Planning and implementation
   a. As soon as diagnosis is made, client should be placed on strict bedrest until surgery; adolescent may use crutches, as long as affected leg is non–weight bearing, but should not sit in a wheelchair, as this may increase the slippage
   b. Reinforce initial bedrest, as adolescents often do not see value of this measure
   c. Provide appropriate diversional activities
   d. Prepare for surgery with pinning or external fixation to stabilize femur head
   e. Provide postoperative care, including frequent neurovascular checks and pain management
   f. Provide adequate nutrition for healing

6. Client and family education
   a. Reinforce ambulation and weight bearing as ordered by surgeon
   b. Contact sports are usually restricted until growth is complete
   c. Reinforce compliance with follow-up visits until epiphyseal plates are closed

7. Evaluation: adolescent is cooperative with activity restrictions and remains free of further injury to hip

C. *Scoliosis*

1. Description
   a. Lateral curvature of spine; may be functional, which occurs as a compensatory mechanism in clients who have unequal leg lengths or poor posture; structural scoliosis is a permanent curvature of spine accompanied by damage to vertebrae

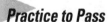

Practice to Pass

Two male clients have been admitted to the pediatric unit, one with slipped capitol femoral epiphysis, and a second with Legg-Calve-Perthes disease. How will the nursing care be different for these two clients?

        b. Structural scoliosis occurs most often during rapid growth spurt in adolescence, 11 to 14 years for females, 13 to 16 years for males

        c. The female-to-male ratio is 5:1 for curves greater than 21 degrees

  2. Etiology and pathophysiology

        a. Structural scoliosis is idiopathic in 70% of cases

        b. There is a familial predisposition for structural scoliosis

        c. Scoliosis is common in diseases where there is unequal muscle balance, such as cerebral palsy, muscular dystrophy, and myelomeningocele

  3. Assessment

        a. A painless and insidious onset is typical

        b. Parent may first notice that skirts hang unevenly, or that bra straps are adjusted unevenly

        c. On examination there are unequal shoulder heights, waist angles, scapula prominences, rib prominences, and chest asymmetry

        d. Screening by school nurse begins in fifth grade as mandated by law in many states

        e. Scoliometer is used to document clinical deformity found on screening

  4. Priority nursing diagnoses

        a. Disturbed Body Image related to bracing

        b. Risk for Injury related to brace

        c. Pain related to surgical experience (spinal fusion)

        d. Ineffective Breathing Pattern related to postoperative discomfort

        e. Impaired Physical Mobility related to brace wear

        f. Deficient Knowledge: Diagnosis and Treatment

        g. Risk for Noncompliance with treatment regimen

  5. Planning and implementation

        a. Prepare adolescent for x-ray to identify extent of curvature and give baseline information for follow-up

        b. If spinal curve is less than 15 to 20 degrees, adolescent is monitored every three to six months for change; exercises to improve posture and muscle tone and increase flexibility of spine are encouraged

        c. If curve is greater than 40 degrees, treatment is rendered by an orthopedic surgeon; if greater than 32 degrees, conservative nonsurgical treatment is warranted with bracing, such as a Milwaukee brace; this brace, and others like it, are made of leather and plastic; it is worn until the adolescent's spinal growth stops; see Client and family education section below

        d. Electrical stimulation may be used for mild to moderate curvatures to cause muscles to contract at regular and frequent intervals, possibly helping to straighten spine

        e. If curvature continues to progress or is greater than 40 degrees, surgery is warranted for spinal instrumentation; instruments such as rods, screws, and wires are placed next to curvature; spine is then fused in correct position; bone from iliac crests may be used to strengthen fusion

          1) See Client and family education section for preoperative teaching

          2) Postoperative care includes ROM exercises, log rolling every two hours, encouraging coughing, deep breathing, and use of incentive spirometry, NPO, nasogastric tube, strict intake and output, frequent VS and neurological checks, monitoring hematocrit, blood transfusions, pain management, antibiotic administration, antiembolism stockings or sequential compression boots, and gradual resumption of activity as ordered

        f. Halo traction may be used for nonsurgical treatment of moderate curves, or postoperatively in severe curves to provide stability for the spine

6. Client and family education

    a. Teaching about use of a Milwaukee or other brace

        1) Brace is worn for 23 hours a day

        2) Brace is off to shower, bathe, and swim

        3) T-shirt should be worn under brace next to skin (for skin protection)

        4) Exercises (such as pelvic tilt and lateral strengthening) are done several times a day while in brace to correct thoracic lordosis

        5) Consistent use of brace will provide maximum benefit

        6) Slight muscle aches may be noticed when first wearing brace

        7) Encourage adolescent to be as active as possible while in brace

    b. Preoperative teaching

        1) Deep breathing, coughing, turning every two hours, use of spirometry

        2) Pain medication

        3) Use of nasogastric tube and NPO status

        4) Range of motion exercises, activity

        5) Possible ICU tour

    c. Discharge teaching

        1) Must not slump in chairs, must not bend or twist the torso or lift over 10 pounds

        2) Complying with activity restrictions, which must be followed for six to eight months

        3) Addressing self-esteem issues

        4) Complying with follow-up visits

7. Evaluation: spine of adolescent with scoliosis is stable; adolescent correctly states activities and care for scoliosis

D. *Muscular dystrophy*

1. Description

    a. Group of disorders characterized by progressive degeneration of skeletal muscles (muscles that are under voluntary control)

    b. All muscular dystrophies are inherited disorders

    c. Duchenne's muscular dystrophy (pseudohypertrophic muscular dystrophy) is most common type, inherited as a sex-linked recessive trait, therefore occurs only in males

    d. Incidence is approximately 1 in 3500 male births

    e. There is progressive muscle weakness, wasting, and contractures, with loss of independent ambulation by 9 to 11 years of age

2. Etiology and pathophysiology

    a. Lack of dystrophin, a protein that is necessary for muscle contraction

    b. Muscle biopsy shows fibrous degeneration and fatty deposits

    c. Disease ultimately affects muscles of respiration, allowing pneumonia to develop easily

    d. Death in Duchenne's muscular dystrophy usually occurs at about 20 years of age from respiratory or heart failure

3. Assessment

    a. Clients generally have a history of meeting motor developmental milestones in earliest years; symptoms become obvious and acute at 3 years of age

    b. Symptoms often begin with a waddling gait, lordosis, difficulty climbing stairs, running or pedaling a bike

    c. As disease progresses, clients have difficulty walking on an even surface and rise from floor only by rolling onto their stomachs, then pushing themselves to their knees, and walk their hands up their legs to stand (Gower's sign)

Practice to Pass

The nurse is caring for a 14-year-old client who is postop day one following a spinal fusion for structural scoliosis. What are the priorities of this client's nursing care?

    d. As disease progresses, muscle weakness becomes more pronounced, and ambulation becomes more difficult, necessitating wheelchair use by 11 or 12 years of age

    e. Muscles feel unusually woody on palpation and look enlarged, called **pseudohypertrophy**

    f. Scoliosis of spine and fractures of long bones may occur from abnormal muscle tension and lack of muscle support

4. Priority nursing diagnoses

    a. Risk for Injury related to disease process

    b. Anticipatory Grieving related to chronic and terminal illness

    c. Impaired Physical Mobility related to wasted muscles

    d. Risk for Constipation related to poor muscle tone

    e. Impaired Gas Exchange related to accumulation of secretions, lack of mobility

    f. Disturbed Self-Esteem related to debilitating disease process

5. Planning and implementation

    a. Care is supportive with physical therapy to prevent disuse atrophy of unaffected muscles; physical therapy should be continued when confined to bed with illness, injury, or surgery, if bedrest extends beyond a few days

    b. Client should be immobilized for as short a period as possible to help prevent disuse atrophy

    c. Frequent rest periods in a recumbent position are helpful to help reduce incidence of scoliosis

    d. Splinting and bracing may help to maintain lower extremity stability and avoid contractures

    e. A daily goal for well clients should be at least three hours of ambulation per day to maintain muscle strength

    f. Encourage a low-calorie, high-protein diet to avoid obesity

    g. Encourage a high-fiber and high-fluid diet to prevent constipation

    h. Infections become increasingly frequent as dystrophic process produces a decrease in vital capacity; even minor upper respiratory infections are treated quickly and vigorously with antibiotics and postural drainage

    i. Certain surgical techniques allow ambulation longer

6. Client and family education

    a. Teach ROM exercises

    b. Reinforce diet to prevent obesity and constipation

    c. Teach how to achieve optimal level of activity within client's limitations

    d. Encourage participation in support groups for parents and client

    e. Teach self-help skills

    f. Provide information on environmental issues that promote mobility and allow for wheelchair use

    g. Refer family members for genetic counseling

7. Evaluation: family states appropriate care of this client to maintain maximum function as long as possible; client exhibits minimal respiratory infections

IV. INFECTIOUS MUSCULOSKELETAL HEALTH PROBLEMS: OSTEOMYELITIS

A. Description

1. **Osteomyelitis** is an infection of bone

2. Can occur at any age; is most common in children between 1 and 12 years

3. Males are affected two to three times more often than females

Practice to Pass

A 15-year-old male is admitted to the adolescent unit with pneumonia. He also has Duchenne's muscular dystrophy. Describe the priorities of his nursing care during this hospitalization.

B. Etiology and pathophysiology
1. May be caused by any microorganism, though usually caused by bacteria; *Staphylococcus aureus* is the offending bacteria most often in older children and *Haemophilus influenza* in younger children
2. Microorganism is carried to bone site through bloodstream from another site of infection or by way of a penetrating wound
3. Infective emboli from focus of infection travel to small end arteries in bone metaphysis, where they set up an infectious process
4. An abscess forms, which spreads along shaft of bone under periosteum, possibly extending to and penetrating bone marrow
5. Edema in area of infection reduces blood supply to bone, causing death of bone tissue

C. Assessment
1. Generally begins with acute symptoms, systemic malaise, fever, irritability, rapid pulse, and possibly dehydration
2. May be a history of trauma to the bone
3. Symptoms include pain, tenderness, swelling, and redness in area of infection; there is also decreased mobility of affected extremity
4. Blood studies reveal an increased white blood cell count, C-reactive protein, and erythrocyte sedimentation rate (ESR); blood cultures will be positive
5. X-ray may not reveal bone changes until 5 to 10 days after beginning of infection; computed tomography may show early-stage bone changes

D. Priority nursing diagnoses
1. Pain related to disease process
2. Impaired Physical Mobility related to disease process
3. Risk for Noncompliance related to long course of antibiotics
4. Deficient Knowledge: Disease Process and Treatment

E. Planning and implementation
1. Limitation of weight bearing on affected extremity; client may be placed on complete bedrest with immobilization of affected extremity
2. Surgery may be needed for incision and drainage; if surgical drainage is carried out, polyethylene tubes are placed in wound—one tube instills antibiotic solution directly into wound, while other provides drainage
3. Strict aseptic technique is used during all dressing changes
4. Diversional activities are important to maintain activity restrictions as client begins to feel better
5. Physical therapy may be instituted to ensure restoration of optimal function

F. Medication therapy
1. Intravenous antibiotics for three to six weeks, initiated in hospital, and then continued at home; length of IV therapy is determined by duration of symptoms, initial response to treatment, and sensitivity of organism
2. Oral antibiotics for two weeks following IV antibiotics

G. Child and family education
1. Compliance with antibiotic treatment
2. Care and maintenance of IV site
3. Activity restrictions ordered by health care professional
4. Providing good food sources of calcium and protein for bone healing
5. Signs and symptoms of infection

H. Evaluation: family and client comply with antibiotic administration

V. ACCIDENTS AND INJURIES CAUSING MUSCULOSKELETAL HEALTH PROBLEMS: FRACTURES

A. Description

1. Growth plate or epiphyseal plate is a common place of injury, and can lead to improper growth if not treated correctly; Salter-Harris classification system is used to describe fractures of growth plate and is based on angle of fracture in relation to epiphysis (see Figure 9-2)
2. Periosteum of a child's bone is thicker and stronger and aids in rapid healing

B. Etiology and pathophysiology

1. Children's bones are more pliable and porous, which allows them to bend, buckle and break in different ways than those of adults (see Figure 9-3)
2. Fractures may result from trauma—falls, motor vehicle accidents, sports injuries or abuse—or may be a result of bone diseases such as osteogenesis imperfecta or cancer that weakens bone

3. Adolescents who limit their intake of calories and calcium and who are involved in sports such as distance running or gymnastics are at risk for stress fractures; these fractures may present with chronic pain that changes in intensity

C. Assessment

1. Complaints of children must be taken seriously; they usually only complain when something is wrong

---

Figure 9-2

Salter-Harris classification
of fractures

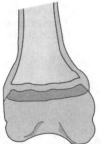

Type I
Common
Growth plate undisturbed
Growth disturbances rare

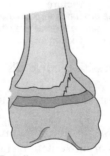

Type II
Most common
Growth disturbances rare

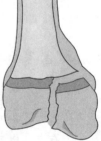

Type III
Less common
Serious threat to growth
   and joint

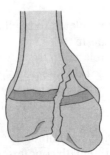

Type IV
Serious threat to growth

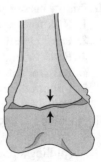

Type V
Rare
Crush injury causes cell death in growth plate,
   resulting in arrested growth and limited
   bone length
If growth plate is partially destroyed, angular
   deformities may result

Figure 9-3

Types of fractures

Source: Hogan, MaryAnn; Brancato, Vera; White, Judy; Falkenstein, Kathleen, *Prentice Hall Reviews & rationales: Child health nursing*, 2nd Ed., ©2007. Reprinted and Electronically reproduced by permission of Pearson Education, Inc. Upper Saddle River, NJ.

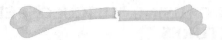

Complete (transverse) fracture
Break across entire section of a bone
at a right angle to the bone shaft resulting
in two or more fragments

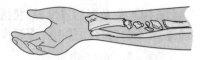

Comminuted fracture
Associated with high impact forces;
bone breaks into three or more segments

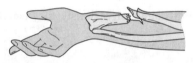

Closed fracture
Broken bone does not
protrude through the skin

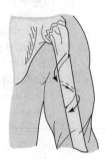

Spiral fracture
Associated with twisting force;
fracture coils around the bone

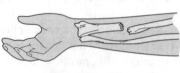

Open fracture
Broken bone protrudes through the
skin leaving a path to the fracture site;
high risk of infection exists

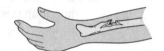

Greenstick fracture
Caused by compression force;
often seen in young children

2. Frequently assess the five "Ps" in affected extremity
   a. Pain and joint tenderness
   b. Pulselessness distal to fracture site
   c. Pallor
   d. Paresthesia distal to fracture site
   e. Paralysis or movement distal to fracture site
3. Assess vital signs, lungs sounds, bowel sounds, and neurological status depending on the cause of fracture
4. Assess blood studies; fracture may cause bleeding or destruction of red blood cells
5. Assess for other associated injuries caused by trauma that caused fracture

D. Priority nursing diagnoses
1. Risk for Impaired Tissue Perfusion related to swelling
2. Pain related to injury or muscle spasm
3. Risk for Impaired Skin Integrity related to traction, cast, or splint
4. Risk for Infection related to loss of skin integrity
5. Impaired Physical Mobility related to cast, splint, or traction
6. Deficient Knowledge: Course of Treatment, Care of Cast, Traction

E. Planning and implementation

1. Treatment of a fracture is to realign and immobilize fractured extremity by **traction** (pulling a body part in one direction with counter-pull in another) or closed manipulation and casting until adequate callus is formed
2. A cast may be applied after closed reduction; a cast may be fiberglass, which dries in 5 to 30 minutes, or plaster, which dries over 24 to 48 hours; various types of casts include short- or long-extremity casts, bilateral long leg cast, shoulder spica cast, single spica, 1½ spica and full spica casts, cylinder cast, bootie cast, and body cast
3. Surgery may be needed for open reduction of fracture using pins, plates, wires, or screws, in order for healing to occur

4. Children are most frequently hospitalized for fractures of femur
5. See Box 9-2 for nursing care of a client in a cast
6. Monitor for complications of fracture reduction: infection with open fractures, neurovascular or vascular injury, malunion or nonunion, and leg length discrepancy
7. Monitor for deep pain unrelieved by analgesics, which may be a symptom of compartment syndrome (a medical emergency); the swelling caused by inflammation and casting reduces blood flow to affected area and can lead to progressive neurological damage; notify physician immediately
8. Traction is used to reduce dislocations and immobilize fractures; it involves pulling on a body part in one direction against a counter-pull exerted in opposite direction
   a. Traction may be straight or running traction (where client's body serves as counter-pull), or suspended or balanced traction (where counter-pull is through weights and pulleys)
   b. Skin traction is used when minimal traction is needed; traction is applied to skin with adhesive materials or straps; foam boots and skin serve as the counter-pull
   c. Skeletal traction is used when a greater strength of traction or a longer period of traction is needed; pull is directly applied to bone by pins or wires surgically placed through distal end of bone
   d. See Box 9-3 for further information about care for a client in traction
9. The following are various kinds of traction
   a. Bryant's traction: used for clients under 3 years of age and weighing less than 35 pounds, who have a fractured femur or congenital hip dysplasia; both legs are placed in skin traction, hips are flexed at a 90-degree angle, with knees extended, and both buttocks are slightly elevated above mattress
   b. Buck's traction: used for knee immobilization or for short-term immobilization of a fracture; this running skin traction keeps leg in extended position without hip flexion
   c. Russell's traction: used for fractures of femur and lower leg; skin traction is placed on lower leg while knee is suspended in a padded sling; hips and knees are slightly flexed; skin care and monitoring of skin resting in the sling is indicated

Practice to Pass

A 23-month-old child is in Bryant's traction for developmental dysplasia of the hip. Describe the nursing care for this child.

Box 9-2	• Assess neurovascular status of involved extremity and compare with unaffected extremity; assess temperature, pallor, pain, tingling sensation, edema, pulse, and capillary refill every 15 minutes for the first hour, hourly for 24 hours, then every 2 to 4 hours.
Nursing Care of a Client in a Cast	• Assess the client's ability to move the fingers or toes and detect sensation in the affected extremity; compare to the unaffected extremity.
	• Report any change in neurovascular status to the physician immediately.
	• Assist with proper drying of a plaster cast (takes 24 to 48 hours) by leaving it exposed to air, turning the client every 2 hours, and using a fan or cool hair dryer.
	• A wet cast is handled only with the palms of the hands to prevent indenting casts and creating pressure areas.
	• Relieve edema by elevating limb and applying ice to the outside of the cast.
	• Assess pain and institute pain management therapies.
	• Provide a well-balanced diet with adequate calories, protein, and calcium.
	• Frequently assess skin around the cast edges for redness and breakdown.
	• Petal the cast edges if rough or broken down by applying strips of adhesive tape over them.
	• Keep the cast dry from water, stool, or urine with the use of plastic wrap.
	• Assess for hot spots felt on the cast surface, which indicate infection underneath. Report any hot spots found.
	• Assist with mobility with use of wagons, wheeled carts, crutches, or wheelchairs.

Box 9-3	**Nursing Interventions for All Types of Traction**

Nursing Care of a Client in Traction	• Assess neurovascular status of involved extremity and compare with unaffected extremity; assess temperature, pallor, pain, tingling sensation, edema, pulse, and capillary refill every 15 minutes for the first hour, hourly for 24 hours, then every 2 to 4 hours.
	• Assess the client's ability to move the fingers or toes and detect sensation in the affected extremity, as compared to the unaffected extremity.
	• Maintain alignment of affected extremity.
	• Ensure that the client is in alignment in bed, and that the head or foot of the bed is elevated as directed for the desired amount of pull and traction.
	• Ensure that the prescribed amount of weight is in place and that weights hang freely and are in a safe location.
	• Assess pain and institute pain management therapies.
	• Provide a well-balanced diet with adequate calories, protein, and calcium.
	• Provide diversional activities appropriate to the client's developmental level.
	• Check beneath the client for small objects.
	• Provide nursing care to prevent complications resulting from immobility.
	  • Assess skin surfaces, provide frequent skin care, and include use of trapeze, air mattress, and sheepskin.
	  • Assess respiratory status and encourage deep breathing, coughing, and incentive spirometry.
	  • Assess urinary elimination, monitor intake and output, and encourage fluids.
	  • Assess bowel function, encourage high-fiber diet.
	  • Encourage range-of-motion exercises.
	  • Anticipate need for antiembolism stockings on unaffected lower extremity.
	
	Additional Nursing Interventions for Skeletal Traction
	• Assess vital signs, especially temperature, every four hours or more often if indicated.
	• Inspect pin insertion sites at least every eight hours for redness, swelling, irritation, or drainage.
	• Obtain culture of pin sites as ordered.
	• Provide pin care according to institution policy.
	• Cover the end of pins with protective padding to prevent injury.
	
	Additional Nursing Interventions for Skin Traction
	• Replace nonadhesive bandages when permitted or when necessary, ensuring that someone maintains traction on the affected limb during the procedure.
	• Assess bandages to ensure that they are correctly applied, neither too loose nor too tight.

Practice to Pass

The nurse is caring for a child who had fractures of the tibia and fibula reduced by closed reduction and just had a fiberglass cast applied. What assessments will be done immediately? Which assessment findings would lead the nurse to call the physician?

    d. Dunlop's traction: used for fractures of humerus; flexed arm is suspended horizontally; this may be applied as skin or skeletal traction

    e. 90-90 traction: skeletal traction used for fractures of femur or tibia; hip and knee are positioned at 90-degree angles, and lower part of extremity is put into a sling or boot cast; ensure skin care to area in boot cast or sling

    f. External fixators: attached to extremity by percutaneous transfixing of pins or wires to bone; these can be used for simple fractures or for complicated fractures or deformities

F. Client and family education: refer back to Box 9-1

G. Evaluation: client's bone heals properly; client's growth and development is not disturbed by fracture; parents state appropriate care of a child in a cast

Case Study

A newborn is found to have developmental dysplasia of the hip prior to being discharged from the birth hospital. You are the nurse caring for this newborn and the new mother prior to discharge.

1. What assessment findings would you expect to find in this newborn?

2. The parents of the newborn ask how this could have happened. How will you respond?

3. What are the priorities of care for this newborn?

4. How will this condition be treated?

5. What teaching needs to be completed with the parents of this newborn prior to discharge?

6. The parents question you about what they can expect regarding long-term consequences. How should you respond?

For suggested responses, see page 354.

POSTTEST

❶ Parents of an unborn infant have just learned that, based on ultrasound, their infant has clubfoot. They ask the nurse how clubfoot is treated. Which treatment should the nurse discuss with the parents?

1. Weekly cast changes with manipulation
2. Probable surgery on the affected limb
3. Abduction device to keep the hip in full abduction
4. Use of a Denis Browne splint to achieve correction

❷ An infant is placed in a Pavlik harness for developmental dysplasia of the hip. The nurse has completed parent teaching, but the parents seem to be overwhelmed by the condition. Which statements made by the parents indicate that more instruction is needed? Select all that apply.

1. "The straps of the harness should be placed next to the skin."
2. "The harness should be worn for six hours a day."
3. "It will take a long time for my child to walk and crawl."
4. "I should not lift the baby by his legs when changing his diaper."
5. "Because my child's defect was caught early, treatment will not usually require surgery."

❸ A 4-year-old child with osteogenesis imperfecta (OI) is admitted to the hospital unit for an unrelated condition. The nurse determines that which nursing diagnosis has the highest priority for this child?

1. Impaired Skin Integrity related to cast
2. Pain related to fractures
3. Risk for Injury related to disease state
4. Disturbed Body Image related to short stature

❹ A child is admitted to the hospital unit with a diagnosis of rule out acute onset of Legg-Calve-Perthes (LCP) disease. The nurse would assess for which symptoms of LCP disease? Select all that apply.

1. Swelling of the involved joint(s)
2. Redness of the involved joint
3. Insidious limp after activities
4. Referred pain to the knee
5. Stiffness in the morning or after rest

❺ A 12-year-old male is admitted to the adolescent unit with a diagnosis of slipped capitol femoral epiphysis. Which activity should not be allowed by the nurse prior to surgical correction?

1. Ambulation with crutches; avoid bearing weight on the affected leg
2. Sitting in a wheelchair
3. Moving on a stretcher
4. Maintaining bedrest

6 An adolescent diagnosed with idiopathic structural scoliosis describes all of the following symptoms. Which one would the nurse conclude is not associated with this diagnosis?

1. Back pain
2. Skirts that hang unevenly
3. Unequal shoulder heights
4. Uneven waist level

7 A 15-year-old who has a diagnosis of scoliosis is being seen in the outpatient clinic. The nurse planning care for this adolescent develops the following nursing diagnoses. Which nursing diagnosis should take highest priority?

1. Disturbed Body Image related to treatment of scoliosis
2. Diversional Activity Deficit related to treatment of scoliosis
3. Anxiety related to outcome of treatment for scoliosis
4. Fear related to treatment and unknown outcomes

8 An adolescent is returning to the hospital unit after surgical spinal fusion for scoliosis. The nurse would include which of the following in the immediate postoperative care of this client? Select all that apply.

1. Oral analgesics for pain
2. Logrolling every two hours as ordered
3. Nasogastric intubation
4. Straight catheterization every four hours
5. Incentive spirometer use every two hours while awake

9 A 3-year-old child is suspected of having Duchenne's muscular dystrophy. Which assessment findings by the nurse would support this diagnosis?

1. A history of delayed crawling
2. Outward rotation of the hips
3. Difficulty climbing stairs
4. Wasted muscle appearance

10 A child is admitted to the hospital with a diagnosis of rule out osteomyelitis. Which serum laboratory value noted by the nurse supports this diagnosis?

1. Decreased white blood cell (WBC) count
2. Elevated erythrocyte sedimentation rate
3. Increased hematocrit (HCT)
4. Increased BUN

➤ *See pages 210–211 for Answers and Rationales.*

ANSWERS & RATIONALES

Pretest

1 **Answer: 1, 3, 5** **Rationale:** Capillary refill should be three seconds or less. The sensation of numbness or tingling is a sign of neurovascular impairment. Neurovascular impairment can lead to nerve ischemia and destruction, with possible permanent paralysis of the extremity. Pain that increases with elevation indicates insufficient circulation from a cast that is possibly too tight and needs to be reported. Edema would need to be reported if it did not resolve with elevation. Warm skin surrounding the cast is a normal finding, as compared to skin that is cool or cold to touch. **Cognitive Level:** Analyzing **Client Need:** Physiological Adaptation **Integrated Process:** Nursing Process: Assessment **Content Area:** Child Health **Strategy:** Determine which findings are abnormal. The wording of the question indicates that more than one option will be correct. **Reference:** Ball, J., Bindler, R., & Cowen, K. (2010). *Child health nursing: Partnering with children and families* (2nd ed.). Upper Saddle River, NJ: Pearson Education, p. 1480.

2 **Answer: 2** **Rationale:** The child with skeletal traction has a pin that passes through the skin into the end of a long bone. This procedure provides an entrance for microorganisms. Frequent monitoring of the pin site, pin care according to institutional policy, and frequent monitoring for signs of infection are important to detect complications. Assessing bowel sounds is a routine assessment. Providing adequate nutrition is important but is a routine care activity that would apply to any client. Providing age-appropriate activities will be important once physiological needs are met. **Cognitive Level:** Analyzing **Client Need:** Physiological Adaptation **Integrated Process:** Nursing Process: Planning **Content Area:** Child Health **Strategy:** The core concept is monitoring for complications of skeletal traction. Consider that skeletal traction is invasive and then consider associated risks to help make the correct selection. **Reference:** Ball, J., Bindler, R., & Cowen, K. (2010). *Child health nursing: Partnering with children and families* (2nd ed.). Upper Saddle River, NJ: Pearson Education, pp. 1481–1482.

3 **Answer: 1** **Rationale:** Slipped capitol femoral epiphysis is a slipping of the femoral head that occurs most frequently before or during the rapid adolescent growth spurt. The onset of symptoms is gradual, and symptoms include limp, holding the leg in external rotation to relieve pain, restricted and painful internal rotation, and knee and hip pain. **Cognitive Level:** Analyzing **Client Need:** Physiological Adaptation **Integrated Process:** Nursing Process: Assessment **Content Area:** Child Health **Strategy:** First, consider the age of the child most frequently seen with this condition. This will rule out one of the responses. Eliminate another as the symptoms are not associated with rotation. **Reference:** Ball, J., Bindler, R., & Cowen, K. (2010). *Child health nursing: Partnering with children and families* (2nd ed.). Upper Saddle River, NJ: Pearson Education, pp. 1453–1454.

4 **Answer: 1** **Rationale:** Antibiotic therapy may continue intravenously for three to six weeks, and orally for another two weeks depending on duration of symptoms, response to treatment, and sensitivity of the organism. Food sources such as calcium and protein should be provided for bone healing. Discharge teaching needs to include care of the IV site. The therapeutic management of the child with osteomyelitis includes limiting weight-bearing on the affected part and immobilization. **Cognitive Level:** Analyzing **Client Need:** Physiological Adaptation **Integrated Process:** Nursing Process: Evaluation **Content Area:** Child Health **Strategy:** The wording of the question indicates the correct answer is an incorrect statement by the parent. Label each statement as either true or false, and select the one that is false as the answer, based on the wording of the question. **Reference:** Ball, J., Bindler, R., & Cowen, K. (2010). *Child health nursing: Partnering with children and families* (2nd ed.). Upper Saddle River, NJ: Pearson Education, pp. 1464–1465.

5 **Answer: 3, 5** **Rationale:** All four of the signs are assessment tests for developmental dysplasia of the hip. The Ortolani and Barlow signs disappear after two to three months. Trendelenburg sign will be seen in the child who is able to stand. Allis sign, shortening of the affected limb on the affected side, is a reliable indicator at 4 months of age. Asymmetric folds would be a positive sign at any age. The child is too young to walk, so a limp would not be observed. **Cognitive Level:** Applying **Client Need:** Physiological Adaptation **Integrated Process:** Nursing Process: Assessment **Content Area:** Child Health **Strategy:** The core concept is the age of the child at the time of diagnosis. Incorrect answers can be eliminated based on age. **Reference:** Ball, J., Bindler, R., & Cowen, K. (2010). *Child health nursing: Partnering with children and families* (2nd ed.). Upper Saddle River, NJ: Pearson Education, p. 1447.

6 **Answer: 3** **Rationale:** Clubfoot is apparent at birth, with the affected foot fixed in an abnormal position. The affected foot is usually smaller, shorter and with an empty heel pad. The affected limb is usually shorter and has some calf muscle atrophy. Temperature remains the same bilaterally. **Cognitive Level:** Applying **Client Need:** Physiological Adaptation **Integrated Process:** Nursing Process: Assessment **Content Area:** Child Health **Strategy:** Recall that clubfoot does not affect circulation to eliminate one option. Next eliminate two options that are very similar. **Reference:** Ball, J., Bindler, R., & Cowen, K. (2010). *Child health nursing: Partnering with children and families* (2nd ed.). Upper Saddle River, NJ: Pearson Education, p. 1443.

7 **Answer: 3** **Rationale:** Children with this disorder have normal calcium and phosphorus levels and abnormal precollagen type I. This prevents the formation of collagen, the major component of connective tissue. The precollagen remains relatively unstable and unable to undergo final transformation into collagen. Vitamin D is not of concern. **Cognitive Level:** Applying **Client Need:** Physiological Adaptation **Integrated Process:** Nursing Process: Assessment **Content Area:** Child Health **Strategy:** Consider that three of the tests listed are common tests, while one is uncommon. **Reference:** Ball, J., Bindler, R., & Cowen, K. (2010). *Child health nursing: Partnering with children and families* (2nd ed.). Upper Saddle River, NJ: Pearson Education, p. 1468.

8 **Answer: 4** **Rationale:** Children with mild OI may be able to participate in sports, and many are able to participate in swimming. There are no current medications that stop this disease process. There are a variety of surgical procedures that may be done to help strengthen the bones; one is the insertion of intermedullary rods to provide for stability. The child with OI may participate in school, though care needs to be provided to protect this child from injury. **Cognitive Level:** Analyzing **Client Need:** Physiological Adaptation **Integrated Process:** Nursing Process: Evaluation **Content Area:** Child Health **Strategy:** The goal of treatment for all children is to promote growth and development. Consider the option that interferes with normal growth and development as the answer based on the negative stem of the question. **Reference:** Ball, J., Bindler, R., & Cowen, K. (2010). *Child health nursing: Partnering with children and families* (2nd ed.). Upper Saddle River, NJ: Pearson Education, p. 1469.

9 **Answer: 4** **Rationale:** Children with muscular dystrophy quickly suffer from complications of immobility. Therefore, when hospitalized, these children should have physical therapy, range-of-motion exercises, and bed-to-chair activity as soon as possible. Children with respiratory infections are treated with vigorous antibiotic therapy, as well as postural drainage and cupping. **Cognitive Level:** Analyzing **Client Need:** Coordinated Care **Integrated Process:** Nursing Process: Planning **Content Area:** Child Health **Strategy:** The core concept is Duchene muscular dystrophy. It is important with these children that function be maintained, so the order that would be questioned would interrupt maintenance of mobility. **Reference:** Ball, J., Bindler, R., & Cowen, K. (2010). *Child health nursing: Partnering with children and families* (2nd ed.). Upper Saddle River, NJ: Pearson Education, p. 1473.

ANSWERS & RATIONALES

10 Answer: 3 Rationale: The Milwaukee brace is worn for scoliosis, when the degree of curve is greater than 20 but less than 40 degrees. It is worn for 23 hours a day. Exercises to increase pelvic tilt, for lateral strengthening, and to correct lordosis should be done several times a day while in the brace. The brace should be worn over a T-shirt to minimize skin irritation. The adolescent may experience muscle aches resulting from new alignment. **Cognitive Level:** Analyzing **Client Need:** Physiological Adaptation **Integrated Process:** Teaching and Learning **Content Area:** Child Health **Strategy:** The goal of therapy is to prevent progression of the scoliosis. To be successful in answering this question, the learner must understand the treatment plan. **Reference:** Ball, J., Bindler, R., & Cowen, K. (2010). *Child health nursing: Partnering with children and families* (2nd ed.). Upper Saddle River, NJ: Pearson Education, pp. 1446, 1457, 1460.

Posttest

1 Answer: 1 Rationale: The initial treatment for clubfoot begins immediately or shortly after birth and consists of weekly cast changes and manipulation. Surgery is completed only if nonsurgical intervention of serial casting is not effective. A Denis Browne splint may be used to maintain correction once it is achieved. Abduction devices are used for hip conditions. **Cognitive Level:** Applying **Client Need:** Physiological Adaptation **Integrated Process:** Teaching and Learning **Content Area:** Child Health **Strategy:** Eliminate one option as it refers to the hip, not the foot. From the remaining options, choose the one that would be used immediately after birth. **Reference:** Ball, J., Bindler, R., & Cowen, K. (2010). *Child health nursing: Partnering with children and families* (2nd ed.). Upper Saddle River, NJ: Pearson Education, p. 1443.

2 Answer: 1, 2, 3 Rationale: Diapers should be placed underneath the straps of a Pavlik harness; a t-shirt should be worn under the straps of the harness. The harness should be worn for 23 hours a day. The child quickly "catches up" once the device is no longer worn if developmental milestones are delayed because of the abduction device. Babies should never be lifted by their legs when changing diapers. Early treatment is usually successful without surgery. **Cognitive Level:** Analyzing **Client Need:** Physiological Adaptation **Integrated Process:** Nursing Process: Evaluation **Content Area:** Child Health **Strategy:** Knowledge of the care of the child in a Pavlik harness will aid in choosing the correct answer. The wording of the question guides you to eliminate responses that are correct information. **Reference:** Ball, J., Bindler, R., & Cowen, K. (2010). *Child health nursing: Partnering with children and families* (2nd ed.). Upper Saddle River, NJ: Pearson Education, p. 1448.

3 Answer: 3 Rationale: Because of their very fragile bones, children with OI experience countless fractures, and the prevention of injury takes highest priority in this child's care. Skin integrity impairment would also not be a

concern unless a fracture actually occurred. Pain would be important if a fracture actually occurs, but the key is prevention of fractures. Disturbed Body Image is not usually a concern for a client of this age. **Cognitive Level:** Analyzing **Client Need:** Physiological Adaptation **Integrated Process:** Nursing Process: Planning **Content Area:** Child Health **Strategy:** Eliminate one option as the child is 4 years old. Of the three remaining, choose the option that would be a concern throughout the care of this child. **Reference:** Ball, J., Bindler, R., & Cowen, K. (2010). *Child health nursing: Partnering with children and families* (2nd ed.). Upper Saddle River, NJ: Pearson Education, p. 1469.

4 Answer: 3, 4, 5 Rationale: Swelling and redness of involved joints is a symptom found in juvenile arthritis, not LCP disease. Stiffness in the morning or after rest, an insidious limp after activities, and referred pain to the knee are all consistent with this diagnosis. **Cognitive Level:** Analyzing **Client Need:** Physiological Adaptation **Integrated Process:** Nursing Process: Assessment **Content Area:** Child Health **Strategy:** Knowledge of the signs and symptoms of LCP disease will help to choose the correct answer. Eliminate symptoms that are not normally seen in LCP. **Reference:** Ball, J., Bindler, R., & Cowen, K. (2010). *Child health nursing: Partnering with children and families* (2nd ed.). Upper Saddle River, NJ: Pearson Education, p. 1452.

5 Answer: 2 Rationale: Wheelchair use should be avoided, as this may increase the amount of slippage. Once the diagnosis is made, the child should be non-weight-bearing on the affected hip, as weight-bearing can increase the amount of slippage. Moving on a stretcher poses no problems to the client. Maintaining bed rest does not put the joint at risk. **Cognitive Level:** Analyzing **Client Need:** Physiological Adaptation **Integrated Process:** Nursing Process: Implementation **Content Area:** Child Health **Strategy:** Knowledge of the care of the client with slipped capital femoral epiphysis will help to answer the question correctly. After noting the critical word *not* in the question, select the option that places the affected joint at risk. **Reference:** Ball, J., Bindler, R., & Cowen, K. (2010). *Child health nursing: Partnering with children and families* (2nd ed.). Upper Saddle River, NJ: Pearson Education, pp. 1453–1454.

6 Answer: 1 Rationale: Back pain is not identified as a symptom of idiopathic structural scoliosis. Skirts that hang unevenly, unequal shoulder height, and uneven waist level are all positive symptoms of this disorder. **Cognitive Level:** Analyzing **Client Need:** Physiological Adaptation **Integrated Process:** Nursing Process: Assessment **Content Area:** Child Health **Strategy:** Determine which options are symptoms of scoliosis. Eliminate these, leaving only the correct answer. **Reference:** Ball, J., Bindler, R., & Cowen, K. (2010). *Child health nursing: Partnering with children and families* (2nd ed.). Upper Saddle River, NJ: Pearson Education, p. 1455.

7 **Answer: 1** **Rationale:** Adolescents are greatly concerned about their physical appearance as part of their growth and development. Unless there is a clear priority based on physiological need, attention to developmental concerns such as body image is important when caring for the adolescent client. Because the client is being treated as an outpatient, there is no evidence of being deprived of diversional activities. Although anxiety may be expected with any health problem, there is no specific evidence that this is a high priority. Since fear is very specific, there is no basis outlined in the scenario pertaining to fear. **Cognitive Level:** Analyzing **Client Need:** Psychosocial Integrity **Integrated Process:** Nursing Process: Planning **Content Area:** Child Health **Strategy:** Eliminate two options because they are so similar. Then, consider the developmental period of the child, which is key to determining the correct response. **Reference:** Ball, J., Bindler, R., & Cowen, K. (2010). *Child health nursing: Partnering with children and families* (2nd ed.). Upper Saddle River, NJ: Pearson Education, pp. 1459–1460.

8 **Answer: 2, 3, 5** **Rationale:** Logrolling must be done every two hours, once allowed, to prevent the accumulation of secretions in the lungs. There is some degree of paralytic ileus following a spinal fusion; therefore, nasogastric intubation is required along with frequent assessment of return of bowel function. Monitoring the child's respiratory status is crucial as is the use of an incentive spirometer. The pain experienced by this client is severe and requires intravenous medication, preferably with patient-controlled analgesia (PCA). Urinary retention is common, and an indwelling catheter is used if present rather than repeated straight catheterization. **Cognitive Level:** Applying **Client Need:** Reduction of Risk Potential **Integrated Process:** Nursing Process: Implementation **Content Area:** Child Health **Strategy:** Look carefully at each option to make sure the option is totally correct.

Eliminate those that are either incorrect or not timely immediately postop. **Reference:** Ball, J., Bindler, R., & Cowen, K. (2010). *Child health nursing: Partnering with children and families* (2nd ed.). Upper Saddle River, NJ: Pearson Education, pp. 1459–1460.

9 **Answer: 3** **Rationale:** Symptoms usually begin at around 3 years of age and include difficulty climbing stairs, running, and pedaling. The child with Duchenne's muscular dystrophy (MD) has a history of meeting early developmental milestones. The appearance of the hips is normal. Duchenne's MD is also called pseudohypertrophic MD because the muscles appear enlarged. **Cognitive Level:** Analyzing **Client Need:** Physiological Adaptation **Integrated Process:** Nursing Process: Assessment **Content Area:** Child Health **Strategy:** Knowledge of Duchenne's muscular dystrophy will aid in choosing the correct answer. Eliminate one option as it is the opposite of the findings of Duchenne's MD. Also, children develop normally until there is onset of symptoms, so another option would be incorrect. **Reference:** Ball, J., Bindler, R., & Cowen, K. (2010). *Child health nursing: Partnering with children and families* (2nd ed.). Upper Saddle River, NJ: Pearson Education, p. 1470.

10 **Answer: 2** **Rationale:** Serum laboratory studies in a child with osteomyelitis will reveal an increased WBC count, C-reactive protein, and sedimentation rate. This disease process does not affect the HCT or BUN. **Cognitive Level:** Analyzing **Client Need:** Reduction of Risk Potential **Integrated Process:** Nursing Process: Assessment **Content Area:** Child Health **Strategy:** First eliminate two options that are not related to inflammation and infection, and then make a final choice by picking the test that elevates with inflammation and infection. **Reference:** Ball, J., Bindler, R., & Cowen, K. (2010). *Child health nursing: Partnering with children and families* (2nd ed.). Upper Saddle River, NJ: Pearson Education, p. 1464.

References

Ball, J., Bindler, R., & Cowen, K. (2012). *Principles of pediatric nursing: Caring for children* (5th ed.). Upper Saddle River, NJ: Pearson Education.

Ball, J., Bindler, R., & Cowen, K. (2010). *Child health nursing: Partnering with children and families* (2nd ed.). Upper Saddle River, NJ: Pearson Education.

Hockenberry, M., & Wilson, D. (2011). *Wong's essentials of pediatric nursing* (8th ed.). St. Louis, MO: Elsevier.

Hockenberry, M., & Wilson, D. (2011). *Wong's nursing care of infants and children* (9th ed.). St. Louis, MO: Elsevier.

London, M., Ladewig, P., Ball, J., Bindler, R., & Cowen, K. (2011). *Maternal & child nursing care* (3rd ed.). Upper Saddle River, NJ: Pearson Education.

Perry, S., Hockenberry, M., Lowdermilk, D., & Wilson, D. (2010). *Maternal child nursing care* (4th ed.). St. Louis, MO: Elsevier.

Pillitteri, A. (2009). *Maternal and child health nursing: Care of the childbearing and childrearing family* (6th ed.). Philadelphia: Lippincott Williams & Wilkins.

Smith, S., Duell, D., & Martin, B. (2012). *Clinical nursing skills: Basic to advanced skills* (8th ed.). Upper Saddle River, NJ: Pearson Education, Inc.

ANSWERS & RATIONALES

10 Integumentary Health Problems

Chapter Outline

NCLEX-RN® Test Prep

Use the accompanying online resource, NursingReviewsandRationales, to test yourself with hundreds of NCLEX®-style practice questions.

Objectives

➤ Identify data essential to the assessment of alterations in health of the integumentary system in a child.
➤ Discuss the clinical manifestations and pathophysiology of alterations in health of the integumentary system of a child.
➤ Discuss therapeutic management of a child with alterations in health of the integumentary system.
➤ Describe nursing management of a child with alterations in health of the integumentary system.

Review at a Glance

bulla fluid-filled lesion greater than 1 cm in diameter

cellulitis inflammation of skin and subcutaneous tissue

dermis highly vascular, inner supportive layer of skin

eczema also known as atopic dermatitis; chronic superficial inflammatory skin disorder characterized by dry scaly patches and pruritus

epidermis tough, outer layer of skin

erythema diffuse skin redness

impetigo highly contagious superficial skin infection caused by group A beta-hemolytic streptococcus or *Staphylococcus aureus*

lichenification large, dry thickened lesions

macule discolored spot on skin that is neither raised nor depressed

papule raised lesion

pediculosis capitis head lice

pruritus itchiness

pustule small, blisterlike elevation that contains pus

scabies skin infestation caused by scabies mite

vesicle small, blisterlike elevation that contains serous fluid

PRETEST

1 What instruction should the nurse provide to a mother of a 3-year-old with atopic dermatitis (eczema) regarding the bath water? Select all that apply.

1. Make it as hot as the child can tolerate.
2. Ensure that it is hot to the touch on the inner wrist.
3. Keep the temperature tepid to the touch.
4. Let the water sit until it is cool.
5. Avoid adding strong or perfumed soap to the water.

2 The nurse explains to the mother that a child who has begun treatment for impetigo with a topical antibiotic can return to daycare in what timeframe?

1. Immediately
2. After 48 hours
3. As soon as crusts are evident
4. When crusts fall off

3 When assessing a child's hair and scalp, the nurse notices what looks like dandruff, but it does not flake off easily. What integumentary problem does the nurse suspect?

1. Scabies
2. Atopic dermatitis
3. *Pediculosis capitis*
4. Impetigo

4 A child has been admitted to the burn unit with a circumferential burn to the right leg. How should the nurse position the client?

1. Flat in bed
2. With the right leg dependent
3. On the left side
4. With the right leg elevated

5 A 3-year-old child is suspected of having atopic dermatitis (eczema). The nurse assesses for which of the following as a major symptom?

1. Pruritus
2. Pustules
3. Vesicles
4. Lichenification

6 A child has been diagnosed with atopic dermatitis. While taking the nursing history, the nurse will assess for a family history of which of the following?

1. Scabies
2. Cellulitis
3. Asthma
4. Impetigo

7 When assessing a child with periorbital cellulitis, the nurse will want to ask the parent about a recent history of which of the following?

1. Nosebleeds
2. Sinusitis
3. Dog bite
4. Sun exposure

8 A child will be treated for cellulitis of the left leg. The nurse will include in the care plan the need for which of the following?

1. Continuing oral antibiotics until the prescription is completed
2. Strict bed rest with the left leg elevated for two weeks
3. Increased fluid intake
4. Limiting visitors to prevent spreading infection

9 There have been several cases of lice in the elementary school. The school health nurse would provide which item of information in an information sheet sent home to parents?

1. All children in the school should be treated with the anti-lice shampoo.
2. Lice readily jump from one head to another, so a large number of children will be affected.
3. Lice can be spread by the family pet.
4. Wearing each other's hats will spread the lice infestation.

10 Permethrin 5% (Elimite) is prescribed for a 10-year-old child diagnosed with scabies. What instructions should the nurse provide for the mother?

1. Apply the lotion liberally from head to toe.
2. Wrap the child in a clean sheet after treatment.
3. Leave the lotion on for 10 minutes, then rinse.
4. Apply lotion only after the child has had a bath and dried thoroughly.

➤ *See pages 226–227 for Answers and Rationales.*

I. OVERVIEW OF ANATOMY AND PHYSIOLOGY OF SKIN

A. Skin structure

1. Layers (see Figure 10-1)
   a. **Epidermis**: tough, outer layer of skin
   b. **Dermis**: highly vascular, inner supportive layer of skin
   c. Subcutaneous fat
2. Accessory structures
   a. Hair
   b. Nails
   c. Glands
      1) Sebaceous: provide sebum into hair follicle
      2) Sweat: provide thermoregulation through sweating

Figure 10-1

Layers and structures of skin

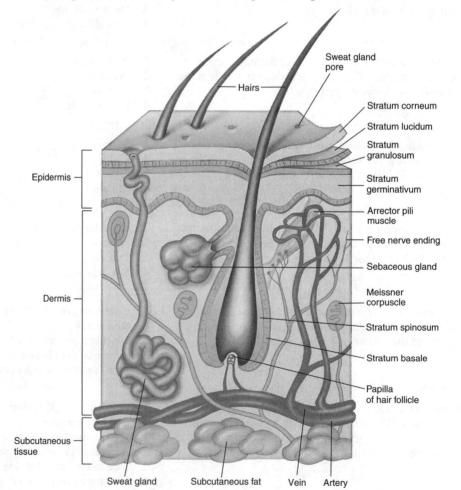

B. Skin functions
1. Sensitivity to pressure, pain, touch, and temperature
2. First line of defense against infectious organisms
3. Thermoregulation through sweating, shivering, and subcutaneous insulation
4. Protects underlying tissues and organs from injury
5. Synthesizes vitamin D
6. Excretes water, salt, and electrolytes
7. Regenerates itself through shedding of old cells and replacing with new cells

C. Pediatric variations in skin
1. Newborns are covered by lanugo, fine, soft hair that is shed in first month of life
2. Newborns have thin skin with little subcutaneous fat that allows rapid heat loss and causes problems with thermoregulation
   a. Leads to increased absorption of harmful chemical substances
   b. Sweat glands are not fully developed until middle childhood
3. Newborns' skin contains more water than older children
4. Dark-colored areas called dermae melanocytosis or Mongolian spots may be present on sacrum or buttocks of Native American, Asian, African-American, or Latino infants

II. DIAGNOSTIC TESTS OF THE SKIN

A. Skin cultures: non-invasive procedure in which a skin sample is obtained with a sterile applicator; used to identify viral, bacterial, or fungal causes of skin lesions

B. Skin scrapings: non-invasive procedure in which epithelial cells are scraped off and examined microscopically to identify viral, bacterial, fungal, or parasitic causes of skin lesions

C. Skin biopsy: invasive procedure in which a skin sample is removed for histological analysis
1. Requires informed consent
2. Apply pressure to site until bleeding stops; sutures may be required
3. Used to identify tumors or persistent dermatitis

III. ACQUIRED INTEGUMENTARY HEALTH PROBLEMS: ECZEMA

A. Description: *eczema* is a superficial inflammatory skin disorder
1. Sometimes called atopic dermatitis (having a hereditary allergic tendency)
2. A chronic, superficial inflammatory skin disorder characterized by severe **pruritus** (itchiness)
3. Affects infants, children, adolescents, and adults
4. Symptoms develop in 60% of affected children during infancy

B. Etiology and pathophysiology
1. Unknown etiology but occurs more frequently in clients when one or both parents have allergies like asthma, hay fever, or contact dermatitis
2. Infantile eczema frequently related to food allergies
3. Eczema in older children often related to allergies to dust mites
4. Intensified by dry skin, detergents, constricting clothing, or perfumed soaps and lotions

C. Assessment
1. In infancy, red **papules** (raised lesions) usually appear first on cheeks and then spread to forehead, scalp and down extensor surfaces of arms and legs
2. Characterized by intense pruritus, which causes excoriation of skin that then leads to exudate and crust formation

3. Childhood stage may follow continuously from infancy or eczema may make first appearance in toddlerhood

4. Childhood eczema characterized by dry, scaly, papular patches of skin on wrists, hands, ankles, antecubital and popliteal spaces

5. In adolescence, exudation is often caused by external irritation or secondary infection

6. Adolescent eczema is characterized by **lichenification** (large, dry, thickened lesions or plaques) on flexor folds, face, neck, back, upper arms, and dorsal aspects of hands, feet, fingers, and toes

7. Diagnosed by family history of allergies and inspection of skin

8. There is no laboratory test that is diagnostic for eczema

D. Priority nursing diagnoses

1. Impaired Skin Integrity
2. Risk for Infection
3. Disturbed Body Image
4. Deficient Knowledge: Disease Process and Treatment

E. Planning and implementation

1. Bathe or shower daily with tepid water using only mild soap on nonaffected areas
2. Do not use bath additives such as baking soda, bubble bath, or bath oils
3. Pat, rather than rub, skin dry
4. Immediately after bath, apply emollient such as Eucerin or Lubriderm
5. Avoid use of perfumed or scented lotions
6. Apply wet wraps to severely affected skin after applying topical medications
7. Use antibacterial soaps for handwashing
8. Keep fingernails clean and short
9. Avoid wool or constricting clothing, which can promote itching or trap perspiration
10. Place cotton gloves or socks over hands of infants or young children to prevent scratching
11. Provide support to client and family during flare-ups and reassurance that lesions do not produce scars unless excessively scratched and secondarily infected

F. Medication therapy

1. Topical steroids (hydrocortisone 1% or triamcinolone 0.1%) are applied to lesions to reduce inflammation during flare-ups
2. Tar preparations are sometimes used during flare-ups when symptoms are mild
3. Antihistamines are used to control itching
4. Oral antibiotics are used only if there is widespread skin breakdown or infection

G. Child and family education

1. Teach appropriate application of creams, ointments, or tar preparations
2. Teach proper application of soaks or compresses
3. Identify foods that exacerbate rash and avoid them
4. Explain need to avoid sunburns
5. Teach need to avoid known or suspected contact allergens, pets, or environmental factors
6. Discuss with family use of antihistamines before naps or bedtimes if sleep deprivation occurs due to itching
7. Explain importance of following treatment plan to promote healing and prevent infections
8. Discuss that condition is not contagious
9. With infants, introduce one new food at a time to identify food allergies

H. Evaluation: skin remains intact and free of secondary infection; client and family express positive image and demonstrate understanding of care during and between exacerbations

Practice to Pass

What comfort measures could the nurse suggest to the mother of an 8-month-old with eczema?

IV. INFECTIOUS INTEGUMENTARY HEALTH PROBLEMS

A. *Impetigo*

1. Description
   a. A highly contagious, superficial skin infection caused by staphylococci or strepto-cocci or both
   b. Accounts for almost 10% of all childhood skin disorders
   c. Most often occurs on face, neck, arms, hands, or legs
2. Etiology and pathophysiology
   a. Impetigo contagiosa (nonbullous) primarily caused by group A beta-hemolytic streptococcus and *Staphylococcus aureus* (*S. aureus*)
   b. Bullous impetigo always caused by *S. aureus*
   c. Causative bacteria are carried in nares and may pass onto skin
   d. Bacteria invade superficial skin in which a break has occurred
   e. Infection can be spread after scratching an affected site
   f. Infection is commonly acquired through contact with infected children who share toys, books, towels, or toiletries
   g. Infection may also be caused by direct skin contact during play or sports
3. Assessment
   a. Lesions are rarely painful but pruritus and burning may be present
   b. Nonbullous impetigo begins as a single erythematous **macule** (nonraised discol-ored spot) 2 to 4 mm in diameter that rapidly progresses to a **vesicle** (small, blis-terlike elevation that contains serous fluid) or **pustule** (small, blisterlike elevation that contains pus); vesicle ruptures leaving a honey-colored crust over superfi-cial erosion
   c. Lesions rapidly spread to adjacent skin showing linear pattern of client's scratching
   d. Mild regional lymphadenopathy may occur
   e. Bullous impetigo lesions are usually less than 3 cm in diameter with little ery-thema that erupt on untraumatized skin
   f. Characterized by **bullae** (fluid-filled lesions greater than 1 cm in diameter) that rupture and leave a varnishlike superficial erosion with little crusting
   g. Tends to spread peripherally
   h. Scraping from lesions show strep or *S. aureus*
4. Priority nursing diagnoses
   a. Impaired Skin Integrity
   b. Risk for Infection
   c. Deficient Knowledge: Prevention of Spread; Treatment
5. Planning and implementation
   a. Soak crusts in warm water
   b. Gently cleanse with antibacterial soap and remove crusts
   c. Do not touch or pick at lesions
   d. Client should wash hands frequently with antibacterial soap
   e. Anyone who touches lesions should wash hands immediately before and after with antibacterial soap
   f. Keep fingernails short and clean to prevent spread of infection from scratching
6. Medication therapy
   a. Apply topical antibiotic ointment such as Neosporin, Polysporin, Bacitracin, or mupirocin (Bactroban) three or four times daily for five to seven days or as ordered
   b. Systemic antibiotic may be ordered, such as dicloxacillin (Dynapen), cephalexin (Keflex), cefaclor (Duricef) or erythromycin, if no response to topical antibiotics in 72 hours

7. Client and family education

> **a.** Infection is communicable for 48 hours after antibiotic treatment is begun
>
> **b.** Client may return to daycare or school after 48 hours of therapy
>
> **c.** Inform school or daycare of infection so other children can be checked and so toys, etc. can be sanitized
>
> **d.** Family members and others in frequent contact with client should be checked for lesions
>
> **e.** Family members should not share towels, washcloths, or clothes
>
> **f.** Linens and clothes of infected client should be washed separately
>
> **g.** Cleanse lesions and treat with antibiotics (topical and/or oral) for full length of prescription

8. Evaluation: improvement at site is seen within 72 hours; infection does not spread; family and client demonstrate safe and effective administration of ointments and oral antibiotics

B. *Pediculosis capitus* (head lice)

1. Description

> **a.** Infestation of hair and scalp with lice
>
> **b.** Highly communicable parasite spread through direct contact (body to body, hair to hair) or indirect contact (clothing, brushes, hats, bedding)

2. Etiology and pathophysiology

> **a.** Lice live and reproduce only on humans
>
> **b.** Eggs (nits) are laid on hair shaft near the scalp
>
> **c.** This is a common problem in child care centers and schools
>
> **d.** Incidence is greatest in school-age children
>
> **e.** Incubation period for nits is 8 to 10 days
>
> **f.** Less common among African-American children because of shape of hair shaft
>
> **g.** Lice can survive for up to 48 hours away from human host
>
> **h.** Nits can survive for 8 to 10 days away from human host
>
> **i.** Lice bites release saliva into the dermis, which causes itching
>
> **j.** Severity of symptoms is usually proportional to the degree of infestation

3. Assessment

> **a.** Look for presence of whitish nits, about 1 mm in diameter, attached to hair shafts near scalp
>
> **b.** Nits are most commonly found behind ears and on crown of head and nape of neck
>
> **c.** Adult lice have six legs and range from light beige to black in color; may be seen on scalp
>
> **d.** Infestation is characterized by intense continuous pruritus on scalp
>
> **e.** Itching may cause erythema, scaling, and skin excoriation
>
> **f.** Secondary infection may occur in excoriated areas

4. Priority nursing diagnoses

> **a.** Health-Seeking Behaviors
>
> **b.** Risk for Infection
>
> **c.** Pain
>
> **d.** Deficient Knowledge: Treatment and Spread of Organisms

5. Planning and implementation

> **a.** Apply about two ounces of pediculicidal agent onto wet hair and add additional water to make a lather
>
> **b.** Allow lather to remain on hair for 10 minutes; do not allow it to remain longer because of toxicity
>
> **c.** Rinse hair thoroughly and apply crème rinse if necessary to facilitate combing of hair

    d. Remove nits from damp hair by dividing hair into 1-inch sections and using a fine-tooth comb

    e. Begin at crown of head first

    f. Pin hair out of the way when a section has been thoroughly combed

    g. Delouse environment by washing all of client's daily clothes and linens in hot water with detergent and drying for at least 20 minutes in a hot dryer

    h. Stuffed toys and bedding that cannot be washed should be sealed in plastic bags for two weeks to make sure any nits are dead

    i. Vacuum all floors, rugs, furniture, and play areas

    j. Combs, brushes, and hair ornaments should be discarded or soaked for one hour in a solution made from anti-lice shampoo or Lysol diluted with water

6. Medication therapy

    a. Over-the-counter pediculicidal agents include permethrin (Nix) or pyrethrum (Rid); also a shampoo containing dimethicone (a synthetic polymer) as an ingredient may be used

    b. After initial treatment, one additional treatment may be needed no sooner than seven days

7. Client and family education

    a. Inform parents to notify child care center or school of lice infestation so other children may be checked

    b. Inform parents that client may return to child care center or school following treatment

    c. Explain to parents that all other persons in household and other contacts should be checked for lice

    d. Teach children not to share hats, combs, hair ornaments, towels, etc.

    e. Explain to client and family that treatment plan must be followed meticulously or live lice or nits may reinfest client and other children

    f. Explain that nit removal is time consuming and may be uncomfortable for client, especially clients with long or thick hair

    g. Teach family members how to examine for and identify lice and nits

    h. Explain that a second treatment with anti-lice shampoo may be recommended 7 to 10 days after first treatment

    i. Explain to family that lice affect children of all socioeconomic levels

    j. Provide support and reassurance to family that may be embarrassed by a lice infestation

8. Evaluation: lice infestation is cleared; secondary infection does not develop; family and client demonstrate safe and effective administration of therapy

C. Scabies

1. Description

    a. Contagious skin condition caused by the mite *Sarcoptes scabiei*

    b. Affects children (and adults) of all ages, socioeconomic levels, and both genders

    c. Rash may have various types of lesions (papules, vesicles, or nodules)

    d. Pruritus is severe, especially at night

2. Etiology and pathophysiology

    a. Transmitted by close personal contact

    b. Mite present on an infected client is attracted to odor and warmth of uninfected client

    c. Female mite burrows into outer layer of epidermis to lay eggs, one to three eggs per day for 15 to 30 days before dying

    d. Larvae hatch in several days and move toward skin surface

    e. After mating males die and females continue reproductive cycle of burrowing, hatching, and mating

Practice to Pass

What measures should the nurse suggest as important to rid the home of lice and nits?

        f. Mite secretions, ova, and feces are highly irritating, so itching begins about one month after infestation

3. Assessment

        a. Intense pruritus, especially at night and nap times

        b. Infants and young children may be irritable, restless, and sleep fitfully

        c. Lesions appear as linear, grayish burrows 1 to 10 cm long ending in a pinpoint vesicle, papule, or nodule

        d. Burrows may be obliterated by excoriation from scratching

        e. In infants and young children, lesions are often found on palms, soles, and axilla

        f. In older children, lesions are often found in webs of fingers, body creases, axilla, waistline, and near genitalia

        g. Skin scraping from a burrow examined under a microscope may reveal mites, ova, or feces

4. Priority nursing diagnoses

        a. Impaired Skin Integrity

        b. Pain

        c. Risk for Infection

        d. Deficient Knowledge: Prevention of Spread; Treatment

5. Planning and implementation

        a. Give client a warm soap and water bath

        b. Apply scabicidal lotion to cool, dry skin over entire body from chin down

        c. Leave on for 8 to 12 hours before washing off

        d. Lotion may be applied to face of clients older than 2 months of age if lesions are present

            1) Do not apply to entire face of infants, only to scalp and forehead if necessary

            2) Pay special attention to application of lotion in skin folds, between fingers and toes, ears, navel, and under fingernails

        e. All family members and close contacts (playmates and caregivers) should be treated

        f. Clothing, bedding, and towels should be changed daily and washed in hot water and dried in a hot dryer

        g. Vacuum floors, carpets, and furniture

        h. Items that cannot be washed should be sealed in plastic bags for four days before use

        i. Provide support to family that may be distressed and believe scabies resulted from poor hygiene or unsanitary conditions

6. Medication therapy

        a. Scabicidal medications include crotamiton (Eurax) and permethrin 5% cream (Elimite); lindane (Kwell) should not be used on infants or young children because of risk of neurotoxicity and seizures

        b. One liberal application should be sufficient

        c. Follow directions precisely

        d. Oral antihistamines may be prescribed to reduce pruritus in older children

        e. Soothing creams or lotions may also be used to reduce pruritus

        f. Antibiotics are only prescribed if secondary infection develops

7. Client and family education

        a. Not all lesions clear immediately and, along with pruritus, may persist for two to three weeks until epidermis is replaced by natural shedding

        b. Inform child care center or school of scabies

        c. Client may return to child care center or school following treatment

        d. All persons in household and close contacts should be treated

        e. Treatment plan should be followed meticulously

Practice to Pass

How will the school nurse differentiate impetigo from scabies?

        f. Teach family how to examine for and identify signs of secondary infection

        g. Scabies does not result from poor hygiene, unsanitary living conditions, or lack of vigilance on part of parents

        h. Explain that children should not share clothes, towels, or hygiene items

    8. Evaluation: scabies infestation is cleared; secondary infection does not develop; family and client describe care of infestation and environment

D. *Cellulitis*

    1. Description

        a. Acute inflammation of skin involving epidermis, dermis, and underlying connective tissue

        b. Occurs in all age groups

        c. Most common site is legs but any area can be affected

    2. Etiology and pathophysiology

        a. History of trauma, impetigo, recent otitis media, or sinusitis

        b. Infecting agents are usually group A beta-hemolytic streptococcus or *S. aureus*

        c. In the skin, these infecting agents produce large amounts of enzyme-spreading factors that break down fibrin networks that usually contain or localize an infection

        d. Onset and spread may be rapid

        e. Cellulitis around eye (periorbital cellulitis) usually results from a recent sinus infection

        f. Facial cellulitis in young children usually results from recent episode of otitis media

    3. Assessment

        a. Clients appear ill and are often febrile

        b. **Erythema** (diffuse redness) or lilac-tinged skin at site of cellulitis

        c. Pitting edema is frequently present over affected area

        d. Warmth and tenderness are present over affected site

        e. Reddish areas of "streaking" away from site may be present

        f. Regional lymph nodes are often enlarged

        g. Pain is present at site

        h. Border of affected area is usually indistinct and not elevated

        i. White blood count is elevated

        j. Blood cultures will identify infectious agent

        k. Fluid aspirated from lesion can be cultured to identify infectious agent

    4. Priority nursing diagnoses

        a. Impaired Skin Integrity

        b. Pain

        c. Deficient Knowledge: Disease and Treatment

    5. Planning and implementation

        a. Hospitalization is needed if cellulitis is on face or covers a large area, otherwise home management is preferred

        b. Administer antibiotics, intravenous if hospitalized or oral if at home

        c. Monitor vital signs, especially temperature

        d. Apply warm compresses to affected area

        e. Elevate affected limb

        f. Maintain bedrest during acute phase

        g. Apply nonocclusive dressing if there is a skin tear or rupture in affected area

    6. Medication therapy

        a. Broad spectrum parenteral antibiotics are administered until infection subsides, then switch to oral; frequently prescribed antibiotics are nafcillin (Nafcil), dicloxacillin (Dynapen), or ceftriaxone (Rocephin)

Practice to Pass

What assessment data will the nurse collect when examining a toddler with what appears to be facial cellulitis?

b. Oral antibiotics are usually prescribed for 10 days; frequently prescribed antibiotics are amoxicillin/clavulanate (Augmentin) or oxacillin (Bactocill)

c. Acetaminophen given for pain or fever

7. Client and family education

a. Teach parents to continue antibiotics for full duration of prescription

b. Explain to parents to continue warm compresses as needed

c. Explain to family to contact health care provider if increased temperature, pain, or swelling occur

d. Explain that marked improvement should be seen in 48 hours

8. Evaluation: infection clears within 10 days; family and client demonstrate safe and effective administration of antibiotics

V. ACCIDENTS AND INJURIES CAUSING INTEGUMENTARY HEALTH PROBLEMS: BURNS

A. Description

1. Injury to skin and possibly subcutaneous tissue, caused by thermal, chemical, electrical, or radioactive causes

2. Injury can range from mild redness and slight tenderness to massive tissue destruction covering a large surface area

3. Second-leading cause of injury or death in clients under age 14

B. Etiology and pathophysiology

1. May be accidental or nonaccidental (adult abuse or neglect)

2. Thermal burns: exposure of skin to flames, scalds, or contact with a hot object

3. Chemical burns: exposure of skin or mucous membranes to chemical or caustic agents

4. Electrical burns: exposure to electrical current in wires or appliances

5. Radioactive burns: exposure of skin to sunlight or radioactive substances

6. Classification of burns based on depth of damage (see Table 10-1)

7. Local and systemic effects are related to extent of damage

a. In partial-thickness (second-degree) burns substantial edema and capillary damage occur at site of injury

b. In full-thickness (third-degree) burns a systemic response occurs of increased capillary permeability, which causes loss of fluid, electrolytes, and plasma proteins

8. Severity of burns is also related to extent of body surface area affected and size and age of child; the Lund and Browder chart identifies extent of burn

a. Minor burns: partial- and full-thickness burns to less than 10% of total body surface area (TBSA) with no other significant injuries; client is more than 5 years old; and no burns on hands, feet, genitalia, face, nor any circumferential burns

Table 10-1	Classification of Burns		
Type of Burn	**Appearance**	**Depth**	**Healing**
Superficial partial thickness	Red, dry skin	Epidermis	3–7 days without scarring
Partial thickness	Bright pink or red skin, moist, blisters	Epidermis and dermis	On own; may be grafted to speed healing if large area
Full thickness	Deep red, brown or black skin, may be charred	Epidermis, dermis, and underlying tissue (subcutaneous fat, perhaps muscle)	Requires grafting unless very small injury

      b. Major burns: full-thickness burns of more than 10% of TBSA; burns of hands, feet, genitalia, face, or any circumferential burns; respiratory tract involvement; fractures or other soft tissue injuries; or deep chemical or electrical burns

  9. The extent of injury is further determined by considering intensity and duration of contact with burn source (lower burn temperatures and shorter duration of contact can cause a more severe burn in a young child than an older one because of thinner skin)

  10. In superficial burns (e.g., sunburn), damaged epithelium peels off in 5 to 10 days without scarring

  11. In partial-thickness burns, crusts form in three to five days, and healing takes place from beneath

  12. In full-thickness burns, healing is slow with thin epithelial covering in about a month; scarring is usual

  13. Systemic effects of severe burns include asphyxia from smoke inhalation that causes edema of respiratory passages; shock from fluid shifts; renal failure from shock; protein loss from open wound; potassium excess from tissue destruction and renal failure

C. Assessment

  1. Calculate TBSA involved

  2. Burns covering more than 10% TBSA usually require fluid replacement

  3. Assess depth of burn injury (refer back to Table 10-1)

  4. Assess involvement of body parts

      a. Hands, feet, face, and perineal area burns have higher potential for functional impairment

      b. Circumferential burns (those surrounding an extremity or trunk) are considered major burns

  5. Pain that may be severe is present in superficial and partial-thickness burns

  6. Full-thickness burns have no pain because nerve endings have been destroyed, though may feel pressure

  7. Younger children have a higher mortality rate than older children with similar burns

  8. Assess renal function and urine output

  9. Perform respiratory assessment including rate, breath sounds, wheezing, hoarseness, smoky breath odor, or accessory muscle use; concurrent inhalation injury possible

  10. Measure vital signs

  11. Record weight, actual or stated

D. Priority nursing diagnoses

  1. Impaired Skin Integrity

  2. Pain

  3. Risk for Infection

  4. Risk for Impaired Tissue Perfusion

  5. Risk for Deficient or Excess Fluid Volume

  6. Risk for Imbalanced Nutrition

  7. Risk for Impaired Mobility

  8. Anxiety

  9. Deficient Knowledge: Treatment of Burn

E. Planning and implementation

  1. Administer analgesics as needed

      a. For major burns, morphine by the IV route is usually prescribed

      b. Administer analgesic about 30 minutes before wound care

Practice to Pass

Describe the clinical manifestations of a partial thickness burn.

2. Fluid replacement
   a. Place a large-bore peripheral IV in nonburned skin
   b. Ringer's lactate is the fluid of choice
   c. Fluid replacement is based on a formula that considers body weight, body surface area, and maintenance needs
3. Insert Foley catheter; monitor intake and output
4. Monitor vital signs
5. Elevate burn site (if practical) to reduce edema
6. Administer tetanus toxoid unless immunization status is known
7. Keep environment warm to minimize heat loss
8. Prevent wound infection
   a. Apply topical antimicrobials to small burns
   b. Major burns may use mafenide (Sulfamylon), silver sulfadiazine (Silvadene), or bacitracin as topical antimicrobials
   c. Use medical and surgical asepsis
   d. Infants and young children may need to be restrained
   e. Use systemic antibiotics as needed
9. Monitor bowel function; major burns may cause paralytic ileus or occult bleeding from stress ulcer
10. Give high-calorie, high-protein, high-carbohydrate diet to promote wound healing
    a. Tube feeding or hyperalimentation (total parenteral nutrition) may be needed in major burns
    b. Vitamin and mineral supplements given as necessary
11. Perform active or passive range of motion (ROM) exercises if possible
12. Debride wound every 8 to 12 hours as prescribed
13. In major burns, prepare for hydrotherapy to cleanse wound
14. Weigh daily to aid in calculation of fluid replacement, medication dosages, and caloric needs
15. Provide care for skin graft and donor sites as ordered if procedure is necessary
16. Work with health care team to plan for occupational and physical therapy, play therapy, child life specialist, rehabilitation, and home care
17. Provide emotional support to client and family who may fear pain and disfigurement

F. **Medication therapy**
1. Analgesics for pain control; opioids (such as morphine sulfate) are drug of choice for major burns
2. Antibiotics for prevention of infection; systemic antibiotics rarely used unless systemic infection present
   a. Mafenide (Sulfamylon) is applied in thin layer over open wound and covered with dressing
   b. Sulfadiazine (Silvadene) is applied in thin layer over open wound and covered with dressing; use with caution when impaired renal function exists; must be washed off and reapplied every 8 to 12 hours
3. H_2-receptor antagonists such as ranitidine (Zantac) or famotidine (Pepcid) are given to prevent stress ulcers in major burns

G. **Evaluation**: pain is controlled; wound infection and systemic complications do not develop; disfigurement is minimized; client and family describe purpose of therapy; client and family describe safe and effective antibiotic administration; client follows through on therapy

Case Study

You are a school nurse. A 7-year-old boy has what looks like impetigo on his right forearm. You call the mother at work at 10:00 a.m. and ask her to come immediately to pick up her son and seek medical attention.

1. What did you see that made you suspect impetigo?

2. Why should the child not be sent home on the bus with a note for the mother?

3. How will the mother be expected to care for her son at home?

4. What are the primary goals in treating impetigo?

5. When do you expect the child to return to school?

For suggested responses, see page 354.

POSTTEST

1 A 4-year-old child was just diagnosed with impetigo. What is the most important action the nurse should take to ensure that it does not spread?

1. Apply bacitracin ointment.
2. Keep it covered.
3. Isolate the child at home.
4. Teach and use good handwashing.

2 The nurse is providing home care instructions for a family with a toddler diagnosed with lice. The nurse includes which of the following instructions in the teaching plan? Select all that apply.

1. Immerse combs and brushes in boiling water for 30 minutes to kill lice.
2. Vacuum floors and furniture to remove hair that might have live nits.
3. Have the mother use a bright light and magnifying glass to check the hair for lice.
4. Launder the child's bedding and clothing in hot water with detergent and dry in a hot dryer for 20 minutes.
5. Teach children to not share combs, brushes, and hats.

3 The emergency department (ED) nurse hears a radio transmission from an ambulance stating that a 10-year-old boy is en route who sustained partial-thickness burns to his right arm and abdomen after tossing gasoline on a fire. On arrival to the ED, the nurse expects the burn site to have which appearance?

1. Smooth and bright red
2. Bright red with numerous blisters
3. White and waxy
4. Dark brown and firm

4 The nurse is working with a teenager diagnosed with atopic dermatitis. To increase compliance with treatment, the nurse will explain which of the following to the client?

1. The appearance of the skin will improve in a few days.
2. Avoiding foods with eggs and milk will speed healing.
3. Scarring is not likely if the treatment plan is followed.
4. This problem will not likely recur past adolescence.

5 When assessing a child with a possible diagnosis of facial cellulitis, the nurse will want to question the parent about a recent history of which of the following?

1. Otitis media
2. Cat scratch
3. Sunburn
4. Dental caries

POSTTEST

6 In teaching a group of school-age children, a nurse would explain that lice on a child can be most easily spread by which mechanism?

1. Sitting close to someone who has lice
2. Sharing hats at recess
3. Riding in the same car
4. Sharing a seat on the same bus

7 The nurse is developing a care plan for a 10-year-old girl with atopic dermatitis (eczema) of the elbows, hands, and face. The nurse would formulate which of the following as an appropriate client goal for this child?

1. Pain will be managed.
2. Infection will not spread.
3. Skin will be well hydrated.
4. Dietary restriction will be maintained.

8 A 5-year-old boy was brought to the emergency department after being burned trying to put out a fire in his closet, where he was playing with matches. What would be the priority nursing assessment for this child?

1. Level of pain
2. Airway patency
3. Psychosocial needs
4. Signs of infection

9 Intravenous (IV) morphine sulfate is ordered for a 13-year-old girl hospitalized with major burns to 30% of her body. A licensed practical nurse (LPN) asks the registered nurse (RN) why the morphine is given by the IV route when the child can talk and swallow. The RN should explain to the LPN that, when given by the IV route, morphine does which of the following?

1. Has a longer half-life
2. Has a predictable absorption rate
3. Prevents ileus
4. Leads to fewer side effects

10 The nurse is providing a teaching session for parents about over-the-counter treatment for head lice. Which of the following would the nurse mention as appropriate for treating this problem?

1. Neosporin
2. Mafenide (Sulfamylon)
3. Silver sulfadiazine (Silvadene)
4. Permethrin (Nix)

➤ *See pages 228–229 for Answers and Rationales.*

ANSWERS & RATIONALES

Pretest

1 **Answer: 3, 5** **Rationale:** Hot water can exacerbate symptoms of atopic dermatitis and increase pruritus. Tepid water feels more comfortable than cool water. Strong or harsh soaps and perfumed products could be irritating to the skin and should not be used. **Cognitive Level:** Applying **Client Need:** Safety and Infection Control **Integrated Process:** Teaching and Learning **Content Area:** Child Health **Strategy:** The wording of the question indicates that more than one option is correct. When you encounter similar options in such a question, they both would be either correct or incorrect. **Reference:** Ball, J., Bindler, R., & Cowen, K. (2010). *Child health nursing: Partnering with children and families* (2nd ed.). Upper Saddle River, NJ: Pearson Education, p. 1508.

2 **Answer: 2** **Rationale:** Impetigo remains contagious for 48 hours after antibiotics are begun. The presence or absence of crusts does not address the issue of contagion. **Cognitive Level:** Applying **Client Need:** Safety and Infection Control **Integrated Process:** Teaching and Learning **Content Area:** Child Health **Strategy:** With many infectious diseases, the client is not considered contagious after 48 hours of antibiotics. **Reference:** Ball, J., Bindler, R., & Cowen, K. (2010). *Child health nursing: Partnering with children and families* (2nd ed.). Upper Saddle River, NJ: Pearson Education, p. 1498.

3 **Answer: 3** **Rationale:** The characteristic appearance of *pediculosis capitis* (lice) is nits that adhere to the hair shaft about 1/4-inch from the scalp. They cannot be easily brushed off as dandruff. Scabies, eczema, and impetigo do not typically appear on the scalp and present as skin lesions elsewhere on the body. **Cognitive Level:** Analyzing **Client Need:** Physiological Adaptation **Integrated Process:** Nursing Process: Assessment **Content Area:** Child Health **Strategy:** The critical words are *dandruff* and *does not flake off easily*. Use this information and knowledge of the various integumentary problems listed to make a selection. **Reference:** Ball, J., Bindler, R., & Cowen, K. (2010). *Child health nursing: Partnering with children and families* (2nd ed.). Upper Saddle River, NJ: Pearson Education, p. 1515–1516.

4 **Answer: 4 Rationale:** The fluid shift that occurs in burns leads to edema, so the burned extremity should always be elevated above the level of the heart. Positioning the client flat in bed does not make use of gravity to reduce edema. An extremity that is in a dependent position is below heart level. While lying on the left side is of some help with a right leg burn, it does not provide the best elevation to reduce the risk of developing edema. **Cognitive Level:** Analyzing **Client Need:** Physiological Adaptation **Integrated Process:** Nursing Process: Implementation **Content Area:** Child Health **Strategy:** Note that two options are opposites, making one of them likely to be the correct answer. Use gravity as the method of making a final selection. **Reference:** Ball, J., Bindler, R., & Cowen, K. (2010). *Child health nursing: Partnering with children and families* (2nd ed.). Upper Saddle River, NJ: Pearson Education, p. 1533.

5 **Answer: 1 Rationale:** Atopic dermatitis in a young child tends to be characterized by dry, scaly crusts that are well circumscribed. Pruritus is always present. Pustules are filled with pus, and this is not characteristic of atopic dermatitis. Vesicles are fluid-filled areas beneath the skin and are not present with atopic dermatitis. Lichenification is the presence of thick, leathery skin that usually results from prolonged rubbing or scratching. **Cognitive Level:** Applying **Client Need:** Physiological Adaptation **Integrated Process:** Nursing Process: Assessment **Content Area:** Child Health **Strategy:** Eliminate any option that describes skin lesions that would not be dry and scaly. **Reference:** Ball, J., Bindler, R., & Cowen, K. (2010). *Child health nursing: Partnering with children and families* (2nd ed.). Upper Saddle River, NJ: Pearson Education, pp. 1504–1505.

6 **Answer: 3 Rationale:** About 60% of children with eczema have a family history of asthma or other allergy. Scabies is caused by contact with a mite; impetigo and cellulitis are bacterial infections. **Cognitive Level:** Applying **Client Need:** Health Promotion and Maintenance **Integrated Process:** Nursing Process: Assessment **Content Area:** Child Health **Strategy:** Note the name atopic dermatitis, and recall the term atopy refers to allergies. Because of this association, the nurse would look for evidence of other allergic disorders in this family history. **Reference:** Ball, J., Bindler, R., & Cowen, K. (2010). *Child health nursing: Partnering with children and families* (2nd ed.). Upper Saddle River, NJ: Pearson Education, p. 1504.

7 **Answer: 2 Rationale:** Sinusitis frequently precedes periorbital cellulitis. Epistaxis or nosebleeds is an unrelated concern. A dog bite could cause cellulitis anywhere. Sun exposure causes a thermal injury. **Cognitive Level:** Applying **Client Need:** Physiological Adaptation **Integrated Process:** Nursing Process: Assessment **Content Area:** Child Health **Strategy:** The suffix *-itis* refers to inflammation, which is often related to infection. Look for an option that suggests another infection in the general area. **Reference:** Ball, J., Bindler, R., & Cowen, K. (2010). *Child health nursing: Partnering with children and families* (2nd ed.). Upper Saddle River, NJ: Pearson Education, p. 1499.

8 **Answer: 1 Rationale:** The only way to eliminate the infectious agent is to complete the prescribed course of antibiotics. Strict bed rest for a prolonged period is not indicated, although the child initially may feel more comfortable resting with the extremity elevated. Fluid intake has no effect on the course of the infection. Cellulitis is not contagious; therefore, visitors do not have to be limited. **Cognitive Level:** Applying **Client Need:** Physiological Adaptation **Integrated Process:** Nursing Process: Planning **Content Area:** Child Health **Strategy:** Consider that any bacterial infection requires completion of the antibiotic therapy. **Reference:** Ball, J., Bindler, R., & Cowen, K. (2010). *Child health nursing: Partnering with children and families* (2nd ed.). Upper Saddle River, NJ: Pearson Education, p. 1499.

9 **Answer: 4 Rationale:** Lice are spread by sharing combs and hats. Only affected children require treatment. Close contact is required as the lice do not jump or fly. Lice are not transmitted via pets. **Cognitive Level:** Applying **Client Need:** Physiological Adaptation **Integrated Process:** Teaching and Learning **Content Area:** Child Health **Strategy:** Eliminate one option considering that healthy children are not treated. Recall how lice are spread to choose correctly from the remaining options. **Reference:** Ball, J., Bindler, R., & Cowen, K. (2010). *Child health nursing: Partnering with children and families* (2nd ed.). Upper Saddle River, NJ: Pearson Education, p. 1517.

10 **Answer: 4 Rationale:** Permethrin is applied to cool dry skin after a bath, but only from the neck down. The child may dress after the lotion is applied. It should be washed off after 8 to 12 hours. A second application is often prescribed for one week later. **Cognitive Level:** Applying **Client Need:** Pharmacological and Parenteral Therapies **Integrated Process:** Teaching and Learning **Content Area:** Child Health **Strategy:** Recall that scabies primarily occur where skin is in contact with skin. It is necessary to remember how long the medication must remain in contact with the skin. Since the scabies burrow into the skin, it would make sense that a longer contact time is needed for treatment. **Reference:** Ball, J., Bindler, R., & Cowen, K. (2010). *Child health nursing: Partnering with children and families* (2nd ed.). Upper Saddle River, NJ: Pearson Education, p. 1519.

ANSWERS & RATIONALES

Posttest

1 **Answer: 4** **Rationale:** Handwashing is always the most important action that a nurse can take to prevent the spread of infection. Merely applying ointment or covering the site does not address the spread of infection, nor does isolation of a child at home. The nurse would teach the family the importance of good handwashing. **Cognitive Level:** Applying **Client Need:** Safety and Infection Control **Integrated Process:** Nursing Process: Implementation **Content Area:** Child Health **Strategy:** Understanding the means of transmission is important in correctly responding to this question. Knowledge of impetigo and the prevention of the spread of infections will aid in choosing correctly. **Reference:** Ball, J., Bindler, R., & Cowen, K. (2010). *Child health nursing: Partnering with children and families* (2nd ed.). Upper Saddle River, NJ: Pearson Education, pp. 1497–1498.

2 **Answer: 2, 3, 4, 5** **Rationale:** Vacuuming floors and furniture may help to trap hair that contains live nits. Live nits can hatch up to 8 to 10 days later, so it is important to remove them from the environment. Each member of the family should be assessed so those infested can be treated. Dry cleaning is not necessary because home washing and drying on hot settings will be sufficient to kill lice and nits. Use of commercial sprays is not recommended. Sharing of hair care material can help to spread lice and should be avoided. Soaking combs in a Lysol or anti-lice shampoo mixture will kill lice or nits. **Cognitive Level:** Applying **Client Need:** Safety and Infection Control **Integrated Process:** Teaching and Learning **Content Area:** Child Health **Strategy:** Knowledge of the spread of lice and the home care necessary to prevent reinfestation is necessary to choose the correct answer. Identify those options that are absolutely incorrect first. Then consider the remaining options. **Reference:** Ball, J., Bindler, R., & Cowen, K. (2010). *Child health nursing: Partnering with children and families* (2nd ed.). Upper Saddle River, NJ: Pearson Education, p. 1518.

3 **Answer: 2** **Rationale:** The anticipated appearance of partial-thickness burns is bright red skin with blisters of varying sizes. A superficial burn typically only has pink or red skin. A full-thickness burn may be dark in color, from deep red to black. **Cognitive Level:** Analyzing **Client Need:** Physiological Adaptation **Integrated Process:** Nursing Process: Assessment **Content Area:** Child Health **Strategy:** Organize the options from the least serious burn injury to the most serious. Since partial thickness falls in the middle of the least serious to most serious, this should allow selection of the right option. **Reference:** Ball, J., Bindler, R., & Cowen, K. (2010). *Child health nursing: Partnering with children and families* (2nd ed.). Upper Saddle River, NJ: Pearson Education, p. 1526.

4 **Answer: 3** **Rationale:** An adolescent can and should be part of the treatment plan. If itching is avoided to prevent excoriation and secondary infection, scarring is unlikely. Improvement is often slow, and the problem may persist into adulthood. Food avoidance will not speed healing although it could prevent a flare if intake of a specific food is known to cause the flare. **Cognitive Level:** Applying **Client Need:** Physiological Adaptation **Integrated Process:** Teaching and Learning **Content Area:** Child Health **Strategy:** The core issue of this question is information to increase treatment compliance. Learning that scarring can be prevented will encourage compliance. **Reference:** Ball, J., Bindler, R., & Cowen, K. (2010). *Child health nursing: Partnering with children and families* (2nd ed.). Upper Saddle River, NJ: Pearson Education, pp. 1508–1509.

5 **Answer: 1** **Rationale:** A recent history of otitis media is often present in children with facial cellulitis. An insect or animal bite can be a cause of cellulitis, but in the case of cellulitis on the face the nurse would question a recent history of an ear infection first if a bite was not obvious. Sunburn would present as more diffuse and widespread redness. Dental caries are unrelated. **Cognitive Level:** Analyzing **Client Need:** Physiological Adaptation **Integrated Process:** Nursing Process: Assessment **Content Area:** Child Health **Strategy:** Knowledge of cellulitis and the etiology and pathophysiology of cellulitis will aid in answering the question. **Reference:** Ball, J., Bindler, R., & Cowen, K. (2010). *Child health nursing: Partnering with children and families* (2nd ed.). Upper Saddle River, NJ: Pearson Education, p. 1499.

6 **Answer: 2** **Rationale:** Lice can only be passed by direct contact because lice do not fly. The usual mode of transmission is sharing of hats, combs, brushes, or hair ornaments. Being close to someone in a classroom, bus, or car does not presuppose direct contact with hair or nits that have been shed on hair. **Cognitive Level:** Applying **Client Need:** Safety and Infection Control **Integrated Process:** Teaching and Learning **Content Area:** Child Health **Strategy:** Select the option that allows for direct contact. The incorrect options do not allow for direct contact of the infected individual or contact with the infected individual's belongings. **Reference:** Ball, J., Bindler, R., & Cowen, K. (2010). *Child health nursing: Partnering with children and families* (2nd ed.). Upper Saddle River, NJ: Pearson Education, p. 1516.

7 **Answer: 3** **Rationale:** Keeping the skin well hydrated will prevent the need to scratch dry skin that can lead to excoriation and secondary infection. Eczema is not infectious, nor is it managed by dietary restrictions. Pruritus, not pain, is associated with eczema. **Cognitive Level:** Analyzing **Client Need:** Physiological Adaptation **Integrated Process:** Nursing Process: Planning **Content Area:** Child Health **Strategy:** Consider the common symptoms of the disease to determine typical client goals. Determine that the correct answer must address the needs of the skin based on disease pathophysiology. **Reference:** Ball, J., Bindler, R., & Cowen, K. (2010). *Child health nursing: Partnering with children and families* (2nd ed.). Upper Saddle River, NJ: Pearson Education, pp. 1508–1509.

8 **Answer: 2** **Rationale:** Because he was in close proximity to the fire and tried to put it out, he is at risk of having inhaled smoke and, therefore, having a compromised airway. Other physiological signs will be of second highest priority, such as pain. Psychosocial concerns are addressed once physiological needs have been met. Infection would be a third priority since it would not happen immediately. **Cognitive Level:** Analyzing **Client Need:** Physiological Adaptation **Integrated Process:** Nursing Process: Assessment **Content Area:** Child Health **Strategy:** Recall that a patent airway is almost always the primary assessment. Assessing pain, psychosocial needs, or for infection occurs only after establishing airway patency. **Reference:** Ball, J., Bindler, R., & Cowen, K. (2010). *Child health nursing: Partnering with children and families* (2nd ed.). Upper Saddle River, NJ: Pearson Education, pp. 1532–1533.

9 **Answer: 2** **Rationale:** The predictable rate of absorption makes IV morphine useful in treating severe pain. As part of the physiological stress response, blood is shunted away from the gastrointestinal tract, making oral absorption rates less predictable. The half-life of the drug is not relevant to the question asked. The IV route will not prevent ileus. The IV route may actually have greater side effects because of rapid onset of action. **Cognitive Level:** Applying **Client Need:** Pharmacological and Parenteral Therapies **Integrated Process:** Communication and Documentation **Content Area:** Child Health **Strategy:** The core concept is the purpose for giving morphine by the IV route. Eliminate two options because they are false. Choose correctly from the remaining two because it directly addressed the purpose of this route. **Reference:** Ball, J., Bindler, R., & Cowen, K. (2010). *Child health nursing: Partnering with children and families* (2nd ed.). Upper Saddle River, NJ: Pearson Education, p. 538.

10 **Answer: 4** **Rationale:** Permethrin is the over-the-counter treatment of choice for head lice. Neosporin is a topical agent for infection. Mafenide would be used topically to treat burns. Silver sulfadiazine is a popular topical treatment for burns. **Cognitive Level:** Applying **Client Need:** Pharmacological and Parenteral Therapies **Integrated Process:** Teaching and Learning **Content Area:** Child Health **Strategy:** Note that three of the medications are antibacterial. The one that is different is the only medication listed for lice. **Reference:** Ball, J., Bindler, R., & Cowen, K. (2010). *Child health nursing: Partnering with children and families* (2nd ed.). Upper Saddle River, NJ: Pearson Education, p. 1517.

References

Adams, M., Holland, L., & Urban, C. (2011). *Pharmacology for nurses: A pathophysiological approach* (3rd ed.). Upper Saddle River, NJ: Pearson Education.

Ball, J., Bindler, R., & Cowen, K. (2012). *Principles of pediatric nursing: Caring for children* (5th ed.). Upper Saddle River, NJ: Pearson Education.

Ball, J., Bindler, R., & Cowen, K. (2010). *Child health nursing: Partnering with children and families* (2nd ed.). Upper Saddle River, NJ: Pearson Education.

Hockenberry, M., & Wilson, D. (2011). *Wong's essentials of pediatric nursing* (8th ed.). St. Louis, MO: Elsevier.

Hockenberry, M., & Wilson, D. (2011). *Wong's nursing care of infants and children* (9th ed.). St. Louis, MO: Elsevier.

London, M., Ladewig, P., Ball, J., Bindler, R., & Cowen, K. (2011). *Maternal & child nursing care* (3rd ed.). Upper Saddle River, NJ: Pearson Education.

Perry, S., Hockenberry, M., Lowdermilk, D., & Wilson, D. (2010). *Maternal child nursing care* (4th ed.). St. Louis, MO: Elsevier.

Pillitteri, A. (2009). *Maternal and child health nursing: Care of the childbearing and childrearing family* (6th ed.). Philadelphia: Lippincott Williams & Wilkins.

ANSWERS & RATIONALES

Chapter Outline

Overview of Anatomy and
Physiology of Immune
System

Diagnostic Tests and
Assessments of Immune
System

Common Nursing Techniques
and Procedures for Immune
System

Congenital Immunologic
Health Problems

Acquired Immunologic Health
Problems

Infectious Immunologic Health
Problems

NCLEX-RN® Test Prep

Use the accompanying online resource,
NursingReviewsandRationales, to test
yourself with hundreds of NCLEX®-style
practice questions.

Objectives

➤ Identify data essential to the assessment of alterations in health of
the immunologic system in a child.

➤ Discuss the clinical manifestations and pathophysiology of
alterations in health of the immunologic system of a child.

➤ Discuss therapeutic management of a child with alterations in
health of the immunologic system.

➤ Describe nursing management of a child with alterations in health
of the immunologic system.

Review at a Glance

anaphylaxis a severe, potentially
fatal hypersensitivity reaction; histamine
is released and leads to respiratory and
vascular changes

antigen a substance that possesses a
unique configuration enabling immune
system to recognize it as foreign; any
substance that causes production of antibodies; antigens are usually large
molecular-weight proteins

antigen-antibody reaction
attachment of an antibody to an antigen
that forms the basis for B-cell-mediated
immunity

antibody a protein produced by
immune system that binds to
specific antigens and eliminates them
from body

autoimmune disease a disease
process where body identifies itself or a
component of itself as foreign and
attacks itself

differential blood count a blood
test that indicates percentages of different
types of white cells present in blood and is
sometimes useful in identifying cause of
an illness

incubation period time between
exposure to an antigen (bacterial or viral
organism) and formation of first general
symptoms of disease

immunity resistance of body to
effects of a harmful organism or its toxin

immunization process of introducing
an antigen into body, allowing immunity
against a disease to develop naturally

period of communicability
period of time when an illness is directly
or indirectly transmittable from one person to another

prodromal period period of time
between initial symptoms and presence
of full-blown disease

sepsis a generalized infection spread
throughout body through blood stream

TORCH an acronym for a complex of
communicable diseases often present at
birth; it stands for T = toxoplasmosis;
O = other (such as syphilis, hepatitis);
R = rubella; C = cytomegalovirus; H = herpes
simplex; this group of viruses can cause
teratogenic effects to unborn fetus

vaccine specific medication given to
stimulate an immune response

PRETEST

1 A 14-year-old client is receiving intravenous antibiotics for an infection. The physician has ordered gentamycin (Garamycin). Because of the side effects of this drug, what would the nurse need to monitor?

1. Temperature
2. Blood pressure
3. Intake and output
4. Breath sounds

2 A 3-year-old client is admitted to the hospital to rule out an infection. Which diagnostic test does the nurse anticipate being ordered that is likely to differentiate an infection from an allergic response?

1. Hemoglobin and hematocrit
2. Red blood cell count
3. White blood cell differential
4. Platelet agglutinization

3 A 2-year-old client has eczema that causes extreme itching. Treatment has not been able to control the rash. It has been determined that the primary allergen is wheat. What would be an appropriate nursing diagnosis?

1. Risk for Infection
2. Imbalanced Nutrition: More Than Body Requirements
3. Ineffective Infant Feeding Behavior
4. Noncompliance

4 A client's mother tells the nurse that her child has been taking prescribed corticosteroids for several months. The nurse considers that which of the following vaccines is contraindicated?

1. Tetanus toxoid
2. Recombinant hepatitis B vaccine
3. Poliovirus vaccine inactivated
4. Rotavirus vaccine

5 A client with severe combined immunodeficiency disorder (SCID) is being discharged from the hospital to home. Client teaching is important to reach client goals. What would an appropriate goal be for the client before and after discharge?

1. Remains well oxygenated
2. Remains free of signs of infection
3. Maintains hydration
4. Avoids contact with other people

6 A client has had several allergic reactions and is to have allergy testing. The nurse would recognize which allergy test that would offer the least risk of anaphylaxis for this client?

1. Prick test
2. RAST test
3. Patch test
4. Intradermal test

7 An infant is born with microcephaly. Part of the infant's assessment includes a TORCH test. In providing client education, the nurse explains to the mother that the TORCH test will assess for which of the following?

1. Presence of the TORCH virus
2. Complications of pregnancy
3. Presence of one or more specific viruses
4. Evidence of thalidomide poisoning

8 A mother tells a nurse she has heard about active and passive immunity and asks how her child can get active immunity to a disease. The nurse would answer that active immunity can be acquired in which way? Select all that apply.

1. From mother while pregnant
2. By having the disease
3. By vaccination with a toxoid
4. Through administration of IVIG
5. By administration of serum

9 A 12-year-old client with positive human immunodeficiency virus (HIV) antibodies is going home from the hospital. Which of the following would be the most important instruction at discharge?

1. Growth and developmental milestones
2. Immunization schedules
3. Lab studies and results
4. Prevention of the spread of HIV

10 A 4-year-old client has been exposed to chickenpox. After the nurse has provided information about chickenpox, the nurse asks the mother to repeat the information. Which statement by the mother indicates a need for additional information?

1. "During the prodromal period, my child will have pox all over his body."
2. "Chickenpox is a viral infection that can be spread to other children."
3. "I should monitor my child for Reye syndrome, which is a complication of chickenpox."
4. "My child should not visit my pregnant sister at this time."

➤ *See pages 245–247 for Answers and Rationales.*

I. OVERVIEW OF ANATOMY AND PHYSIOLOGY OF IMMUNE SYSTEM

A. Nonspecific *immunity* (resistance of body to a harmful organism)
1. Functional at birth
2. First line of defense
3. Reacts similarly to all invaders
4. Includes phagocytosis of foreign material by white blood cells (WBCs)
   a. Polymorphonuclear leukocytes or granulocytes, which include basophils, eosinophils, and neutrophils, are the most common type of WBCs and are involved in acute inflammatory process
   b. Monocytes migrate to tissues where they become macrophages and have great phagocytic ability, functioning to eliminate foreign invaders and other material
   c. Lymphocytes include B lymphocytes (B cells) and T lymphocytes (T cells), which are responsible for specific immune response as well as NK cells (Natural Killer cells) concerned with viral control as well as autoimmune responses
5. "Inflammatory response" is a nonspecific response to any tissue injury aimed at maintaining homeostasis; chemicals are released from injured cells, which cause blood vessels to dilate, bringing large numbers of neutrophils and macrophages to area for phagocytosis of injured cells and foreign material, allowing healing to occur

B. Specific immune response
1. Second line of defense
2. Not functional at birth, must be learned by body
3. Not fully functional until a child is 6 years old
4. Humoral immunity depends upon antibody-producing abilities of B cells
   a. In response to **antigens** (foreign substances that trigger an immune response), B cells convert into plasma cells and secrete specific **antibodies** (immune system proteins) to assist body in eliminating foreign proteins
   b. Five classes of antibodies with different functions
      1) IgG is antibacterial and antiviral antibody found in large quantities in all body fluids; this antibody can cross placenta; maternal IgG provides passive immunity for first 6 months of infant's life
      2) IgA is found in saliva, tears, bronchial secretions, mucous secretions of small intestine, vagina, and in breast milk; IgA is not present at birth and reaches normal levels at 6 to 7 years of age
      3) IgM is body's primary antibody response to an antigen; IgM levels are low at birth and reach adult levels by 1 year of age
      4) IgD's role is unknown but seems to be related to B cell differentiation
      5) IgE is normally found in very small amounts and is associated with allergic reactions; elevated levels of IgE are found in individuals with an allergy and clients infected with intestinal parasites; IgE is not present at birth

Practice to Pass

Compare and contrast nonspecific immunity and specific immunity.

5. Cellular response
   a. T cells are produced in thymus and function to protect individual from intracellular organisms, viruses, and slow-growing bacteria
   b. Responsible for rejection of foreign grafts
   c. Specialized types of T cells include killer T cells, suppressor T cells, and helper T cells
   d. Killer T cells kill virus infected cells and depend upon IgG being bound to cell
   e. Suppressor T cells inhibit activities of other T and B cells
   f. Helper T cells help regulate actions of B cells
6. Complement
   a. Enzyme that responds to **antigen-antibody reactions** causing inflammation and destruction of foreign cells
   b. Plays a role in **autoimmune diseases** (body attacks itself)
   c. Levels of proteins lower in newborns than older children and adults

II. DIAGNOSTIC TESTS AND ASSESSMENTS OF IMMUNE SYSTEM

A. **Bone marrow aspiration**: fluid-containing bone marrow cells are aspirated from iliac crest to provide information about hematologic and immunologic disorders
   1. Usually performed under local anesthesia
   2. Postprocedure complications include bleeding and infection
B. **White blood cell differentials (differential blood count)**
   1. There are five types of white blood cells, which include neutrophils, eosinophils, basophils and monocytes, and lymphocytes; see Table 11-1
   2. Values or amounts for each type are reported as percentages of total, thus as one cell type increases in number, other cell types decrease in number
   3. Determining types of WBCs present can help to diagnose type of infection
      a. Neutrophils rise in response to inflammation, acute bacterial infections, and a few malignancies; neutrophils can be further divided into segmented neutrophils (segs), which are mature, and bands (which are immature neutrophils); bands rise when the body is attempting to produce many neutrophils quickly
      b. Elevations in eosinophils are associated with allergies and parasitic infections as well as skin diseases such as eczema and psoriasis
      c. Basophil counts may rise in response to chronic infection and stress; these WBCs contribute to inflammatory process and allergic reactions because they store histamine
      d. Monocytes are active in chronic infection
      e. Lymphocytes are increased in several infections

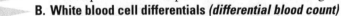

Table 11-1 White Blood Cell Differentials

Test and Type of Cell Evaluated	Action	Implication of Increased or Decreased Levels
Neutrophil (54–62%)	Phagocytic cell that defends against bacteria	↑ in bacterial infection, inflammatory processes, some malignancies
Eosinophil (1–3%)	Associated with antigen-antibody reaction	↑ in allergic reaction; ↓ in children receiving corticosteroids
Basophils (0–3%)	Phagocytic cell; involved in immediate hypersensitivity reaction; stores histamine and has receptor sites for IgE	↑ in leukemia; ↓ in allergy, acute infection, collagen and chronic diseases
Monocytes (4–9%)	Phagocytic cell active in chronic infection	↑ in tuberculosis, protozoan infection, monocytic leukemia
Lymphocytes (T, B, non-B/non-T [NK]) (25–33%)	Major components of immune system	↑ in many infections; ↓ in children with immune deficiency

Source: London, Marcia L,; Ladewig, Patricia W.; Ball, Jane W.; Bindler, Ruth C.; Cowen, Kay J., *Maternal & child nursing care*, 3rd Ed., ©2011. Reprinted and Electronically reproduced by permission of Pearson Education, Inc. Upper Saddle River, NJ.

Practice to Pass

Describe the preparation of the client needed prior to bone marrow aspiration, WBC and differential, and allergy testing.

C. Allergy testing

1. Determines reactions to specific antigens
2. Four types of tests available; stop antihistamines three days prior to skin tests
   a. Scratch tests can test many antigens at once; although less sensitive than other allergy tests, results can be obtained in about 30 minutes
   b. Patch test is a painless method that involves placing suspected allergen on a gauze pad and taping it to skin for a period of 24 to 48 hours
   c. Intradermal testing injects antigen into dermis; reactions are noted by redness and swelling

   d. Radioallergosorbent testing (RAST) looks for allergen-specific IgE antibodies in a blood sample; it is no more sensitive than other methods but does not involve risk of **anaphylaxis** or other allergic reactions

III. COMMON NURSING TECHNIQUES AND PROCEDURES FOR IMMUNE SYSTEM

A. Immunity from disease can be acquired either from exposure to disease or by **immunization** (introducing an antigen into body)

1. Active immunity involves body's formation of antibodies in response to exposure to an antigen
2. Passive immunity is temporary immunity achieved by administration of antibodies produced by another individual; when antibodies pass from mother to the fetus, passive immunity is acquired

B. Vaccines contain antigens to specific diseases; they cause body to respond with development of antibodies and active immunity

1. Vaccines may contain killed virus, live virus, or toxoids; live vaccines have weakened virus but still carry risk of infection; killed virus and toxoid vaccines do not carry this risk; live vaccines should be avoided in immunocompromised or pregnant client
2. Infant/child vaccinations are currently recommended to prevent infections with hepatitis A and B, rotovirus, *meningococcus*, *pneumococcus*, diphtheria, tetanus, pertussis, *hemophilus influenzae B*, *poliovirus*, influenza, measles, mumps, rubella, and varicella
3. Older child/adolescent vaccines include human papillomavirus (HPV), MCV-4
4. Vaccination schedules allow initial vaccination to occur after passive immunity from mother has disappeared; some vaccinations do not provide lifelong immunity and should be repeated

Practice to Pass

How does the nurse ensure practicing according to the current vaccine recommendations?

5. The American Academy of Pediatrics (AAP) and Centers for Disease Control and Prevention (CDC) provide current recommendations on vaccination schedule (see Chapter 1)
6. Prior to administering vaccinations, verify absence of allergic reaction history
7. Instruct parents to maintain vaccination schedule; if vaccinations are delayed, follow recommendations outlined for completing vaccination program

IV. CONGENITAL IMMUNOLOGIC HEALTH PROBLEMS

A. Severe combined immunodeficiency disease

1. Description
   a. Severe combined immunodeficiency disease (SCID) is most severe of several different congenital disorders of immune system yielding susceptibility to infections
   b. Other forms of immunodeficiency include B cell and T cell deficiencies
2. Etiology and pathophysiology
   a. SCID occurs as a result of X-linked recessive or autosomal recessive inheritance, as well as because of a spontaneous mutation
   b. Characterized by absence of both humoral and cellular immunity

    c. Maternal antibodies may protect infant for a short period of time, but chronic infections become apparent around 3 months of age

    d. Death usually occurs within first 2 years of life

3. Assessment

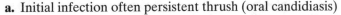

    a. Initial infection often persistent thrush (oral candidiasis)

    b. Followed by chronic infections

    c. Organisms causing infection may include cytomegalovirus and *Pneumocystis carinii*

    d. Failure to thrive also accompanies diagnosis

    e. Leukocyte counts are usually reduced

4. Priority nursing diagnoses

    a. Risk for Infection related to immunodeficiency

    b. Delayed Growth and Development

    c. Imbalanced Nutrition: Less Than Body Requirements

    d. Risk for Ineffective Coping

5. Planning and implementation

    a. Protecting child from infection is of primary importance; careful hand hygiene is essential, as well as preventing contact with infected individuals

    b. Live plants and fresh flowers should be avoided as they harbor mold and bacteria

    c. While hospitalized, care should be taken in planning room assignment to reduce exposure to infection

    d. Bone marrow transplant offers best hope for survival

6. Medication therapy

    a. Intravenous immune globulin (IVIG) (see Box 11-1)

Box 11-1	**General Information and Use**
Nursing Considerations for Administration of Intravenous Immune Globulin (IVIG)	• Intravenous globulin is prepared from pools of multiple samples of human plasma and contains globulin (primarily IgG). • It is used in idiopathic thrombocytopenic purpura, Kawasaki disease, HIV infection, and other disorders. • Specific types of immune globulin are administered intramuscularly and are effective against specific diseases such as hepatitis A and B and varicella.

Side Effects

- Local inflammatory reaction includes malaise, fever, nausea, vomiting, arthralgia.
- Hypersensitivity reaction is manifested by fever, chills, anaphylactic shock.
- Infusion reaction is associated with nausea, flushing, chills, headache, difficulty breathing, pain in back or abdomen.

Nursing Implications

- Have emergency drugs and equipment readily available to treat hypersensitivity reaction or infusion reaction.
- Child may be treated with antipyretic or antihistamine before the infusion.
- Follow manufacturer directions for reconstitution, dilution, and intravenous infusion rates. Do not mix with other medications for infusion.
- Monitor vital signs throughout infusion. Stop infusion immediately and notify physician for any signs of hypersensitivity.
- Activate emergency system as needed.
- Have family instruct health care providers about IVIG therapy because immunization recommendations will be altered.

Source: Bindler, Ruth C.; Ball, Jane W.; Cowen, Kay J., *Clinical handbook for child health nursing: Partnering with children and families*, 2nd Ed., ©2010. Reprinted and Electronically reproduced by permission of Pearson Education, Inc. Upper Saddle River, NJ.

> **b.** Immunizations should be administered 14 days prior to or 3 months after IVIG administration
>
> **c.** Antibiotic therapy when indicated; monitor for overgrowth of nonsusceptible organisms
>
> **d.** Maintain intact skin and mucous membranes

7. Client and family education

a. Teach family ways to protect child from infection

b. Provide emotional support and support group referrals

c. Genetic counseling provides family with information about transmission

8. Evaluation: client remains free of infection; family demonstrates appropriate coping methods related to diagnosis and prognosis

V. ACQUIRED IMMUNOLOGIC HEALTH PROBLEMS

A. Allergies

1. Description

a. Hypersensitivity to a foreign protein

b. Antigen-antibody reaction causes release of histamine and other chemicals into body; chemicals are responsible for allergic symptoms

c. Broad group of disorders; symptoms vary dependent on body cell that has been sensitized

2. Etiology and pathophysiology

a. First exposure to antigen causes production of antibodies (usually IgE)

b. Subsequent exposure to same antigen causes an antigen–antibody reaction with cell damage causing release of histamine and other chemicals

c. Chemicals travel through bloodstream causing allergic symptoms

d. Most allergens are large molecular weight proteins

1) Common inhalant allergens include mold, pollen, house dust, and pet dander

2) Common food allergens include cow's milk, eggs, wheat, chocolate, citrus fruits

3) Common drug allergies can include oral and injectable medications

4) Animal serum/venom and insect stings may be allergens

5) Contact allergens include plants, dyes, and chemicals

3. Assessment

a. Family history of allergies

b. History of reactions: allergy symptoms can be numerous

1) Respiratory system: allergic rhinitis, asthma, serous otitis media, allergic croup

2) Skin: eczema, atopic dermatitis, angioedema, urticaria

3) Gastrointestinal system: diarrhea, constipation, colic

4) Neurologic system: headache, tension-fatigue, convulsions

5) Genitourinary system: dysuria, enuresis

6) Miscellaneous: serum sickness and anaphylaxis

c. Elevated eosinophil counts

d. Allergy testing: Skin or RAST test

1) Skin testing can involve a scratch or intradermal injection of small amounts of suspected allergens; scratch test is often an initial diagnostic tool as it allows for testing a large number of allergens quickly with results in about 30 minutes; if the child is allergic to allergen, a reddened wheal will form in 15 to 30 minutes; anaphylaxis is a rare but potential problem

2) The RAST test is a blood test looking for the specific IgE antibodies; used in individuals who have a history of a strong reaction, as this test allows no opportunity for anaphylaxis during testing; it is more expensive and felt to be less sensitive

4. Priority nursing diagnoses
   a. Risk for Injury
   b. Risk for Shock
   c. Impaired Skin Integrity
   d. Diarrhea
   e. Deficient Knowledge, Parental (reduction of allergen exposure)
5. Planning and implementation
   a. Interventions are aimed at reducing exposure to allergen
      1) Food: once food allergens are identified, read all labels of prepared food carefully to avoid allergens
      2) Environment: create surface that is easily cleaned; focus in particular on child's bedroom; no carpet, bedroom curtains and bedding should be washable; avoid dust-collecting items in bedroom; avoid live plants and flowers; keep animals out of bedroom; no stuffed toys in bedroom
      3) Inhalant: avoid cigarette smoking in child's presence and environment
   b. Immunotherapy aims at increasing child's tolerance of allergen; also called hyposensitization or allergy shots, this therapy provides for introduction of the allergen in small but increasing amounts by subcutaneous injections
      1) Injections are given in controlled environment because of risk of systemic reaction or anaphylaxis
      2) Keep child in controlled environment for 15 minutes postinjection to allow for monitoring of side effects
      3) Emergency treatment must be readily available in case anaphylaxis occurs
6. Medication therapy
   a. Antihistamines are given prior to or early in reactive phase; antihistamines compete with histamine on receptor sites, therefore will be ineffective if given late in reaction
   b. Bronchodilators may be given for lower respiratory symptoms
   c. Corticosteroids may be administered systemically or topically, depending upon symptoms
   d. Epinephrine is administered for anaphylaxis (Epi-Pen Junior for up to 65 pounds and Epi-Pen Adult if over 65 pounds)
7. Client and family education
   a. Teach parents and child to manage symptoms, control environmental exposure, and recognize medical emergencies
   b. Obtain medic alert bracelets, especially for drug allergies
   c. Safe administration of medications
8. Evaluation: child and parents verbalize medication understanding, demonstrate their use correctly, and verbalize environmental control of allergens

Practice to Pass

When a child develops an allergy, what kinds of life changes may need to be made?

VI. INFECTIOUS IMMUNOLOGIC HEALTH PROBLEMS

A. TORCH

1. Description
   a. **TORCH** is an acronym for a group of infections, which when acquired in utero, cause teratogenesis (fetal harm)
      1) T is for toxoplasmosis: toxoplasmosis is an infectious disease caused by organism *Toxoplasma gondii* and is usually contracted from cat feces and undercooked meats
      2) O is for other, which includes syphilis and hepatitis; congenital syphilis is caused by spirochete *Treponema pallidum*
      3) R stands for rubella; also called German measles

        4) C refers to cytomegalovirus or CMV, a member of herpes family

        5) H is for herpes simplex virus

  2. Etiology and pathophysiology

    a. Maternal exposure to organism allows fetal exposure through placenta

    b. The earlier in gestation that infection occurs, the greater the damage that may occur

    c. Mother may be asymptomatic during pregnancy and syndrome may not be recognized until after the baby is born

  3. Assessment

    a. Assessment of newborn is comprehensive, reviewing all systems

    b. Maternal history during pregnancy

    c. Intrauterine growth retardation may be apparent at birth

    d. Symptoms including hydrocephalus, blindness, microcephaly, mental retardation, as well as failure to thrive, suggest TORCH infection; depending upon organism involved, infant may also display jaundice, rash, deafness, cardiac defects

    e. Serologic blood sampling for toxoplasmosis, rubella, CMV, and herpes; VDRL for syphilis and a hepatitis profile

  4. Priority nursing diagnoses

    a. Imbalanced Nutrition: Less Than Body Requirements

    b. Risk for Impaired Parent Attachment

    c. Risk for Delayed Development

  5. Planning and implementation

    a. Isolate child as virus may be shed for up to a year after birth; pregnant women are at increased risk

    b. Parents may grieve at loss of normal newborn; emotional support must be available

    c. Physical care supporting infant's needs will be individualized

    d. Nutritional support will be needed to support intake of food; child may require a nasogastric or gastric tube or utilize a "preemie" nipple to make sucking easier

  6. Medication therapy

    a. Depends upon infectious organism

    b. For toxoplasmosis, an extended course of pyrimethamine (Daraprim) and sulfadiazine (generic) may be given; folic acid supplement will be used to prevent anemia

    c. Treatment for congenital syphilis is usually a 10- to 14-day course of penicillin

    d. Acyclovir (Zovirax) is used to treat infants with congenital herpes infection

  7. Client and family education

    a. Parents are educated to meet the physical needs of their handicapped infant; nutrition support is of primary importance

    b. Infant stimulation to promote physical development of child; special instructions need to be given to assist parents working with blind or deaf child

    c. Instructions must be given about potential viral shedding; parents are instructed to avoid contact with pregnant women

  8. Evaluation: parents verbalize and demonstrate appropriate child care measures including nutritional support; parents express confidence in their ability to care for their child; parents demonstrate safe medication administration

B. Sepsis

  1. Description: **sepsis** is systemic bacterial infection spread through bloodstream

  2. Etiology and pathophysiology

    a. Neonates are at high risk because of inability to localize an infectious organism; prematurity and low birth weight is a risk factor for sepsis

    b. Immunocompromised children at high risk

    c. Children with skin defects/injuries or with invasive devices at high risk

    d. Organisms involved include *Escherichia coli*, pseudomonas, enterococcus, staphylococcus

3. Assessment
   a. Monitor clients for risk factors for sepsis
   b. Hypothermia or hyperthermia
   c. Lethargy, poor feeding
   d. Jaundice or hepatosplenomegaly
   e. Respiratory distress
   f. Vomiting
   g. Hypoglycemia or hyperglycemia, metabolic acidosis
   h. CBC will indicate infection; blood culture will determine organism and sensitivities; spinal tap may be done to rule out meningitis
4. Priority nursing diagnoses
   a. Hypothermia
   b. Hyperthermia
   c. Ineffective Infant Feeding Pattern
5. Planning and implementation
   a. Maintain temperature within normal range with antipyretics as ordered, tepid sponge bath, appropriate clothing
   b. Monitor blood glucose; support nutrition; lethargy, hypoglycemia, and hyperthermia can all contribute to poor feeding
   c. Maintain antibiotic therapy on schedule, monitor for side effects
6. Medication therapy
   a. Antibiotic therapy based on culture and sensitivity
   b. Antipyretics such as acetaminophen (Tylenol) for elevated temperature
7. Client and family education
   a. Teach parents how to monitor temperature and means of maintaining a neutral body temperature
   b. Instruct parents on purpose of antibiotics and potential side effects
8. Evaluation: harmful sequelae of sepsis will be prevented; parents are able to describe purpose of antibiotics and identify side effects for which child is being monitored

C. **Acquired immunodeficiency syndrome (AIDS)**
1. Description: results from infection with retrovirus human immunodeficiency virus (HIV)
2. Etiology and pathophysiology
   a. Virus transmitted through blood and body fluids of infected person
   b. Most common source of infection in children is perinatally, from an infected mother to her infant
      1) Across placenta
      2) At time of birth
      3) Possibly through breast milk
   c. Also could be contracted from transfusions with infected blood or blood products
   d. Once in body, HIV enters T lymphocytes, particularly CD4 cell
   e. CD4 cell begins synthesis of HIV DNA
   f. Leads to death of CD4 cell
   g. Infected child is susceptible to infection caused by deficiency in cell-mediated and humoral immunity
3. Assessment
   a. Diagnostic tests for HIV start at birth; child of HIV-positive mother is followed up to 18 months before infection can be determined; tests are divided into early (birth, 3, and 6 months) and later (12, 15, and 18 months)
   b. Early tests include HIV antigen (p24 antigen), HIV (HIV culture and polymerase chain reaction [PCR])
   c. After maternal antibodies have disappeared, ELISA (enzyme-linked immunosorbent assay) test is done
   d. CBC and CD4 levels

    e. Presenting symptoms include chronic diarrhea, failure to thrive, delayed development

    f. Frequent infections including candidiasis, *Streptococcus pneumoniae*, *Hemophilus influenzae*, *Staphylococcus aureus*, and herpes simplex

    g. Opportunistic infections including *pneumocystis carinii*

4. Priority nursing diagnoses

    a. Risk for Infection related to immunosuppression secondary to HIV infection

    b. Imbalanced Nutrition: Less Than Body Requirements

    c. Risk for Impaired Parental Attachment

5. Planning and implementation

    a. Focus on preventing infection

        1) Normal health precautions include hand hygiene, avoiding contact with infected persons, maintaining nutritional status, good skin care, promoting a hygienic environment

        2) Give immunizations on schedule; child may be given live virus vaccines if CD4 count is adequate

        3) Follow medical orders regarding prophylactic drugs

    b. Management of symptoms

        1) Diarrhea management, monitoring hydration and nutrition status, maintaining skin integrity

        2) Monitoring for infection including pneumonia, meningitis, otitis media, and others

        3) Support of family coping

            a) Encourage participation in parent support groups

            b) Demonstrate acceptance of child during everyday contact

            c) Utilize communication skills to allow parents to verbalize feelings

6. Medication therapy

    a. Prophylaxis treatment

        1) Against HIV: zidovudine (AZT)

        2) Against *pneumocystis carinii*: trimethoprim-sulfamethoxazole (Bactrim or Septra)

        3) Against bacterial infections: intravenous immune globulin (IVIG)

    b. Infections: appropriate antimicrobial therapy; for antibiotic therapy, see Table 11-2

7. Client and family education

    a. Information is presented on preventing spread of HIV to other members of household and those having contact with child

    b. Parents are taught to maintain a clean home environment and ways to reduce bacterial exposure

    c. Information about nutritional support, diarrhea, and skin management as well as medication regimen is given

    d. Developmental stimulation information is shared with parents

    e. Infection monitoring information is given to parents

8. Evaluation: parents verbalize medication regimen, describe safety measures to prevent infection, identify symptoms of infection to be reported to physician, discuss their concerns about caring for this child, and join a support group

D. Childhood communicable diseases

  1. Description: a group of diseases common during childhood

  2. Etiology and pathophysiology

    a. Variety of diseases spread from person to person

    b. Infectious organism often viral

    c. Mode of transmission describes how organism moves from one individual to another

    d. Incubation period describes time between exposure to disease and disease outbreak; during this time, child may be contagious

    e. Period of communicability is time period when organism can move from host to another individual

Table 11-2 Antibiotic Therapy

Classification and Examples	Mechanism	Common Side Effects	Nursing Responsibilities & Additional Comments
Penicillins Four generations including natural penicillins (Penicillin G, Pen Vee K); Penicillinase resistant (Methicillin, Dynapen); Extended spectrum (Ampicillin, Amoxicillin); and Antipseudomonal (Ticar, Pipracil)	Inhibits cell wall synthesis; indicated for Gram-positive and Gram-negative infections	Allergic—rash, anaphylaxis; loss of normal flora—black, furry tongue, diarrhea; hematologic—hemolytic anemia or leukopenia; electrolyte imbalances	First antibiotic; first cases of antibiotic resistance occurred when bacteria began forming penicillinase, which deactivates penicillin
Cephalosporins (Keflin, Ancef, Ceclor, Mandol)	Prevents production of enzymes which make cell wall rigid; use for Gram-positive and Gram-negative infections	Allergy; may be neurotoxic and cause seizures in clients with preexisting renal disease	Use caution, many cephalosporins have similar names (keflex, keflin; cefoxitin sodium, ceftizoxime sodium) but are not the same drug or generation of cephalosporin
Aminoglycosides (Neomycin, Kanamycin, Gentamicin)	Gram-negative infections	Ototoxicity; nephrotoxicity	Not absorbed well through the GI tract, usually administered IM or IV; contraindicated with renal impairment or hearing disorders; peak and trough levels are usually ordered to monitor for toxicity; when concomitantly administered with penicillin, separate by time and use separate IV lines
Vancomycin (Vancocin)	Inhibits cell wall synthesis; used for Gram-positive infection, staphylococcus and *clostridium difficile*	Ototoxicity, nephrotoxicity, hypotension (red man syndrome)	Not given IM; give IV slowly to prevent hypotension and "red man syndrome"; if hypotension occurs, stop drug and notify MD; after administration of antihistamine, may slowly restart drug
Macrolides (Erythromycin)	Bacteriostatic; use is similar to narrow-spectrum penicillin	Hepatotoxicity, ototoxicity, phlebitis	CDC has reported a possible link between erythromycin and pyloric stenosis; monitor infant for symptoms; inhibits metabolism of theophyllin—may lead to theophyllin toxicity
Quinolones (Cipro, Floxin)	Broad-spectrum; soft-tissue infections	Nausea, headache, dizziness, confusion	Cautious use with clients under 17; interferes with theophyllin and coumadin
Streptogramins (Synercid)	One of two new classes of antibiotics; bacteriostatic; effective against methicillin and vancomycin-resistant organisms	Thrombophlebitis, rash, arthralgia, elevated bilirubin levels	Incompatible with saline and heparin flush solutions—flush with D5W; use with caution in clients with liver disease
Oxazolidinone (Zyvox)	Newer class of antibiotics; indicated for vancomycin- and methicillin-resistant organisms	Thrombocytopenia	Assess for signs of bleeding; monitor platelet count as ordered

(continued)

Table 11-2   **Antibiotic Therapy (Continued)**

Classification and Examples	Mechanism	Common Side Effects	Nursing Responsibilities & Additional Comments
Sulfonamides (Gantrisin, Bactrim, Septra)	Deprive bacteria of folate products used in protein synthesis	Allergic rash, Stevens-Johnson syndrome, crystalluria	Not recommended for children under two months of age (elevated bilirubin)
Lipopeptides (Cubicin)	Inhibits protein, DNA, and RNA synthesis	GI disturbances, Bell's palsy	Released in 2003; indicated for severe skin infections caused by resistant organisms; measure creatine phosphokinase weekly
Tetracyclines (Vibramycin, terramycin)	Inhibit protein synthesis	Increased skin sensititivity to sunlight	Teratogenic; causes discoloration of developing teeth
Tigecycline (Tygacil)	Derived from and similar activity to tetracyclines	N & V, *clostridium difficile* pseudomembraneous colitis	Not recommended for children under 18; similar nursing implications to tetracyclines

3. Assessment
   a. Nurses in contact with children should be constantly alert to appearance of symptoms associated with childhood diseases and take measures to prevent spread of infection to other children
   b. Client history will include record of vaccinations as well as history of exposure to children with communicable diseases
   c. Regardless of reason child is seeking treatment, assess all children for symptoms of communicable diseases including rashes, temperature, and swollen glands
   d. Period of time between initial symptoms and presence of full-blown disease is called **prodromal period**
4. Priority nursing diagnoses
   a. Hyperthermia
   b. Risk for Injury secondary to complications of childhood diseases
   c. Disturbed Body Image
   d. Risk for Impaired Skin Integrity related to scratching secondary to itch
   e. Social Isolation
5. Planning and implementation
   a. Immediate steps are taken to reduce exposure of other children to the possibly infected child
   b. Monitor temperature and use temperature control measures to reduce hyperthermia
      1) Tepid baths
      2) Limit clothing and bed coverings
      3) Give NSAIDs as ordered; avoid aspirin as aspirin intake with a viral infection may contribute to development of Reye syndrome
      4) Increase liquid intake
   c. Provide skin care to prevent breakdown
      1) If child is scratching, keep nails short, and use topical anti-itch medications
      2) If skin is intact but dry, apply moisturizers
   d. Bedrest is usually recommended during prodromal and/or febrile phases of the infectious diseases
      1) Provide activities that allow quiet play
      2) Activities that include socialization are preferred over solo activities
   e. Monitor child for signs of complications of specific illness (see Table 11-3)

Table 11-3 **Childhood Communicable Diseases**

Disease Information	Clinical Manifestations	Clinical Management	Potential Complication
Rubeola: Red measles *Causal agent*: Virus *Transmission*: Direct or indirect contact with droplets *Incubation*: 10–20 days *Communicability*: Several days before rash appearance to 5 days after rash appearance *Immunity*: From vaccination or disease	*Prodromal*: Fever and lethargy, cough, and coryza; photophobia; koplik spots on buccal mucosa *Acute*: Red, flat rash (lasting about a week) begins behind ears, spreads to face, trunk, and extremities	Manage temperature, keep room dim, vaporizer may improve respiratory secretions	Pneumonia: monitor lung sounds; otitis media: monitor ear pain; encephalitis: monitor for headache, vomiting, seizures
Rubella: German or 3-day measles *Causal agent*: Virus *Transmission*: Droplets *Incubation*: 2–3 weeks *Communicability*: 1 week before to 5 days after onset of rash *Immunity*: From vaccination or disease	*Prodromal*: Low-grade temperature, headache, sore throat and cough *Acute*: Flat red rash begins on face and spreads to rest of body; rash lasts 3 days	Nonaspirin antipyretics; encourage fluid; recommend to avoid contact with all pregnant women; nonimmune females should be immunized before reaching childbearing age	Usually benign childhood disease; greatest risk to fetus, especially in 1st trimester
Parotitis: Mumps *Causal agent*: Virus *Transmission*: Droplet or direct contact *Incubation*: 2 to 3 weeks *Communicability*: 1 week before parotid swelling until 1 week after swelling begins *Immunity*: From vaccination or disease	*Prodromal*: Fever, headache, earache that worsens with chewing *Acute*: Swelling of parotid glands	Nonaspirin antipyretics; fluids and soft liquids are easier to swallow; avoid sour foods	Orchitis: monitor for testicular swelling; encephalitis: monitor for headache and vomiting; deafness: monitor for signs of hearing loss
Varicella: Chickenpox *Causal agent*: Virus *Transmission*: Direct contact and airborne *Incubation*: 2–3 weeks *Communicability*: Day(s) before rash to 1 week after first lesions crust over *Immunity*: From vaccination or disease	*Prodromal*: Mild fever and malaise for 24 hours *Acute*: Rash that progresses from macule to vesicle to crusts; eruption lasts up to 5 days and lesions of all types will be present at one time	Acyclovir may be administered or IVIG may be administered to high-risk child; nonaspirin antipyretics, calamine lotion topically, oral antihistamines, oatmeal and Aveeno™ baths; keep nails short, discourage scratching	Encephalitis: Monitor for headaches and vomiting; Reye syndrome: monitor for vomiting and mental confusion—seek medical treatment immediately if seen

6. Medication therapy
   a. Antibiotic therapy usually not recommended unless secondary bacterial infection occurs
   b. Antipyretics, analgesics, and anti-inflammatory drugs may be ordered; aspirin is usually contraindicated in acute viral infections

▶ **Practice to Pass**

Discuss the four stages of a communicable disease.

7. Client and family education
   a. Provide instructions regarding available vaccines to prevent development of childhood contagious diseases
   b. Provide information regarding isolation precautions for illness
   c. Parents should be aware of symptoms that indicate development of complications of specific illness
8. Evaluation: client receives vaccinations on schedule; client develops no complications of childhood communicable disease; parents describe isolation precautions for their child with a communicable disease

Case Study

A 5-year-old child is admitted to the clinic with symptoms of elevated temperature, cough, and rhinitis. He also exhibits one small round red spot on his abdomen.

1. What diagnostic tests does the nurse prepare to do?

2. During the nursing assessment, what specific information does the nurse ask for?

3. What are three priority potential nursing diagnoses?

4. Discuss three nursing interventions appropriate for this child.

5. What criteria would guide the evaluation of this client?

For suggested responses, see pages 354–355.

POSTTEST

① The nurse has explained allergy-proofing the home to the mother of a child with dust allergies. Which statement(s) by the mother indicates a clear understanding of appropriate allergy proofing? Select all that apply.

1. "I'm going to replace the cotton curtains on the window with blinds."
2. "The only toys allowed in his bedroom are his stuffed toys."
3. "I should store his out-of-season clothes in his bedroom."
4. "The mattress and box springs both need to be enclosed in a thick plastic cover."
5. "I will try to clean and vacuum the bedroom frequently to limit dust collection."

② A client is in the clinic for a scratch test for allergy. Because of the risk of anaphylaxis, the nurse has which medication available for emergency treatment?

1. Epinephrine (Adrenalin)
2. Prednisone (Deltasone)
3. Naloxone (Narcan)
4. Cromolyn sodium (Intal)

③ A mother brings a 3-year-old child to the clinic for a well-child checkup. The child has not been to the clinic since 6 months of age. The nurse determines that which of the following is the priority care for this client?

1. Assess growth and development.
2. Begin dental care.
3. Update vaccinations.
4. Complete hearing screening.

④ The mother of a 1-year-old child says that breastfeeding her infant is sufficient to provide immunity. She does not want to sign the permit for immunizations. What is the nurse's best approach in working with this client?

1. Discuss active and passive immunity.
2. Tell her immunizations are legally mandatory.
3. Ask about the mother's diet.
4. Give the immunization without her permission.

⑤ A hospital pediatric unit has had a recent outbreak of bacterial diarrhea. None of the children were admitted for diarrhea, but the nurse is aware that they may be exposed. After assessing assigned clients, the nurse determines that which child would be most susceptible to developing diarrhea?

1. Toddler with severe combined immunodeficiency disease
2. Preschooler in traction for a fractured femur
3. School-age child with atopic dermatitis
4. Adolescent with frequent stools secondary to malabsorption syndrome

6 A child is admitted to the hospital with an allergic reaction. The physician orders a complete blood count (CBC) with differential. The nurse would expect to see an elevated result in which test?

1. Red blood cells (RBCs)
2. Hemoglobin
3. Leukocytes
4. Eosinophils

7 An infant is being discharged from the infant and children's unit with a positive TORCH titer. Parents should be informed of which of the following? Select all that apply.

1. The child may shed the virus for a year.
2. TORCH is a genetic disorder.
3. Pregnant women should avoid contact with the baby.
4. Since the infant is asymptomatic at birth, there will be no residual effect.
5. The earlier in pregnancy that TORCH occurred, the greater the risk to the embryo.

8 An infant with acquired immunodeficiency syndrome (AIDS) will be attending daycare. The day care staff is concerned about spreading the human immunodeficiency virus (HIV). The public health nurse consulting with the staff should teach which of the following precautions?

1. Store all of this infant's supplies separately from those of the other children.
2. Wear gloves when changing the child's diapers.
3. Always wear gloves and isolation gowns when handling the infant.
4. Minimize contact with the infant when it is febrile.

9 A mother overhears two nurses discussing a measles outbreak. The nurses are talking about the incubation period. The mother asks the nurses why it is important to know the incubation period for a childhood disease. The nurse would include which information about the incubation period of a disease in the reply?

1. Describes a period when the child might be contagious
2. Determines the severity of the infection
3. Varies depending on the age of the child
4. Is a period of time when medications can prevent the development of symptoms

10 An infant with numerous congenital defects and a diagnosis of rule out TORCH syndrome is admitted from the birth hospital directly to the pediatric hospital. The father tells the pediatric nurse that he and his wife had planned a beautiful birth experience and can't believe what's happened. The nurse would formulate which of the following nursing diagnoses as a priority for this family at this time?

1. Risk for Caregiver Role Strain
2. Situational Low Self-Esteem
3. Risk for Impaired Parent–Infant Attachment
4. Parental Role Conflict

➤ *See pages 247–248 for Answers and Rationales.*

ANSWERS & RATIONALES

Pretest

1 **Answer: 3** **Rationale:** One of the most common side effects of gentamycin is nephrotoxicity. The nurse can monitor kidney function by monitoring intake and output. Monitoring specific gravity of the urine would also be appropriate. Although a child who has an infection may have a fever, a change in body temperature is not a side effect of gentamycin. A change in blood pressure is not a side effect of gentamycin. Development of adventitious breath sounds is not a side effect of gentamycin. **Cognitive Level:** Applying **Client Need:** Pharmacological and Parenteral Therapies **Integrated Process:** Nursing Process: Evaluation **Content Area:** Child Health **Strategy:** Recall that gentamycin is a member of the aminoglycoside group of antibiotics, all of which are nephrotoxic and ototoxic. **Reference:** Ball, J., Bindler, R., & Cowen, K. (2010). *Child health nursing:*

Partnering with children & families (2nd ed.). Upper Saddle River, NJ: Pearson, p. 1227.

2 **Answer: 3** **Rationale:** White blood cells are one component of the general nonspecific immune response. They are among the first responders stimulated by a pathogenic organism. A white cell differential can often determine if the elevation is of bacterial, viral, or allergic origin. Hemoglobin and hematocrit evaluate the oxygen carrying potential of the blood and the percentage of blood that is red blood cells. Red blood cell count is another measure of the oxygen carrying property of the blood. Platelet agglutinization evaluates the clotting ability of the blood. **Cognitive Level:** Analyzing **Client Need:** Physiological Adaptation **Integrated Process:** Nursing Process: Assessment **Content Area:** Child Health **Strategy:** Recall that a WBC count can determine infections. The WBC with differential can also determine if an allergic reaction has occurred. **Reference:** Ball, J., Bindler, R., & Cowen, K. (2010). *Child health nursing: Partnering with children & families* (2nd ed.). Upper Saddle River, NJ: Pearson, p. 1028.

3 **Answer: 1** **Rationale:** Because of the itching, the client will be scratching. Intense scratching can break the skin, and the client might develop a bacterial infection secondary to the skin trauma. Imbalanced Nutrition: More Than Body Requirements does not clearly state the problem with the food allergies, nor does ineffective infant feeding behavior. There is no evidence of noncompliance, and infant feeding would not be a diagnosis for a 2-year-old. **Cognitive Level:** Analyzing **Client Need:** Basic Care and Comfort **Integrated Process:** Nursing Process: Diagnosis **Content Area:** Child Health **Strategy:** Critical words are *itching*, *rash*, and *wheat*. Use knowledge of the immune response and risks associated with interrupting the skin as a line of defense to make a selection. **Reference:** Pillitteri, A. (2010). *Maternal & child health nursing: Care of the childbearing & childrearing family* (6th ed.). Philadelphia: Lippincott Williams & Wilkins, p. 1251.

4 **Answer: 4** **Rationale:** A live virus includes an organism that has been weakened, but is still alive and could cause disease in immunosuppressed individuals, such as those taking corticosteroids. A toxoid is not an organism and, therefore is incapable of causing disease. Recombinant means the vaccine contains an organism that has been genetically altered, so it is incapable of causing disease. An inactivated virus is a killed organism and, therefore it cannot cause disease. **Cognitive Level:** Analyzing **Client Need:** Health Promotion and Maintenance **Integrated Process:** Nursing Process: Implementation **Content Area:** Child Health **Strategy:** Consider that the client taking corticosteroids is immunosuppressed and then consider which vaccine has the risk of being most harmful to one in this state. **Reference:** Ball, J., Bindler, R., & Cowen, K. (2010). *Child health nursing: Partnering with children & families* (2nd ed.). Upper Saddle River, NJ: Prentice Hall, p. 621.

5 **Answer: 2** **Rationale:** Care of the immunocompromised client focuses on preventing infection. Remaining free

of signs of infection is the best goal as the nursing diagnosis would be Risk for Infection. Goals would be developed related to assessment findings. The client with SCID has no unusual problems with oxygenation if there is no infection. The client with SCID has normal fluid requirements. Avoiding contact with other people would be an action by the client, but is not a goal. Furthermore, the client does not need to avoid contact with all others, but limiting contact or avoiding those with infection should be sufficient. **Cognitive Level:** Analyzing **Client Need:** Health Promotion and Maintenance **Integrated Process:** Nursing Process: Planning **Content Area:** Child Health **Strategy:** Recognize that a client with an immunodeficiency will not be able to fight infections, so prevention is important. **Reference:** Pillitteri, A. (2010). *Maternal & child health nursing: Care of the childbearing & childrearing family* (6th ed.). Philadelphia: Lippincott Williams & Wilkins, p. 1239.

6 **Answer: 2** **Rationale:** The RAST test involves a blood draw and a laboratory evaluation for IgE. There is no risk of anaphylaxis. The prick test injects potential allergens under the skin and includes a risk of anaphylaxis. Although the allergen is not being injected into the skin with a patch test, there is still a small risk of anaphylaxis. The prick test can also be called an intradermal test or scratch test. **Cognitive Level:** Analyzing **Client Need:** Reduction of Risk Potential **Integrated Process:** Nursing Process: Assessment **Content Area:** Child Health **Strategy:** Remember, the more internal the test, the greater the risk. **Reference:** Pillitteri, A. (2010). *Maternal & child health nursing: Care of the childbearing & childrearing family* (6th ed.). Philadelphia: Lippincott Williams & Wilkins, p. 1243.

7 **Answer: 3** **Rationale:** The TORCH acronym refers to a specific variety of organisms (toxoplasmosis, other [syphilis, hepatitis], rubella, cytomegalovirus, and herpes simplex virus) that cause fetal anomalies. It is a study of common viruses that cause significant fetal damage. There is no virus called the TORCH virus. Microcephaly is a fetal complication, but this is not the best answer. TORCH is not associated with thalidomide. **Cognitive Level:** Applying **Client Need:** Physiological Adaptation **Integrated Process:** Teaching and Learning **Content Area:** Child Health **Strategy:** Recall the meaning of the acronym TORCH to answer this question correctly. **Reference:** Chapman, L., & Durham, R. (2009). *Maternal-newborn nursing: The critical components of nursing care.* Philadelphia: F.A. Davis Company, p. 124.

8 **Answer: 2, 3** **Rationale:** When a child has a disease, the body produces antibodies against the organism which is *active immunity*. The body will produce antibodies against the toxoid, which is a form of active immunity. *Passive immunity* is immunity acquired from antibodies produced by another. Receiving immunity from the mother is a form of passive immunity. Intravenous immunoglobulins are antibodies produced by others. It provides passive immunity. Serum is not used frequently, but provides passive immunity. **Cognitive Level:** Applying **Client Need:** Physiological Adaptation **Integrated Process:** Nursing Process: Implementation **Content Area:** Child Health **Strategy:** Remember passive immunity is not produced by the person while active immunity is produced by the person. **Reference:** Ball, J., Bindler, R., & Cowen, K. (2010). *Child health nursing: Partnering with children & families* (2nd ed.). Upper Saddle River, NJ: Prentice Hall, p. 615.

9 **Answer: 4** **Rationale:** Protection of others is of primary importance. Families need to know that casual contact cannot spread HIV. However, basic infection control practices must be maintained to prevent exposure through body fluids. Growth and development milestones are routine elements of teaching, and are therefore not as high a priority for this client as infection control. Immunization schedules would be an ongoing component of routine teaching for a 12-year-old client. The parents would be told of lab results prior to discharge. This is not a component of the discharge instructions. **Cognitive Level:** Analyzing **Client Need:** Safety and Infection Control **Integrated Process:** Teaching and Learning **Content Area:** Child Health **Strategy:** Consider that the spread of infection would be a concern for this child whether at home or at the hospital. **Reference:** Ball, J., Bindler, R., & Cowen, K. (2010). *Child health nursing: Partnering with children & families* (2nd ed.). Upper Saddle River, NJ: Prentice Hall, p. 995.

10 **Answer: 1** **Rationale:** The prodromal period refers to the period of time between the initial symptoms and the presence of the full-blown disease. The rash would not be apparent during this time. All the other statements are correct. **Cognitive Level:** Analyzing **Client Need:** Physiological Adaptation **Integrated Process:** Nursing Process: Evaluation **Content Area:** Child Health **Strategy:** The wording of the question indicates that the correct option contains incorrect information. Understanding the meaning of the term *prodromal* to select the correct response. **Reference:** Pillitteri, A. (2010). *Maternal & child health nursing: Care of the childbearing & childrearing family* (6th ed.). Philadelphia: Lippincott Williams & Wilkins, p. 1268–1269.

Posttest

1 **Answer: 4, 5** **Rationale:** Cloth items hold in dust. Only essential items should be stored in the child's bedroom, and those should be in drawers or closets. Stuffed animals retain dust and should be removed from the bedroom. Cotton curtains would be preferred over blinds because cotton curtains can be washed frequently. Both the mattress and the bed should be enclosed in special plastic covers to eliminate a source of dust. **Cognitive Level:** Analyzing **Client Need:** Health Promotion and Maintenance **Integrated Process:** Nursing Process: Evaluation **Content Area:** Child Health **Strategy:** Consider what objects would hold dust and eliminate them from the environment. **Reference:** Ball, J., Bindler, R., & Cowen, K. (2010). *Maternal & child*

health nursing: Care of the childbearing & childrearing family* (6th ed.). Philadelphia, PA: Lippincott Williams & Wilkins, p. 1016.

2 **Answer: 1** **Rationale:** Epinephrine is an adrenergic. When given for anaphylaxis, epinephrine will inhibit the release of mediators of immediate hypersensitivity reactions from mast cells. Prednisone is a corticosteroid, which serves as an anti-inflammatory, but does not provide immediate relief from anaphylaxis. Naloxone would be given to reverse the central nervous system depressant effects of opioid analgesics. Cromolyn sodium is a mast cell inhibitor used to reduce the incidence of asthmatic attacks. **Cognitive Level:** Applying **Client Need:** Pharmacological and Parenteral Therapies **Integrated Process:** Nursing Process: Planning **Content Area:** Child Health **Strategy:** Eliminate naloxone immediately after associating it with narcotic overdose. The other three drugs are related to allergies, but the correct answer is one that will work quickly and have a systemic response rather than a local one. **Reference:** Ball, J., Bindler, R., & Cowen, K. (2010). *Child health nursing: Partnering with children & families* (2nd ed.). Upper Saddle River, NJ: Prentice Hall, p. 1015.

3 **Answer: 3** **Rationale:** Updating vaccinations is the priority intervention. The child is behind in the vaccination schedule. Although growth and development is important, assessing it is not the priority nursing intervention. Dental care should already be begun, but if not the nurse should teach the mother about dental care as a routine intervention. Hearing screenings are not usually done at this age; therefore it is not a priority. **Cognitive Level:** Analyzing **Client Need:** Health Promotion and Maintenance **Integrated Process:** Nursing Process: Planning **Content Area:** Child Health **Strategy:** The critical word in this stem is *the priority nursing action*. While all these activities must be completed, consider which is the most important to the client's well-being. **Reference:** Pillitteri, A. (2010). *Maternal & child health nursing: Care of the childbearing & childrearing family* (6th ed.). Philadelphia: Lippincott Williams & Wilkins, p. 948.

4 **Answer: 1** **Rationale:** Discussing active and passive immunity provides the mother with information she needs to make an informed decision. Infants receive passive immunity, which lasts three to four months, through the placenta or breast milk. Active immunity lasts long term and is acquired by exposure to disease or immunizations. Parents have the right to make decisions for their children regarding immunizations. The mother's diet will have little effect on the child's immunity. Giving the immunization without permission could put the nurse in legal jeopardy. **Cognitive Level:** Analyzing **Client Need:** Health Promotion and Maintenance **Integrated Process:** Nursing Process: Implementation **Content Area:** Child Health **Strategy:** Eliminate one option that does not constitute good practice. Eliminate another that is irrelevant, leaving only two options to choose between. **Reference:** Ball, J., Bindler, R., & Cowen, K. (2010). *Child health nursing: Partnering with* *children & families* (2nd ed.). Upper Saddle River, NJ: Prentice Hall, pp. 630–633.

5 **Answer: 1** **Rationale:** The immunocompromised child would be the one at greatest risk for acquiring an infectious organism. The other children would be at less risk for acquiring the gastrointestinal infection. **Cognitive Level:** Analyzing **Client Need:** Safety and Infection Control **Integrated Process:** Nursing Process: Diagnosis **Content Area:** Child Health **Strategy:** The ability to fight infection is related to the immune system. Select the child with a disease of the immune system. **Reference:** Perry, S., Hockenberry, M., Lowdermilk, D., & Wilson, D. (2010). *Maternal child nursing care* (4th ed.). St. Louis, MO: Mosby, pp. 1519–1520.

6 **Answer: 4** **Rationale:** Eosinophils are the type of white blood cell that is associated with allergic reactions. Hemoglobin is present in red blood cells (RBCs), and RBCs carry oxygen to tissues. Leukocytes fight infection. **Cognitive Level:** Applying **Client Need:** Reduction of Risk Potential **Integrated Process:** Nursing Process: Assessment **Content Area:** Child Health **Strategy:** First eliminate two options that are not related to the immune system. Choose between the remaining two to select the type of WBC that is associated with allergies. **Reference:** McKinney, E., James, S., Murray, S., & Ashwill, J. (2009). *Maternal-child nursing* (3rd ed.). St. Louis, MO: Saunders, p. 1044.

7 **Answer: 1, 3, 5** **Rationale:** Many of the viruses associated with TORCH may be shed for an extended period. The fetus of the pregnant woman may become infected if the woman is in contact with this child. The more immature the fetus when exposed, the greater the risk. TORCH is the acronym for a group of viral diseases known to cause fetal anomalies and illness, and include toxoplasmosis, syphilis, hepatitis, rubella, cytomegalovirus, and herpes simplex. Identification of all the effects of the TORCH viruses may take a period of time. **Cognitive Level:** Analyzing **Client Need:** Safety and Infection Control **Integrated Process:** Teaching and Learning **Content Area:** Child Health **Strategy:** Recall what the acronym TORCH stands for in order to answer the question correctly. **Reference:** Chapman, L., & Durham, R. (2009). *Maternal-newborn nursing: The critical components of nursing care.* Philadelphia: F.A. Davis Company, pp. 124–130.

8 **Answer: 2** **Rationale:** The virus is found in blood and body fluids, so gloves should be worn when changing the diaper. The HIV virus is fairly fragile and does not survive long on objects. The HIV virus cannot be acquired through casual contact. The child may spread the organism causing the fever, but the HIV virus is acquired only through blood and body fluids. **Cognitive Level:** Applying **Client Need:** Safety and Infection Control **Integrated Process:** Nursing Process: Implementation **Content Area:** Child Health **Strategy:** Recall that the virus responsible for AIDS is a blood-borne pathogen. The correct answer is the one that represents standard precautions, which are sufficient to prevent the acquisition of a blood-borne pathogen. **Reference:** Pillitteri, A. (2010). *Maternal & child health nursing: Care of the childbearing & childrearing family* (6th ed.). Philadelphia: Lippincott Williams & Wilkins, p. 1238.

9 **Answer: 1** **Rationale:** The incubation period is the time between exposure and outbreak of the disease. It is often a period when the child can be contagious without others being aware of the possible exposure. **Cognitive Level:** Applying **Client Need:** Safety and Infection Control **Integrated Process:** Teaching and Learning **Content Area:** Child Health **Strategy:** To answer this question correctly, it is necessary to understand the concept of the incubation period. **Reference:** Pillitteri, A. (2010). *Maternal & child health nursing: Care of the childbearing & childrearing family* (6th ed.). Philadelphia: Lippincott Williams & Wilkins, p. 1260.

10 **Answer: 3** **Rationale:** With the birth of a less-than-expected infant, the parents may have difficulty accepting the child. In addition, the anticipated longer hospitalization and separation from the parents inhibit bonding, which could lead to altered attachment. **Cognitive Level:** Analyzing **Client Need:** Psychosocial Integrity **Integrated Process:** Nursing Process: Diagnosis **Content Area:** Child Health **Strategy:** Two options that have no evidence in the stem can be eliminated first. Choose between the remaining options by choosing the option that includes all of the clients in the question. **Reference:** Chapman, L., & Durham, R. (2009). *Maternal-newborn nursing: The critical components of nursing care.* Philadelphia: F.A. Davis Company, pp. 256–257.

References

Adams, M., Holland, L., & Urban, C. (2011). *Pharmacology for nurses: A pathophysiological approach* (3rd ed.). Upper Saddle River, NJ: Pearson Education.

Ball, J., Bindler, R., & Cowen, K. (2012). *Principles of pediatric nursing: Caring for children* (5th ed.). Upper Saddle River, NJ: Pearson Education.

Ball, J., Bindler, R., & Cowen, K. (2010). *Child health nursing: Partnering with children and families* (2nd ed.). Upper Saddle River, NJ: Pearson Education.

Hockenberry, M., & Wilson, D. (2011). *Wong's essentials of pediatric nursing* (8th ed.). St. Louis, MO: Elsevier.

Hockenberry, M., & Wilson, D. (2011). *Wong's nursing care of infants and children* (9th ed.). St. Louis, MO: Elsevier.

London, M., Ladewig, P., Ball, J., Bindler, R., & Cowen, K. (2011). *Maternal & child nursing care* (3rd ed.). Upper Saddle River, NJ: Pearson Education.

Perry, S., Hockenberry, M., Lowdermilk, D., & Wilson, D. (2010). *Maternal child nursing care* (4th ed.). St. Louis, MO: Elsevier.

Pillitteri, A. (2009). *Maternal and child health nursing: Care of the childbearing and childrearing family* (6th ed.). Philadelphia: Lippincott Williams & Wilkins.

Cellular Health Problems

12

Chapter Outline

Introduction to Alterations in
    Cellular Health

Congenital Cellular Health
    Problems: Neuroblastoma

Acquired Cellular Health
    Problems

Objectives

➤ Identify data essential to the assessment of alterations in cellular
  health in a client.
➤ Discuss the clinical manifestations and pathophysiology related to
  alterations in cellular health in a client.
➤ Discuss therapeutic management of a client with alterations in
  cellular health.
➤ Describe nursing management of a client with alterations in cellular
  health.

NCLEX-RN® Test Prep

Use the accompanying online resource,
NursingReviewsandRationales, to test
yourself with hundreds of NCLEX®-style
practice questions.

Review at a Glance

anemia a reduction in number of
circulating RBCs

biopsy procedure for obtaining a
representative tissue sample for
microscopic examination

chemotherapy treatment of a
disease with chemical agents that have
specific toxicity on disease process

debulk process of surgically removing
part of a neoplasm when complete
excision is impossible

infratentorial below tentorium
cerebelli; area containing the cerebellum

metastasis a secondary growth in a
distant location arising from a primary
malignancy

nadir lowest point, such as blood
count after chemotherapy

neutropenia abnormally small
numbers of neutrophils in blood

palliation treatment intended to
relieve or reduce intensity without cure

radiation therapy use of ionizing
rays for therapeutic purposes in cancer
therapy

staging process of classifying tumors
with respect to degree of differentiation,
potential for responding to treatment and
client prognosis

supratentorial above tentorial notch:
containing the cerebral hemispheres

thrombocytopenia a reduction in
number of circulating platelets

PRETEST

1 An 18-month-old client is brought in for a well-child visit. The parent reports feeling a lump to the right of the "bellybutton" during bathing. Initial assessments should include which of the following? Select all that apply.

1. Measuring weight and height
2. Palpation of the area
3. Routine urine testing
4. Vital signs
5. Questioning the parents about abuse

2 The parent of a client with neuroblastoma verbalizes regret at not coming in earlier for the client's complaints. What would be an appropriate response by the nurse?

1. "This tumor may be diagnosed early because of obvious symptoms."
2. "This is a silent tumor, which is difficult to diagnose early."
3. "This is a very common brain tumor in children."
4. "I know you feel guilty about not being more observant, but you shouldn't blame yourself."

3 A 4-year-old is diagnosed with acute lymphocytic leukemia (ALL). Following teaching about the testing and therapy, the nurse evaluates the family's understanding of the problem. Which statement indicates the family has appropriate knowledge?

1. "This will determine the extent of the tumor growth and the possible need to use only comfort measures."
2. "This will help determine whether chemotherapy as a treatment option is needed."
3. "This will determine whether surgery would be an appropriate way to treat the cancer."
4. "This will determine the extent of the cancer and find out what state it has advanced to."

4 The school health nurse has seen a child several times with the same complaints. The school health nurse would suspect a brain tumor after noting the presence of which symptoms that are compatible with this health problem?

1. Hyperactivity and irritability
2. Papilledema and positive red reflex
3. Early morning headache and vomiting
4. Fever and seizures

5 A 17-year-old client is being admitted for an amputation related to a bone tumor. The nurse is developing a nursing care plan and determines the most appropriate age-related diagnosis is which of the following?

1. Risk for Disuse Syndrome
2. Disturbed Body Image
3. Self-Care Deficit
4. Activity Intolerance

6 A client has been treated with chemotherapy for cancer. The nurse anticipates that neutropenia is an expected consequence and teaches the parents to have the child avoid which of the following?

1. Contact sports
2. Crowded spaces
3. Spicy foods
4. All immunizations

7 A client diagnosed with Ewing's sarcoma is being treated with chemotherapy. The results of a complete blood count (CBC) indicate severe thrombocytopenia. Nursing interventions related to this finding would include which of the following? Select all that apply.

1. Encouraging foods high in iron
2. Limiting physical contact with the client
3. Removing fresh flowers from the client's room
4. Clearing the floor of the client's room to prevent falls and bruises
5. Minimizing needle sticks and intrusive procedures

8 The parents of a client with neutropenia secondary to chemotherapy have been taught protective isolation behaviors. The nurse evaluates that the parents require further education when the parents do which of the following?

1. Bring the child toys from home.
2. Encourage friends to visit by phone rather than in person.
3. Pull the client in a wagon around the nursing unit for entertainment.
4. Wash their hands before entering the client's room but not upon exiting the room.

9 Following diagnosis of Wilms' tumor, the client undergoes removal of the affected kidney. In the postoperative period, priority nursing assessments should focus on which of the following?

1. The incision
2. Lung sounds
3. Temperature
4. Kidney function

10 A client will be undergoing chemotherapy. The nurse discusses the issue of hair loss with the client and family before chemotherapy begins. Later, the family asks the nurse why this information was given to the client at this time. The nurse's response will include which of the following?

1. Hair loss is a symptom of toxic blood levels of chemotherapy, so the client should be watching for this phenomenon.
2. The presence or absence of hair is related to body image. Strategies for handling hair loss should precede the event.
3. It is the nurse's legal responsibility to discuss this issue with the client.
4. Hair loss can be prevented with appropriate nursing interventions.

➤ *See pages 265–266 for Answers and Rationales.*

I. INTRODUCTION TO ALTERATIONS IN CELLULAR HEALTH

A. Normal cell reproduction
1. Life of a cell is described as cell cycle, beginning with its formation and ending with division of cell into two daughter cells
2. Different tissues have different lengths of cell cycles, varying from 16 hours to 400 hours; some cells, including neurons, never enter cell cycle and thus never reproduce

B. Development of neoplasms
1. Any group of cells can develop abnormal growth and reproduction; this abnormal reproduction of cells is termed neoplasia; immune system normally protects body against reproduction of these abnormal cells
2. Definitive causative agents for development of neoplasms are unknown
   a. Numerous factors have been labeled as contributing to development of a neoplasm, but exact relationship between these factors and neoplasm development remains unknown
   b. Factors implicated in development of neoplasms include genetics, radiation, exposure to power lines, the effect of cigarette smoking, viruses, and certain chemicals and drugs
3. Neoplasms can be either benign or malignant
   a. Benign neoplasms typically do not metastasize and tend not to recur when surgically removed; they do not destroy tissue except secondarily by interfering with blood flow; benign tumors can be serious and even fatal if they interfere with vital functions
   b. Malignant neoplasms are those that tend to recur after removal and metastasize to distant tissues and organs; tissue is destroyed by invasion of these tumors and growth tends to be rapid

4. Treatment for neoplasms includes surgery, radiation, and chemotherapy, alone or in combination
   a. Cure of tumor occurs when treatment removes all evidence of tumor permanently
   b. **Palliation** (treatment intended to relieve or reduce intensity without cure) reduces size of tumor, thus decreasing symptoms and making client more comfortable

II. CONGENITAL CELLULAR HEALTH PROBLEMS: NEUROBLASTOMA

A. Description
1. Solid tumor outside cranium originating in primitive neural crest cells, which give rise to adrenal medulla, paraganglia, and sympathetic nervous system of cervical sympathetic chain and thoracic chain
2. Is most common tumor in children located outside cranium
3. Usual age at onset is 22 months of age
4. Prognosis is based on client age and **staging** of tumor (process of classifying tumors with respect to degree of differentiation, potential for responding to treatment and patient prognosis); children under one year of age have a better prognosis

B. Etiology and pathophysiology
1. Cause is unknown although environmental factors, such as prenatal drug exposure, may be implicated
2. Oncogenes have been found to be present in neuroblastoma cells; the DNA sequence responsible for this is called *N-myc*; high *N-myc* levels are associated with rapid progression of disease and poorer prognosis
3. Tumor is often silent leading to late diagnosis and poor prognosis

C. Assessment
1. Symptoms are representative of location and stage of the disease
   a. A peritoneal tumor may present as an abdominal mass or may be evidenced by bowel and bladder dysfunction
   b. Typical signs include weight loss, abdominal fullness, irritability, fatigue, and fever
   c. Mediastinal tumors cause dyspnea and lead to neck and facial edema if the tumor is large
   d. Bone metastasis may lead to limp, fever, and malaise; ptosis and ecchymosis of the eyes can also occur
2. Computed tomography (CT) of skull, neck, chest, abdomen, and bone are done to locate tumor
3. Bone marrow aspiration helps to locate mass and determine **metastasis** (a secondary growth in a distant location arising from a primary malignancy)
4. Urine testing is done to detect breakdown of products of adrenal catecholamines (epinephrine and norepinephrine), since some tumors secrete them; these breakdown products are vanillylmandelic acid (VMA) and homovanillic acid (HVA)

D. Priority nursing diagnoses
1. Deficient Knowledge (parental) of disease process and treatment modalities
2. Acute Pain
3. Interrupted Family Processes

E. Planning and implementation
1. Surgery is used for tumor removal following **biopsy** (procedure for obtaining a representative tissue sample for microscopic examination)
2. **Radiation therapy** (use of ionizing rays for therapeutic purposes in cancer therapy) is used in more advanced cases in addition to surgery and as palliation to reduce symptoms of metastasis

Figure 12-1

Chemotherapy protocol
decision tree

Protocol = Map or plan
of action

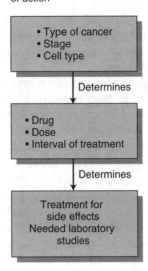

* Type of cancer
* Stage
* Cell type

Determines

* Drug
* Dose
* Interval of treatment

Determines

Treatment for
side effects
Needed laboratory
studies

3. **Chemotherapy**
   a. Is defined as treatment of a disease with chemical agents that have specific toxicity on disease process
   b. Is a primary form of treatment for cancer; see Figure 12-1 for chemotherapy protocol

   c. Drug classifications, sample drugs, and side effects are identified in Table 12-1

Table 12-1 **Classes of Chemotherapy, Commonly Used Examples, and Side Effects**

Drug Classes with Selected Examples	Common Side Effects
I. Cell-cycle nonspecific drugs	
Alkylating Drugs	
Cyclophosphamide (Cytoxan)	Bone marrow depression (BMD), hemorrhagic cystitis, alopecia, and stomatitis; Mesna (Mesnex) is given with cyclophosphamide to counteract hemorrhagic cystitis
Antibiotics	
Doxorubicin (Adriamycin)	BMD, stomatitis, nausea, and vomiting
Hormones	
Prednisone (Meticorten)	Hyperglycemia, gastrointestinal upset, increased appetite, moon face, and increased risk for infection
II. Cell-cycle specific	
Antimetabolites	
6-Mercaptopurine (Purinethol)	BMD, stomatitis, nausea and vomiting, and anorexia
Cytarabine (Ara-C)	BMD, nausea and vomiting, and diarrhea
Methotrexate (Folex)	BMD, nausea and vomiting, and diarrhea
	(Note: leucovorin rescue—use of leucovorin, an analogue of folic acid—may be used to reduce normal cell kill due to methotrexate)
Plant Alkaloids	
Vincristine (Oncovin)	BMD, nausea and vomiting, fever, and neurologic toxicity (includes constipation)
Enzymes	
Asparaginase (Elspar)	Allergic reaction, fever, nausea and vomiting, and anorexia
III. Miscellaneous	
Biologic Response Modifiers	
Interferon	Flu-like symptoms

        d. Combination drug regimens allow for better cell kill with minimal toxicity and also decrease resistance of cancer cells

        e. Central venous access has facilitated safer drug administration of chemotherapeutic agents; it is important to check for blood return before, during, and after administration to prevent infiltration of vesicant drugs that will destroy infiltrated tissue

    4. If surgery is performed, monitor surgical site for hemorrhage and infection; use temperature as most accurate measure of infection

    5. Monitor skin integrity at radiation site; see Table 12-2 for nursing care related to radiation therapy

    6. Monitor mucous membrane integrity; use appropriate nursing interventions to prevent and treat mouth ulcers

    7. Minimize exposure to infection

        a. All visitors and staff should use good hand hygiene before contact

        b. Private room may be indicated during the period of **nadir** (lowest point, such as blood counts) after chemotherapy

        c. Monitor temperature

        d. Avoid live attenuated immunizations

    8. Monitor bleeding

        a. Take vital signs as ordered

        b. Test all stools and body fluids for occult blood

        c. Avoid rectal temperatures, intramuscular injections, and hard tooth brushes

        d. Avoid vigorous activities and contact sports

Table 12-2 **Nursing Care of the Child Receiving Radiation Therapy**

Nursing Diagnosis	Nursing Care
Risk for Impaired Skin Integrity	Instruct the child to wear loose-fitting clothing.
	Use mild soap to wash and gently pat dry the area.
	Avoid lotions; may use water-soluble lubricant for dry desquamation.
	Use water-soluble lubricant or moist compresses for itching.
	Antihistamines may be ordered by health care provider.
	Keep site protected from rubbing, scratching, and sun exposure.
Risk for Impaired Oral Mucous Membranes	Monitor oral mucosa at least daily.
	Offer oral hygiene after meals and snacks.
	Use soft toothbrush and mild toothpaste.
	Rinse mouth frequently; may use plain water or alcohol-free mouthwash.
	Child may suck on hard candy to stimulate saliva and remove bad taste.
	Health care provider may order medicated mouth rinse to reduce pain of mouth ulcers.
	Offer bland food and fluids, and avoid extremely hot or cold food and beverage temperatures.
Risk for Infection	Restrict contact with infected health care workers, family, and friends.
	Use good personal hygiene; keep nails short and clean.
	Remove sources of infectious organisms, including fresh flowers and vegetables; maintain clean environment.

Practice to Pass

The parents of a 6-month-old with neuroblastoma are visiting their child in the hospital. They are tearful, protective, and insist on doing all personal care. How would you assess the family process?

F. Client and family education

1. Teach family about disease process and treatment modalities

2. Instruct family about blood dyscrasias and actions they can take to improve client's condition

3. Give family information about need for good nutrition and management of nausea

G. Evaluation: family displays appropriate coping mechanisms and actively participates in client's care; family describes disease process and lists side effects of medications client is receiving

III. ACQUIRED CELLULAR HEALTH PROBLEMS

A. Leukemia

1. Description

  a. Cancer of blood-forming tissues; a proliferation of immature, abnormal WBCs

  b. Most common malignancy of childhood

  c. Peak age of development is 4 years; boys are affected more frequently than girls

  d. Classification is based on type of WBC that becomes neoplastic and immaturity of neoplastic cell

    1) Acute lymphocytic leukemia (ALL), which has a better prognosis

    2) Acute non-lymphocytic leukemia (ANLL) or acute myelogenous leukemia (AML), which has the poorer prognosis

    3) Chronic leukemias are rare in children

2. Etiology and pathophysiology

  a. Although etiology is unknown, genetics is implicated by increased incidence in identical twins; chromosomal factors are implicated by increased risk in children with chromosomal abnormalities such as Down syndrome and Fanconi's syndrome

  b. Unrestricted proliferation of immature WBCs occurs

  c. Bone marrow infiltration crowds out stem cells that normally produce red blood cells and platelets; **anemia** (a reduction in number of circulating RBCs) and **thrombocytopenia** (reduction in number of circulating platelets) occur; WBCs that are produced are immature and incapable of fighting infection

  d. Spleen, liver, and lymph nodes become infiltrated and enlarged

  e. Central nervous system (CNS) is at risk for infiltration

  f. Clinical manifestations are directly related to area of involvement, such as bone pain from marrow proliferation

  g. Prognosis is based on initial WBC count; prognosis is more favorable if initial WBC count is below $50,000/mm^3$; children have a better prognosis if they are between ages of 2 and 10 at time of diagnosis; a better prognosis is given for ALL than for ANLL

  h. Overall prognosis has improved; majority of newly diagnosed children who receive multi-agent treatment will survive

3. Assessment

  a. History, physical, and peripheral blood smear are performed

    1) Peripheral blood count reveals anemia, thrombocytopenia, and **neutropenia** (abnormally small numbers of neutrophils in the blood)

    2) Leukemic blasts (immature white blood cells) may be seen on smear

  b. Bone marrow aspiration is definitive test

    1) Usually obtained from iliac crest

    2) Anemia, thrombocytopenia, and neutropenia

    3) Normal marrow contains less than 5% blasts

    4) Leukemic marrow has much higher percentage of blasts, often 60 to 100%

      c. Other diagnostic tests may include spinal tap to determine if there is CNS involvement

      d. Physical assessments

        1) Monitor temperature

        2) Observe for evidence of new bleeding, such as bruises, bleeding gums, and blood in stool

        3) Observe level of consciousness; note and record irritability, vomiting, and lethargy which may be related to CNS infiltration

4. Priority nursing diagnoses

    a. Risk for Infection

    b. Risk for Injury

    c. Activity Intolerance

    d. Anxiety

    e. Risk for Compromised Family Coping

    f. Acute Pain

5. Planning and implementation

    a. Aim of treatment is to induce a remission using combinations of chemotherapy; remission refers to absence of all signs of leukemia including less than 5% blasts in bone marrow; once induction of remission is achieved, client is placed on maintenance therapy, which may last two to three years

    b. Relapses occur when symptoms of leukemia return; reinduction places client back into remission; relapse may occur at any time but probability of occurrence decreases over time; bone marrow transplant may be utilized on clients who have returned to remission after a relapse

    c. Sanctuary therapy (CNS prophylaxis) is frequently administered during initial period of treatment; presence of leukemic cells in CNS fluid leads to CNS involvement; most chemotherapy drugs do not cross blood–brain barrier; failure to treat the leukemic cells in CNS may allow disease to return after remission appears to be achieved; CNS treatment can include radiation therapy to brain and spinal cord or administration of chemotherapy drugs into CSF

    d. Nursing care is directed toward managing symptoms of leukemia as well as preventing/treating side effects of chemotherapy

    e. Supportive care for anemia includes protection of body from injury to prevent trauma to RBCs present; client will need rest periods to combat fatigue associated with anemia; activity intolerance will require organization of nursing care to allow for adequate rest; adequate nutrient intake will be necessary for production of new RBCs

    f. Platelet deficiency means client will be prone to bleeding

      1) Use a soft toothbrush or gauze over a finger for oral care to reduce bleeding of gums

      2) Avoid alcohol-containing mouthwashes to prevent drying of oral mucous membranes

      3) Keep environment clear to avoid risk of client bumping into objects and sustaining falls that lead to bruises

      4) Avoid rectal temperatures and test all stools for occult blood

    g. Although WBC count may be high initially, the WBCs present are immature and unable to fight infections; ensure good hand hygiene by all who have contact with client to protect client from infection; prevent individuals with infections from coming in contact with client; do not allow fresh flowers or fruits in client's room because of presence of mold and fungus on these items

    h. Monitor vital signs, intake and output, weight and urine specific gravity

    i. Monitor for constipation

j. Inspect oral mucous membranes daily

k. Monitor level of consciousness, degree of irritability, and overall behavior

l. Manage pain with medications and other alternative interventions

m. See Table 12-3 for nursing interventions to treat side effects of chemotherapy

6. Medication therapy

a. Combinations of chemotherapy drugs are used to enhance tumor cell death and reduce side effects; drugs are chosen that use different mechanisms to cause cell death; protocols often vary among institutions

b. The chemotherapy treatment can be divided into three phases

   1) Induction, which is designed to achieve remission

   2) Intensification, which serves to maintain remission

   3) Maintenance, during which chemotherapy may be continued for two to three years; CNS prophylaxis may be used to eliminate leukemic cells in CNS

Practice to Pass

A 10-year-old with acute lymphocytic leukemia refuses all morning hygiene. What would you recommend to his parents when they seek your guidance on what to do?

Table 12-3	**Nursing Care of the Child Receiving Chemotherapy**
Nursing Diagnosis	**Nursing Care**
Risk for Infection	Perform careful handwashing.
	Avoid contact with infectious individuals.
	Avoid crowds.
	Eliminate fresh flowers and potted plants from the child's room.
	Cook all fruits and vegetables to reduce risk of introducing organisms into the environment.
	Protective isolation may be needed if white cell count drops significantly.
Risk for Injury	Keep environment uncluttered to reduce bumping into objects and subsequent falls.
	Use soft toothbrush or gauze over finger to provide oral care.
	Avoid alcohol-containing mouthwash, which dries the mouth.
	Select toys that do not pose a risk of injury to the child.
Imbalanced Nutrition: Less Than Body Requirements	Provide antiemetics in anticipation of nausea.
	Allow parents to provide home-cooked foods if desired.
	Encourage foods of high nutrient value instead of non-nutritious snacks.
	Make meals pleasant; allow social meals.
	Keep environment aesthetically pleasant.
	Avoid visual reminders of vomiting, including keeping the emesis basin close but out of sight during meals.
Risk for Altered Oral Mucous Membranes	Rinse mouth frequently throughout the day with water.
	Avoid drying mouthwashes.
	Avoid foods that have high acidic content.
	Avoid spicy foods.
	Seek medical intervention for pain control for mouth ulcers.
Disturbed Body Image related to hair loss	Discuss possibility with child and family before it occurs.
	Plan with child for camouflage if desired; purchase wigs, hats, and scarves before hair loss occurs.
	Provide emotional support for hair loss.
	Avoid excessive hair combing/brushing.

      c. Induction: induces remission, lasts four to six weeks and uses prednisone (Meticorten), vincristine (Oncovin), asparaginase (Elspar), with or without doxorubicin (Daunomycin)

      d. Intensification or consolidation: further decreases tumor burden and includes use of such drugs as asparaginase (Elspar) and methotrexate (Folex)

      e. CNS prophylaxis adds intrathecal chemotherapy consisting of methotrexate, cytarabine (Ara-C), and hydrocortisone (Cortef) during other phases of treatment

      f. Maintenance lasts two and a half to three years and includes oral 6-mercaptopurine (Purinethol) and weekly intramuscular methotrexate

      g. Reinduction is used for relapses and adds drugs not previously used

      h. Bone marrow transplants are not usually used for ALL until a second relapse occurs

      i. Hematopoietic stem cell transplantation may be used to treat leukemia as well as other malignancies and some nonmalignant conditions

   7. Client and family education

      a. Explain disease process and treatment modalities to family

      b. Provide client and family with information to assist them in reducing symptoms related to blood dyscrasias

      c. Teach family about side effects of chemotherapy and means of reducing client's discomfort

      d. Promote nutrition by providing information about nausea control

      e. Explain need for good physical hygiene; explain means of protecting client from infection

   8. Evaluation: client remains free of side effects of chemotherapy; blood values remain within normal limits; family demonstrates appropriate coping mechanisms

B. Brain tumors

   1. Description

      a. Most common solid tumor in children

      b. Over half of brain tumors in children are **infratentorial** (below tentorium cerebelli, the area containing the cerebellum), primarily in cerebellum and brainstem

      c. The remaining are **supratentorial** (above tentorial notch containing the cerebral hemispheres) and are mainly in cerebrum (see Figure 12-2)

      d. The terms benign and malignant are of little value since benign brain tumors can be fatal

   2. Etiology and pathophysiology

      a. Cause is unknown although radiation and environmental factors have been implicated

      b. Supporting cells of brain, such as glias and astrocytes, frequently account for pediatric brain tumors

   3. Assessment

      a. Symptoms depend upon location of tumor and age of client

      b. Since an infant's sutures are open, symptoms may be found late

      c. Increased intracranial pressure (ICP) occurs with brain tumors because of presence of tumor and obstructions in flow of CSF; symptoms related to increased ICP include headache, especially on awakening, and vomiting unrelated to eating

      d. Visual symptoms include diplopia and papilledema

      e. Supratentorial tumors give rise to symptoms that include personality changes and seizures

      f. Infratentorial tumor symptoms include ataxia, visual disturbances, delayed or precocious puberty, and growth failures

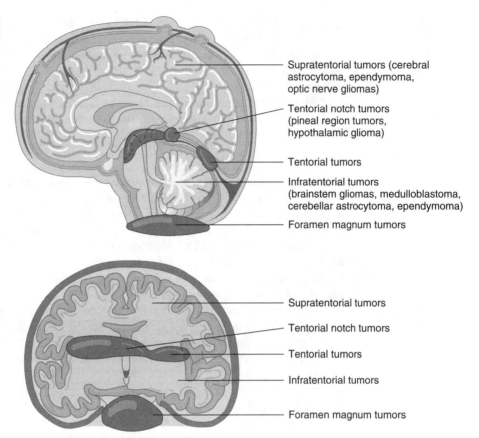

Figure 12-2

Sites of Pediatric Brain Tumors: Infratentorial tumors account for over half of all pediatric tumors

Supratentorial tumors (cerebral astrocytoma, ependymoma, optic nerve gliomas)

Tentorial notch tumors (pineal region tumors, hypothalamic glioma)

Tentorial tumors

Infratentorial tumors (brainstem gliomas, medulloblastoma, cerebellar astrocytoma, ependymoma)

Foramen magnum tumors

Supratentorial tumors

Tentorial notch tumors

Tentorial tumors

Infratentorial tumors

Foramen magnum tumors

    g. Diagnosis is based on results of MRI, CT scans, and radiographic studies with IV contrast; angiography is done when CT scans are positive; biopsy as a diagnostic procedure is done during surgery

  4. Priority nursing diagnoses

    a. Acute Pain

    b. Risk for Imbalanced Nutrition

    c. Impaired Walking

    d. Anxiety

    e. Risk for Compromised Family Coping

  5. Planning and implementation

    a. Surgery is used for biopsy (diagnosis), to completely remove a tumor, or to **debulk** an unremovable tumor (surgically remove part of a neoplasm when complete excision is impossible); surgery may also be performed to restore the patency of the ventricles

    b. Laser surgery can be used for more sensitive areas, where greater precision is needed

    c. Radiation therapy may be used at site postoperatively

    d. Chemotherapy is commonly used, sometimes intrathecally; an Ommaya Reservoir may be surgically implanted under scalp to administer chemotherapy directly into central nervous system

    e. Complications such as hydrocephalus, seizures, sensorimotor deficits, and endocrine disorders may also need management

    f. Maintain nutritional support; if client vomits from increased ICP, provide hygiene and refeed; often act of vomiting reduces ICP

g. Monitor level of consciousness (LOC) and observe for signs of increased ICP; monitor fluid status to prevent rises in ICP; observe for seizures and provide nursing care should they occur; protect client from injury and have suction and oxygen available at bedside

h. Monitor intake and output and measure urine specific gravity

i. Postoperatively, position of head may be critical
  1) With an infratentorial incision, position head flat and on either side with neck slightly extended
  2) With supratentorial incision, elevate head; the physician orders degree of head elevation, often 30 degrees

j. If a ventriculoperitoneal shunt is placed to restore ventricle patency, nursing care includes maintaining suture line and skin integrity over shunt

k. Provide eye care because swelling of eyes may occur postoperatively

l. Monitor pain and provide relief; avoid medications that sedate client, as it is difficult to determine LOC when client is sedated

m. Assess sensory-perceptual status and assist with loss of function

n. Assess surgical site for hemorrhage and infection

6. Client and family education
  a. Reinforce information provided by the physician about diagnosis and treatment; prepare client and family for surgical procedure, including need to shave head and to expect ecchymosis of eyes, which is common following craniotomy
  b. Teach family activities that can reduce client's pain preoperatively and postoperatively
  c. Encourage client and family to talk honestly about diagnosis and their feelings
  d. If diabetes insipidus occurs secondary to brain tumor, teach client and family about medication to control symptoms

7. Evaluation: client's nutritional status is optimized; client's pain is managed at an acceptable level; family describes care of ventriculoperitoneal shunt; family safely and accurately describes side effects of client's medications

C. Wilms' tumor

1. Description
  a. Intrarenal tumor that is also called a nephroblastoma
  b. Common abdominal tumor during childhood
  c. Occurs between 1 and 5 years of age but is most common between ages 18 months and 3 years

2. Etiology and pathophysiology
  a. A small proportion of Wilms' tumors show a genetic basis with family members being at increased risk of development
  b. Tumor may be unilateral or bilateral; bilateral tumors have poorer prognosis
  c. Tumor is often encapsulated until relatively late
  d. It metastasizes to lungs and liver
  e. Prognosis is based on stage of disease; over 75% of children have a five-year survival rate

3. Assessment
  a. Usually asymptomatic
  b. Most frequent admitting symptom is an abdominal mass; parent often finds mass, which is located to one side of midline of abdomen
  c. Pain and hematuria may be present in some children
  d. Hypertension is present in approximately 25% of children because of increased renin production
  e. Diagnosis is made by ultrasound or CT scan of abdomen
  f. CT scan and MRI of lungs detect metastasis

g. Avoid palpating abdomen preoperatively to reduce risk of rupturing capsule and causing tumor spillage; a sign is often placed over client's bed with the instruction, "No abdominal palpations"

4. Priority nursing diagnoses
   a. Risk for Impaired Urinary Elimination
   b. Acute Pain
   c. Risk for Compromised Family Coping

5. Planning and implementation
   a. Unless bilateral tumors are present, surgery is performed to remove affected kidney and look for metastasis
   b. Radiation to abdomen and chemotherapy can be used before and/or after surgery
   c. Postoperatively, monitor functioning of remaining kidney
      1) Measure intake and output
      2) Monitor daily weight and urine specific gravity
      3) Monitor fluid levels, IV infusions, and blood pressure
   d. Complete pain assessment when measuring vital signs; provide pain relief with pharmaceuticals and nursing interventions; in addition to incisional pain, pain may result from postoperative shift of internal organs to compensate for the loss of kidney
   e. Assess bowel sounds, abdominal distention, and bowel movements
   f. Monitor for infection, observing surgical wound and body temperature

6. Client and family education
   a. Explain to family the need to avoid unnecessary palpation of abdomen prior to surgical removal
   b. Provide parents with information they need to provide care to their child, including nature of disease, treatment options, and therapeutic and side effects of chemotherapy in use
   c. Explain to parents and client the need to protect remaining kidney; teach signs and symptoms of urinary tract infections, and to avoid contact sports, during which injury to kidney might occur

7. Evaluation: client and family describe disease process and treatment options; client denies pain; family members identify successful coping strategies; client and family identify means of protecting remaining kidney

D. Bone tumors

1. Osteogenic sarcoma
   a. Description: a tumor that arises from a bone cell, probably the osteoblast
      1) Most common bone cancer in children
      2) Most frequently affects metaphysis of long bones
   b. Etiology and pathophysiology
      1) Osteogenic sarcoma usually occurs in adolescent boys; tumor growth is detected at time of rapid bone growth
      2) Most frequently affects distal portion of femur, proximal tibia and proximal humerus
      3) Is a malignant tumor that frequently metastasizes to lungs; metastasis may be present at time of diagnosis
      4) Etiology is unknown except for increased incidence noted in children who have had retinoblastoma; an abnormal gene may also be implicated, as osteogenic sarcoma has been found in several members of same family
   c. Assessment
      1) Pain and swelling are initial symptoms
      2) Chronic cough is often a symptom of metastasis at the time of diagnosis

Practice to Pass

The parents of your client with Wilms' tumor are confused by your finding of hypertension. They state that the child is too young and maybe you could repeat the check. How would you explain this finding to them?

        3) X-rays following traumatic injury may be first indication of disease

        4) Follow-up assessments will include CT or MRI imaging to detect areas of metastasis

    d. Priority nursing diagnoses

        1) Acute Pain

        2) Anxiety

        3) Risk for Injury

        4) Compromised Family Coping

        5) Risk for Disturbed Body Image

        6) Impaired Walking

    e. Planning and implementation

        1) Treatment may include radical resection or amputation

        2) Selected clients may have limb-salvaging procedures with prosthetic replacement

        3) Thoracotomy may be performed for metastasis to lung

        4) Chemotherapy may be administered pre- and postoperatively

        5) Emotional support of client is important both pre- and postoperatively, as the client and family deal with a life-threatening disease where treatment involves body image as well as mobility issues

        6) Employ a straightforward approach when amputation is indicated; allow for verbal expression of feelings

        7) Postoperative care includes sterile incision care and special bandaging as ordered

        8) Elevate limb for 24 hours, if prescribed, but avoid prolonged elevation

        9) Maintain body alignment

        10) Perform range of motion to joints above amputation

        11) Assist with early ambulation; assist with temporary prosthesis use

        12) Teach appropriate use of assistive devices

        13) Encourage early interaction with peers

    f. Client and family education

        1) Teach client and family about disease process and treatment options

        2) Teach client and family residual limb care

        3) Demonstrate safe use of prosthesis; teach client to monitor condition of limb

        4) Discuss with client and family phantom limb pain and its management

    g. Evaluation: client demonstrates appropriate limb care; client ambulates safely with prosthesis and ambulation assistive devices; client and family demonstrate appropriate coping strategies; client demonstrates positive body image by making positive comments about himself; client maintains relationships with peers

2. Ewing's sarcoma

    a. Description

        1) Ewing's sarcoma is a malignant, small, round cell tumor

        2) Usually involves diaphysial (shaft) portion of long bones; commonly found in femur, pelvis, tibia, fibula, ribs, scapula, humerus, and clavicle

    b. Etiology and pathophysiology

        1) Tumor arises in marrow spaces of bone

        2) Tends to occur between ages of 4 and 25

        3) Is a highly malignant tumor that metastasizes to lungs

    c. Assessment

        1) Pain

        2) Soft tissue mass

        3) Secondary symptoms of anorexia, malaise, fever, fatigue, and weight loss

Practice to Pass

The parents of a 5-year-old have been told their child's tumor has not responded to treatment and the child is terminally ill. The child is later heard to be asking what happens when someone dies. The family asks the nurse how they should respond to the child's questions. What would you tell the parents?

        4) Diagnosed with x-rays of affected area

        5) Radionuclide bone scans and CT scans of chest assess for metastasis

     d. Priority nursing diagnoses

        1) Acute Pain

        2) Compromised Family Coping

        3) Risk for Injury

        4) Impaired Walking

     e. Planning and implementation

        1) Amputation is usually not recommended

        2) Treatment includes extensive radiation along with chemotherapy

        3) Emotional support of client is important, as radiation therapy can affect appearance and mobility of extremity

        4) Encourage mobility of extremity as tolerated

        5) Refer to Tables 12-1, 12-2, and 12-3 for information on chemotherapy and radiation therapy

        6) Allow open communication with client and family about disease and prognosis

     f. Client and family education

        1) Discuss with client and family the disease process and treatment options

        2) Teach skin care related to radiation therapy

     g. Evaluation: client and family demonstrate adequate coping behaviors; client's skin remains intact; client maintains mobility of extremity

Practice to Pass

A pediatric patient has been diagnosed with a brain tumor, and after years of treatment, death is near. The mother has reached the stage of bereavement where she is calm and accepting. The father expresses anger at the doctors and nurses for their failure to save his child. How would you support this family?

Case Study

A 6-year-old is being admitted to your pediatric unit for the first round of chemotherapy in treating newly diagnosed acute lymphocytic leukemia (ALL). You are assigned this admission and are to prepare the client and family for insertion of a central venous access device and the subsequent chemotherapy.

1. What physical assessments would you make of the child?

2. What emotional assessments are relevant to the situation?

3. What priorities of care should be addressed?

4. What education would the child and family need?

5. How would you respond when the parents ask if they will be able to go to Disney World as planned in two weeks?

For suggested responses, see page 355.

For suggested responses, see page 355.

POSTTEST

POSTTEST

1 A 6-year-old client is being admitted for surgical removal of a brain tumor. The nurse anticipates that which of the following nursing assessment data will be present during the preoperative period?

  1. Bulging fontanels
  2. Vomiting
  3. Drainage from the ear or nose
  4. Elevated blood glucose levels

---

2 A client is receiving chemotherapy to induce remission in acute leukemia. When considering common side effects of chemotherapy, the nurse would write which appropriate nursing diagnoses early in the course of therapy? Select all that apply.

  1. Disturbed Sleep Pattern
  2. Impaired Oral Mucous Membranes
  3. Risk for Infection
  4. Risk for Impaired Tissue Perfusion: Peripheral
  5. Imbalanced Nutrition: Less Than Body Requirements related to nausea and vomiting

3 A client is to begin radiation therapy after the removal of a Wilms' tumor. Which statement by a parent indicates to the nurse a lack of understanding of related skin care?

1. "Use loose-fitting clothes on our child."
2. "Protect our child from sun exposure."
3. "Keep the area moist with petrolatum jelly."
4. "Prevent our child from scratching the site."

4 An adolescent receiving cyclophosphamide (Cytoxan) for acute lymphocytic leukemia (ALL) asks the nurse to come quickly to evaluate "blood in my urine." What is the most important action by the nurse?

1. Explain this is normal for these drugs.
2. Measure intake and output.
3. Decrease fluids to reduce bladder irritation.
4. Recognize that this is untoward and report the event.

5 A pediatric client who is known to have cancer is being admitted for mild neutropenia and a severe oral monilial infection. The nurse should assign the client to which room?

1. A semi-private room with a medical patient
2. A semi-private room with a surgical patient
3. A private room without further precautions
4. A private room with protective isolation

6 The nurse is assigned to the postoperative care of an adolescent client with a below-the-knee amputation for osteogenic sarcoma. The nurse plans to include which of the following in nursing care of the client?

1. Maintain bedrest until able to use permanent prosthesis.
2. Keep residual limb elevated continuously until prosthesis applied.
3. Apply a dressing to the residual limb that allows continuous viewing of the distal area.
4. Encourage early visits from friends.

7 The nursing diagnosis for a client undergoing chemotherapy for leukemia is Imbalanced Nutrition: Less Than Body Requirements related to nausea and anorexia. The nurse would formulate which appropriate goal for this client?

1. Administer antiemetics PRN.
2. The child's caloric intake will be (specify caloric range within normal range).
3. The child does not complain of nausea.
4. Intake and output are approximately equal.

8 A client is to receive chemotherapy with a vesicant drug by the intravenous (IV) route. The nurse can ensure safe administration of this drug by doing which of the following?

1. Administering the drug using a positive pressure infusion pump
2. Checking for blood return before, during, and after administration of the drug
3. Maintaining the infusion site below the level of the heart
4. Delivering the infusion as rapidly as possible

9 A client with leukemia has developed pancytopenia. The nurse would institute which measures designed to reduce stomatitis and improve nutritional intake in this client during the course of chemotherapy? Select all that apply.

1. Using alcohol-based mouthwash to reduce oral organisms
2. Drinking through a straw
3. Increasing intake of citrus juices, such as orange juice, that contain vitamin C
4. Rinsing the mouth several times a day with plain water
5. Brushing the teeth twice a day with a firm-bristled toothbrush

10 During rounds, the interdisciplinary team is discussing a client with leukemia who has just been diagnosed as terminal. The nurses describe the mother's behavior as angry, claiming the nurses are not providing care for her child. The team leader then focuses on which of the following as most likely the cause of the mother's anger?

1. Poor care on the part of the nurses
2. Lack of attention for the mother's needs
3. Overwhelming guilt for having caused the leukemia
4. A stage of bereavement over the anticipated loss of the child

➤ *See pages 266–268 for Answers and Rationales.*

ANSWERS & RATIONALES

Pretest

1 **Answer: 1, 3, 4** **Rationale:** Height and weight are evaluated on every well-child visit. Routine urine testing is done on well-child visits. Since Wilms' tumor is a cancer of the kidney, it important to assess kidney function. Vital signs are a part of every routine well-child visit. Since Wilms' tumor is a cancer of the kidney, blood pressure may be elevated due to increased renin production. This is the usual presentation of Wilms' tumor (nephroblastoma), and palpating the area may cause the tumor to spread. There is not evidence of abuse, so questioning the parents would be inappropriate. **Cognitive Level:** Applying **Client Need:** Physiological Adaptation **Integrated Process:** Nursing Process: Assessment **Content Area:** Child Health **Strategy:** Consider what conditions are common in the abdomen of toddlers. All normal assessments would be performed as well as assessments related to the possible condition. Knowledge of Wilms' tumor and the contraindication for palpating the abdomen will also help to identify the correct answers. **Reference:** London, M., Ladewig, P., Ball, J., Bindler, R., & Cowen, K. (2011). *Maternal & child nursing care* (3rd ed.). Upper Saddle River, NJ: Prentice Hall, p. 1498.

2 **Answer: 2** **Rationale:** This statement is accurate, giving the parents information they need to lessen their guilt. Symptoms are vague and depend on location. Symptoms of neuroblastoma tend to be generalized and difficult to identify in its early stages. Neuroblastoma is not a brain tumor but a tumor of the sympathetic nervous system. It arises out of embryonic neural crest cells and, therefore, is usually found in the adrenals or retroperitoneal sympathetic chain. Telling someone not to blame themselves is never beneficial. Providing correct information would be more helpful. **Cognitive Level:** Analyzing **Client Need:** Physiological Adaptation **Integrated Process:** Communication and Documentation **Content Area:** Child Health **Strategy:** Look for a therapeutic response that addresses the parent's comment. Eliminate the answers that are not therapeutic and only convey information. Knowledge of neuroblastoma and therapeutic communication will aid in choosing the correct answer. **Reference:** Hockenberry, M., & Wilson, D. (2009). *Wong's Essentials of pediatric nursing* (8th ed.). St Louis, Missouri: Mosby, p. 997.

3 **Answer: 4** **Rationale:** Acute lymphocytic leukemia (ALL) is staged at diagnosis to determine treatment. Following diagnosis, further testing is performed to stage the cancer and determine involvement of organs other than the bone marrow. The goal is remission, which is usually accomplished using chemotherapy. Palliative treatment is designed to reduce uncomfortable symptoms but not to affect a cure. This is not the treatment for ALL. ALL is a cancer that responds to chemotherapy.

The goal of treatment is to achieve a remission. This is not a solid mass tumor so there is no solid tumor that can be removed by surgery. **Cognitive Level:** Analyzing **Client Need:** Physiological Adaptation **Integrated Process:** Nursing Process: Evaluation **Content Area:** Child Health **Strategy:** The core concepts to correlate are leukemia tumor staging. Knowledge of ALL and the use of tests to diagnose the disease will aid in choosing the correct answer. **Reference:** Ward, S., & Hisley, S. (2009). *Maternal-child nursing care: Optimizing outcomes for mothers, children, & families.* Philadelphia: F.A. Davis Company, p. 1107.

4 **Answer: 3** **Rationale:** The most commonly reported symptoms of brain tumors in children are headache, especially upon awakening, and vomiting that is unrelated to eating. Both are related to increased intracranial pressure. Irritability would be a symptom of a brain tumor but hyperactivity would not be a symptom. Children with brain tumors have papilledema but a positive red reflex is seen in any child who does not have cataracts. Seizures may be a symptom of a late-stage brain tumor or a tumor arising above the tentorium of the brain, but fever is not a symptom of a brain tumor. Meningitis would be more suggestive here. **Cognitive Level:** Analyzing **Client Need:** Physiological Adaptation **Integrated Process:** Nursing Process: Assessment **Content Area:** Child Health **Strategy:** Remember that the earliest symptoms of brain tumors in school-age children are often due to the inability of the skull to expand; select symptoms accordingly. **Reference:** London, M., Ladewig, P., Ball, J., Bindler, R., & Cowen, K. (2011). *Maternal & child nursing care* (3rd. ed.). Upper Saddle River, NJ: Prentice Hall, p. 1493.

5 **Answer: 2** **Rationale:** Bone tumors usually occur in otherwise healthy children. Given the interruption of normalcy and the developmental tasks of the adolescent, body image disturbance can occur when a limb is lost because the amputation will render this individual different from his or her peers. The limb will be amputated. This is not failure to use the limb. There is no information in the stem as to the limb to be amputated; there may or may not be a self-care deficit. There is no indication of intolerance of activity. **Cognitive Level:** Analyzing **Client Need:** Psychosocial Integrity **Integrated Process:** Nursing Process: Diagnosis **Content Area:** Child Health **Strategy:** The critical words in the stem of the question are *age-related*. Body image is a concern for all adolescents even without physical problems. Knowledge of the clinical management of a bone tumor will also aid in identifying the correct answer. **Reference:** Perry, S., Hockenberry, M., Lowdermilk, D., & Wilson, D. (2010). *Maternal child nursing care* (4th ed.). St. Louis, MO: Mosby, p. 1706.

6 **Answer: 2** **Rationale:** Neutropenia refers to diminished numbers of WBCs and thus the inability to fight infections effectively. Diminished platelets and/or diminished clotting factors would be a reason to avoid contact sports. Spicy foods might need to be avoided if there were oral mucosa lesions but is not related to neutropenia. Neutropenia is a reduced white blood count, which increases the risk for infection. Only live immunizations would need to be avoided. Immunizations of killed viruses or toxoids could still be given. **Cognitive Level:** Applying **Client Need:** Safety and Infection Control **Integrated Process:** Teaching and Learning **Content Area:** Child Health **Strategy:** Knowledge of the side effects of chemotherapy and how to manage the resultant neutropenia aids in answering the question correctly. **Reference:** Perry, S., Hockenberry, M., Lowdermilk, D., & Wilson, D. (2010). *Maternal child nursing care* (4th ed.). St. Louis, MO: Mosby, p. 1509.

7 **Answer: 4, 5** **Rationale:** Thrombocytopenia is a decrease in the platelet count. Without platelets, the client may bleed excessively from a small injury. Because of the risk of bleeding, minimizing needle sticks and intrusive procedures would be appropriate. The question stem does not indicate any anemias so promoting iron intake is not specifically indicated. Placing the client on protective isolation would be appropriate for neutropenia, not thrombocytopenia. Fresh flowers may carry bacteria. This choice would be appropriate for neutropenia, not thrombocytopenia. **Cognitive Level:** Analyzing **Client Need:** Physiological Adaptation **Integrated Process:** Nursing Process: Implementation **Content Area:** Child Health **Strategy:** Recall which blood cell is deficient in thrombocytopenia and choose options that take corrective measures. **Reference:** Lewis, S., Dirksen, S., Heitkemper, M.. Bucher, L., & Camera, I. (2011). *Medical-surgical nursing: Assessment and management of clinical problems* (8th ed.). St. Louis, MO: Mosby, pp. 678–684.

8 **Answer: 3** **Rationale:** Children in hospitals may carry a number of infectious organisms. Hospitalized neutropenic children should be protected from exposure to other children whenever possible. These toys carry little risk of exposing the client to organisms. Limiting the number of visitors will reduce the client's risk of acquiring an infection. Telephone contacts allow for the peer support the client needs. The concern is introducing organisms to the client, not the spread of organisms from the client. Handwashing before contact with the client is the important intervention. **Cognitive Level:** Analyzing **Client Need:** Safety and Infection Control **Integrated Process:** Nursing Process: Evaluation **Content Area:** Child Health **Strategy:** Knowledge of neutropenia and the care of the client will aid in choosing the answer that indicates a need for further teaching of the parents. Consider the activity that would have the highest exposure to organisms. **Reference:** Perry, S., Hockenberry, M., Lowdermilk, D., & Wilson, D. (2010). *Maternal child nursing care* (4th ed.). St. Louis, MO: Mosby, pp. 1509–1510.

9 **Answer: 4** **Rationale:** All of these assessments look at possible postoperative complications. Since the client is left with only one kidney, failure of that kidney due to inadequate blood flow, infection, or any other cause could be fatal. **Cognitive Level:** Analyzing **Client Need:** Physiological Adaptation **Integrated Process:** Nursing Process: Planning **Content Area:** Child Health **Strategy:** Although respiratory is often the response in prioritizing assessments, in this specific case, the learner should recognize the importance of the remaining kidney. **Reference:** Ward, S., & Hisley, S. (2009). *Maternal-child nursing care: Optimizing outcomes for mothers, children, & families.* Philadelphia: F.A. Davis Company, p. 1113.

10 **Answer: 2** **Rationale:** Body image is very important in the client's development. Planning for the event can lessen the concerns if it should happen. Hair loss is related to the specific chemotherapy agent used in treatment. Acknowledging a legal responsibility does not explain why this knowledge will benefit the client. At this time, no preventive measures for hair loss have been found to be effective. **Cognitive Level:** Analyzing **Client Need:** Psychosocial Integrity **Integrated Process:** Nursing Process: Planning **Content Area:** Foundational Sciences **Strategy:** Knowledge of the effect of hair loss on the client and the need to prepare the client prior to this stressful event to facilitate coping will help to identify the correct answer. **Reference:** Ward, S., & Hisley, S. (2009). *Maternal-child nursing care: Optimizing outcomes for mothers, children, & families.* Philadelphia: F.A. Davis Company, p. 1124.

Posttest

1 **Answer: 2** **Rationale:** Vomiting is due to increased intracranial pressure which would be a symptom of a brain tumor. Fontanels normally close between 12 and 18 months. This client is 6 years old. The meninges are intact and there would be no drainage of fluid from the ear or nose. Drainage from the ear or nose might indicate a basilar skull fracture, not a brain tumor. Some brain tumors display the symptom of diabetes insipidus, not diabetes mellitus, thus the symptom would be dilute urine rather than elevated blood glucose. **Cognitive Level:** Applying **Client Need:** Physiological Adaptation **Integrated Process:** Nursing Process: Assessment **Content Area:** Child Health **Strategy:** Consider two items in answering the question: normal growth and development of the school-age child, and typical symptoms of a brain tumor. **Reference:** Perry, S., Hockenberry, M., Lowdermilk, D., & Wilson, D. (2010). *Maternal child nursing care* (4th ed.). St. Louis, MO: Mosby, p. 1572.

2 **Answer: 1, 2, 3, 5** **Rationale:** Nausea and vomiting, anorexia, mouth sores, sleep disorders, constipation, and pain are early and common side effects of chemotherapy. Bone marrow suppression reaches its peak 7 to 10 days after induction. Peripheral tissue perfusion is not related to the question. **Cognitive Level:** Applying **Client Need:** Pharmacological and Parenteral Therapies

Integrated Process: Nursing Process: Diagnosis **Content Area:** Pharmacology **Strategy:** The core concept is early side effects of chemotherapy. Recall that chemotherapy drugs kill rapidly growing and dividing cells to help select the options that pertain to rapidly growing cells that line the gastrointestinal tract. **Reference:** Kee, J., Hayes, E., & McCuistion, L. (2012). *Pharmacology: A nursing approach* (7th ed.). St. Louis, MO: Saunders, pp. 519–520.

3 **Answer: 3** **Rationale:** Self-care during external radiation therapy includes loose-fitting clothes, gentle washing with mild soap, avoiding sun exposure, and avoiding scratching and other irritation. Any lubricant must be water-soluble, not oil-based such as petrolatum jelly. **Cognitive Level:** Analyzing **Client Need:** Physiological Adaptation **Integrated Process:** Nursing Process: Evaluation **Content Area:** Child Health **Strategy:** The critical words in the question are *lack of understanding*. Eliminate those responses that would be appropriate skin care for a client receiving radiation. **Reference:** Lewis, S., Dirksen, S., Heitkemper, M., Bucher, L., & Camera, I. (2011). *Medical-surgical nursing: Assessment and management of clinical problems* (8th ed.). St. Louis, MO: Mosby, p. 285.

4 **Answer: 4** **Rationale:** Hematuria is an adverse effect of the commonly used cancer medication cyclophosphamide (Cytoxan) and should be reported. Hematuria is not a normal finding, even with a chemotherapeutic drug. Measuring intake and output should be done routinely on all clients and is not specific to managing this complication. Fluids are usually encouraged prior to administration, and the bladder is emptied frequently to prevent hematuria. **Cognitive Level:** Analyzing **Client Need:** Pharmacological and Parenteral Therapies **Integrated Process:** Nursing Process: Implementation **Content Area:** Child Health **Strategy:** Eliminate two options that are normal activities for all clients receiving chemotherapy. Determine the correct response from the remaining two considering that hematuria is not a normal finding. **Reference:** Kee, J., Hayes, E., & McCuistion, L. (2012). *Pharmacology: A nursing approach* (7th ed.). St. Louis, MO: Saunders, pp. 519–520.

5 **Answer: 3** **Rationale:** A private room assignment is indicated for clients with chemotherapy-related neutropenia. Careful hand hygiene is also an essential element to reduce the risk of infection. Because the neutropenia is mild at this time, the client does not require neutropenic precautions and does not require full protective isolation. However, neutropenic precautions could be instituted later if the client's neutrophil count continues to decline. **Cognitive Level:** Analyzing **Client Need:** Management of Care **Integrated Process:** Nursing Process: Implementation **Content Area:** Child Health **Strategy:** This oral infection is spread by direct contact, so the infection itself would not prevent the client from sharing a room. However, the neutropenia would require the client not to share a room. Note the critical word *mild* to determine that neither neutropenic precautions nor protective isolation are needed at this

time. **Reference:** Berman, A., & Snyder, S. (2012). *Kozier & Erb's fundamentals of nursing: Concepts, process, and practice* (9th ed.). Upper Saddle River, NJ: Prentice Hall, pp. 682–685.

6 **Answer: 4** **Rationale:** Adolescents need their peer group as their support system. The client will be fitted with a temporary prosthetic as soon as possible. He or she also can be out of bed in a wheelchair for short periods of time. Keeping the residual limb elevated continuously would lead to contracture in the hip joint. The dressing applied to the residual limb is occlusive and also used to help shape it for the prosthetic. **Cognitive Level:** Applying **Client Need:** Psychosocial Integrity **Integrated Process:** Nursing Process: Implementation **Content Area:** Child Health **Strategy:** To answer correctly, consider appropriate stump care and eliminate those options as incorrect, leaving only the psychological response. **Reference:** Perry, S., Hockenberry, M., Lowdermilk, D., & Wilson, D. (2010). *Maternal child nursing care* (4th ed.). St. Louis, MO: Mosby, p. 1706.

7 **Answer: 2** **Rationale:** The client's goal should be stated in terms of behaviors of the client that demonstrate the problem is solved. Interventions are not goals. Absence of nausea does not guarantee adequate intake. Equal intake and output indicates fluid balance but does not indicate adequate nutrition. Only the caloric intake adequately addresses the outcome needed by this client. **Cognitive Level:** Analyzing **Client Need:** Physiological Adaptation **Integrated Process:** Nursing Process: Planning **Content Area:** Child Health **Strategy:** Consider which response best answers the problem of imbalanced nutrition. The correct option would likely be addressing caloric intake or maintaining/gaining weight. **Reference:** London, M., Ladewig, P., Ball, J., Bindler, R., & Cowen, K. (2011). *Maternal & child nursing care* (3rd. ed.). Upper Saddle River, NJ: Prentice Hall, p. 1483.

8 **Answer: 2** **Rationale:** A vesicant drug can cause significant tissue damage if the IV line infiltrates. Checking for blood return on a regular basis during administration allows for early recognition should the catheter escape the vein. A positive pressure pump will continue to pump the drug into the tissues when the IV route is infiltrated. This will not prevent the vesicant drug from entering tissues. Delivering the infusion as rapidly as possible does not protect the tissues from extravasation. **Cognitive Level:** Applying **Client Need:** Pharmacological and Parenteral Therapies **Integrated Process:** Nursing Process: Implementation **Content Area:** Pharmacology **Strategy:** The core concept in this question is the vesicant property of the drug and safe administration. Eliminate two options because they are excessive or extreme. Choose correctly between the remaining two because it directly addresses the issue of proper IV catheter placement in the vein. **Reference:** Berman, A., & Snyder, S. (2012). *Kozier & Erb's fundamentals of nursing: Concepts, process, and practice* (9th ed.). Upper Saddle River, NJ: Prentice Hall, p. 1500.

9 **Answer: 2, 4** **Rationale:** Drinking through a straw provides a degree of comfort while drinking if lesions are present. Rinsing the mouth several times a day with plain water has been found to be very effective in preventing stomatitis. Alcohol-based mouthwashes would dry the oral mucosa and are not recommended. Citrus juices are acidic and would be uncomfortable. Firm bristled toothbrushes should be replaced with soft bristles or if that is too painful, simply wrapping a gauze strip around the finger and using that to "brush" the teeth. **Cognitive Level:** Applying **Client Need:** Physiological Adaptation **Integrated Process:** Nursing Process: Implementation **Content Area:** Child Health **Strategy:** Consider the pain of stomatitis to determine the appropriate activities. Choose the options that relieve discomfort or prevent irritation as the correct care measures. **Reference:** Perry, S., Hockenberry, M., Lowdermilk, D., & Wilson, D. (2010).

Maternal child nursing care (4th ed.). St. Louis, MO: Mosby, pp. 1513–1514.

10 **Answer: 4** **Rationale:** The stages of grief and bereavement include denial, anger, bargaining, depression, and acceptance. The anger expressed may often be displaced and directed toward persons who have a role in the loss. Nurses and other healthcare personnel must be aware of this in order to help the family cope with the impending loss. **Cognitive Level:** Analyzing **Client Need:** Psychosocial Integrity **Integrated Process:** Nursing Process: Diagnosis **Content Area:** Fundamentals **Strategy:** Most of the options include information not provided in the stem. Only one option is complete with the stem information. **Reference:** Berman, A., & Snyder, S. (2012). *Kozier & Erb's fundamentals of nursing: Concepts, process, and practice* (9th ed.). Upper Saddle River, NJ: Prentice Hall, p. 1101.

References

Adams, M., Holland, L., & Urban, C. (2011). *Pharmacology for nurses: A pathophysiological approach* (3rd ed.). Upper Saddle River, NJ: Pearson Education.

Ball, J., Bindler, R., & Cowen, K. (2012). *Principles of pediatric nursing: Caring for children* (5th ed.). Upper Saddle River, NJ: Pearson Education.

Ball, J., Bindler, R., & Cowen, K. (2010). *Child health nursing: Partnering with children and families* (2nd ed.). Upper Saddle River, NJ: Pearson Education.

Hockenberry, M., & Wilson, D. (2011). *Wong's essentials of pediatric nursing* (8th ed.). St. Louis, MO: Elsevier.

Hockenberry, M., & Wilson, D. (2011). *Wong's nursing care of infants and children* (9th ed.). St. Louis, MO: Elsevier.

London, M., Ladewig, P., Ball, J., Bindler, R., & Cowen, K. (2011). *Maternal & child nursing care* (3rd ed.). Upper Saddle River, NJ: Pearson Education.

Perry, S., Hockenberry, M., Lowdermilk, D., & Wilson, D. (2010). *Maternal child nursing care* (4th ed.). St. Louis, MO: Elsevier.

Pillitteri, A. (2009). *Maternal and child health nursing: Care of the childbearing and childrearing family* (6th ed.). Philadelphia: Lippincott Williams & Wilkins.

Gastrointestinal Health Problems

13

Chapter Outline

Overview of Anatomy and Physiology of Gastrointestinal System

Assessment of Gastrointestinal System

Congenital Gastrointestinal Health Problems

Acquired Gastrointestinal Health Problems

Infectious Gastrointestinal Health Problems

Objectives

➤ Identify data essential to the assessment of alterations in health of the gastrointestinal system of a child.

➤ Discuss the clinical manifestations and pathophysiology of alterations in health of the gastrointestinal system of a child.

➤ Discuss therapeutic management of a child with alterations in health of the gastrointestinal system.

➤ Describe nursing management of a child with alterations in health of the gastrointestinal system.

NCLEX-RN® Test Prep

Use the accompanying online resource, NursingReviewsandRationales, to test yourself with hundreds of NCLEX®-style practice questions.

Review at a Glance

acholic free of bile

anicteric without jaundice

cachexia a state of ill health, malnutrition, and wasting

dehiscence bursting open or separation

fecalith solidified feces

hematemesis vomiting of blood

icteric with jaundice

McBurney's point point of tenderness in acute appendicitis, situated between umbilicus and right anterosuperior iliac spine

omentum a double fold of peritoneum attached to stomach which connects to certain abdominal viscera

peristalsis a progressive, wavelike muscular movement that occurs involuntarily

reflux a return or backward flow

steatorrhea increased fat in stools

PRETEST

1 An 18-month-old child with a history of cleft lip and palate has been admitted for palate surgery. The nurse would provide which explanation about why a toothbrush should not be used immediately after surgery?

1. The toothbrush would be frightening to the child.
2. The child no longer has deciduous teeth.
3. The suture line could be interrupted.
4. The child will be NPO.

2 The nurse instructs the parents about postoperative feeding after their infant's pyloromyotomy. The nurse evaluates that the parents understand the instructions when the parents state that they will do which of the following?

1. Avoid bubbling the baby after feeding to prevent vomiting.
2. Rock the baby to sleep after feeding to keep the infant calm.
3. Slowly increase the volume offered according to the physician's orders.
4. Maintain the infant on antiemetics to prevent vomiting.

3 Immediately after the delivery of an infant with an omphalocele, the nurse would take which action?

1. Weigh the infant.
2. Insert an orogastric tube.
3. Call the blood bank for two units of blood.
4. Cover the sac with moistened sterile gauze.

4 While gathering admission data on a 16-month-old child, the nurse notes all the following abnormal findings. Which finding is directly related to a diagnosis of Hirschsprung's disease? Select all that apply.

1. Bile-stained vomitus
2. Child not toilet trained yet
3. Poor weight gain since birth
4. Intermittent sharp pain
5. Alternating constipation and diarrhea

5 A 6-week-old infant is brought into the pediatrician's office with a history of frequent vomiting after feedings and failure to gain weight. The diagnosis of gastroesophageal reflux is made. While planning teaching on feeding techniques with the parents, the nurse should include instructions to do which of the following?

1. Dilute the formula.
2. Delay burping to prevent vomiting.
3. Change from milk-based formula to soy-based formula.
4. Position the infant at a 30- to 45-degree angle after feedings.

6 A client is being treated for gastroesophageal reflux disease. The physician is planning on starting the client on medications. The nurse would expect which medication to be ordered?

1. Omeprazole (Prilosec)
2. Amoxicillin (Amoxil)
3. Simethicone
4. Belladonna alkaloid and phenobarbital (Donnatal)

7 The nurse has completed discharge teaching on the dietary regimen of a child with celiac disease. The nurse evaluates that client education has been successful when the mother states that the child must comply with the gluten-free diet for how long?

1. Throughout life
2. Until the child has achieved all major developmental milestones
3. Only until all symptoms are resolved
4. Until the child has reached adolescence

8 An appropriate nursing assessment of an infant suspected of having necrotizing enterocolitis would be which of the following?

1. pH of the stomach contents every four hours
2. Neurological status every two hours
3. Rectal temperature every two hours
4. Abdominal girth every four hours

9 The nurse is developing a teaching plan for the parents of an infant diagnosed with hepatitis A. Which instruction would the nurse include to reduce the risk for transmission of this disease?

1. Disinfect all clothing and eating utensils on a daily basis.
2. Tell family members to wash their hands frequently.
3. Spray the yard to eliminate infected insects.
4. Vacuum the carpets and upholstery to rid the house of the infectious host.

10 Which of the following signs would the nurse recognize as an indication of moderate dehydration in a preschooler?

1. Sunken fontanel
2. Diaphoresis
3. Dry mucous membranes
4. Decreased urine specific gravity

➤ *See pages 297–299 for Answers and Rationales.*

I. OVERVIEW OF ANATOMY AND PHYSIOLOGY OF GASTROINTESTINAL SYSTEM

A. Development
1. The gastrointestinal (GI) system begins to develop during third week of gestation
2. Primitive gut is initially formed and then divides into foregut, midgut, and hindgut; structures continue to develop in an intricate fashion to become digestive tract and accessory organs

B. Structure: GI tract extends from mouth to anus; includes organs of digestion and accessory organs such as liver, gallbladder, and pancreas
1. The mouth serves as entryway into GI tract; tongue senses taste and texture of food; submandibular, parotid, and sublingual glands secrete saliva; fetus will begin swallowing amniotic fluid as early as 20 weeks' gestation
2. Esophagus transports food from mouth to stomach by **peristalsis** (waves of gut movement); upper esophageal sphincter prevents air from being swallowed while breathing; lower esophageal sphincter (LES) prevents reflux of gastric contents into lower esophagus
3. Stomach is a food reservoir that receives partially processed food and drink funneled from mouth and esophagus and gradually releases it into small intestine
4. Small intestine's primary function is absorption of nutrients (carbohydrates, fats, proteins, minerals, and vitamins) into systemic circulation; after appropriate absorption of nutrients, small intestine is left with initial fecal liquid
5. Large intestines receive this fecal material from small intestine; water is removed from stool, which is stored for a short period of time
6. Rectum receives fecal material and defecation ensues

C. Gastrointestinal functions: primary functions of GI tract are digestion and absorption of nutrients and water, secretion of various substances, and elimination of waste products
1. Digestion
   a. Mouth serves as principal site for initial preparation of food for body to use
   b. Two basic activities are involved in digestive process
      1) Muscular activity, which produces GI movement; three types of muscles contribute to motility and are controlled by CNS

         a) Circular muscles churn and mix food particles

         b) Longitudinal muscles propel food bolus

         c) Sphincter muscles control passage of food from one segment to next segment

2) Enzymatic activity, which results from stimulation of GI tract and aids in food breakdown and the utilization process; enzymatic and chemical process of digestion involves many types of GI secretions; there are enzymes for degradation of nutrients, hormones to stimulate or inhibit GI secretions, hydrochloric acid to produce pH necessary for enzyme activity, mucus for lubrication and protection of GI tract, and water and electrolytes to transport nutrients for digestion and absorption

2. Absorption of nutrients primarily occurs in small intestine
   a. Large intestine completes process of absorption and functions primarily to absorb sodium and additional water
   b. Several mechanisms of absorption include passive diffusion, carrier-mediated diffusion, active energy-driven transport, and engulfment

II. ASSESSMENT OF GASTROINTESTINAL SYSTEM

A. Medical history
   1. Assess for presence of pain (location, type, duration, quality, aggravating or alleviating factors)
   2. Identify normal bowel habits (frequency, consistency, color, associated pain, medications, or enemas)
   3. Obtain data regarding constipation and diarrhea (client's definition, frequency, and treatment)
   4. Assess for changes in appetite
   5. Identify thirst level (increased or decreased desire for liquids)
   6. Identify food intolerances (which foods, symptoms, and treatment)
   7. Assess for belching, vomiting, heartburn, flatulence (when, frequency, quality, treatments)
   8. Identify feeding routine (what, when, amount, toleration)
   9. Past medical history related to GI system (illnesses, surgeries, accidents or injuries, family history)

B. Physical assessment
   1. Assess weight and height
   2. Determine hydration status (skin turgor, mucous membranes, peripheral pulses, and tears)
   3. Inspect abdomen (contour, visible peristalsis, rash, lesions, asymmetry, masses, enlarged organs, or pulsations)
   4. Auscultate bowel sounds (normal is 5 to 20/minute)
   5. Palpate (light and deep)
   6. Assess for rebound tenderness
   7. Assess rectal patency

C. Common diagnostic studies related to GI function
   1. Serum chemistry study, liver profile, lipid profile, erythrocyte sedimentation rate (ESR), C-reactive protein (CRP), thyroid function
   2. Stool examination for ova and parasites, blood, WBCs, pH; stool culture; Clinitest for reducing substances
   3. Fecal fat collection for 72 hours to rule out fat malabsorption
   4. Bowel studies: upper GI series, barium enema, biopsy, rectosigmoidoscopy
   5. Abdominal radiographs
   6. Abdominal and pelvic ultrasound

III. CONGENITAL GASTROINTESTINAL HEALTH PROBLEMS

A. Cleft lip and cleft palate

1. Description
   a. Cleft lip is a congenital anomaly involving one or more clefts in upper lip; degree of cleft varies from a small notch to a complete separation (see Figure 13-1)
   b. Cleft palate is a congenital anomaly consisting of a cleft ranging from soft palate involvement alone to a defect including hard palate and portions of maxilla in severe cases
2. Etiology and pathophysiology
   a. Causes include hereditary, environmental, and teratogenic factors
   b. Cleft lip occurs in approximately 1 in every 1000 births; it is more common in boys than girls
   c. Cleft palate occurs in 1 in 2500 births; incidence in girls is double that in boys
   d. These defects occur during embryonic development; cleft lip results from failure of fusion of lateral and medial tissues forming upper lip occurring around 7 weeks' gestation; cleft palate is a failure of fusion of tissues forming palate which occurs around 9 weeks' gestation
3. Assessment
   a. These defects are readily apparent at birth
      1. Cleft lip involves a notched upper lip border, nasal distortion, and may include unilateral or bilateral involvement
      2. Cleft palate is an opening between mouth and nose and may be unilateral or bilateral; may involve only soft palate or may involve both hard and soft palates
   b. Careful physical assessment should be performed to rule out other midline birth defects
4. Priority nursing diagnoses
   a. Ineffective Airway Clearance
   b. Impaired Parental Attachment
   c. Imbalanced Nutrition: Less Than Body Requirements
   d. Deficient Knowledge (parental) of disease process, medical management, feeding behaviors

Figure 13-1

A. Unilateral cleft lip,

B. Bilateral cleft lip.

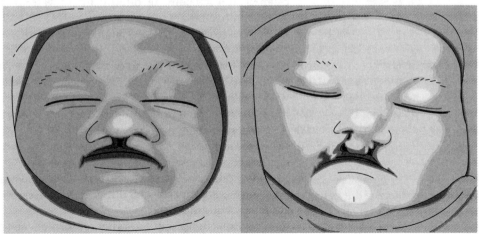

A   B

5. Planning and implementation
    a. Depending on severity of defect and general health of child, surgical correction of cleft lip typically is done at 1 to 2 months; cleft palate is generally repaired between age 6 and 18 months; cleft palate may be corrected through several operations performed in stages
    b. Early correction of cleft palate enables development of more normal speech patterns; delayed closure of large defects may require use of orthodontic devices
    c. Preoperative nursing care
        1) Assess respiratory status continuously during feedings
        2) Feed infant in upright position
        3) Feed the infant slowly and burp frequently
        4) Use ESSR method (Enlarged nipple, Stimulate suck by rubbing nipple on lower lip, Swallow, Rest after each swallow to allow for complete swallowing)
        5) Use alternate feeding devices such as elongated nipple (lamb's nipple), asepto syringe or breck feeder (large syringe with soft rubber tubing).
        6) Assess degree of cleft and ability to suck
        7) Encourage parents to verbalize fears, concerns, and negative emotions
        8) Facilitate grief responses of shock, denial, anger, and mourning
        9) Encourage touching, holding, cuddling, and bonding
        10) Provide parents with pictures of other children before and after repair
        11) Discuss infant's positive characteristics
        12) Refer to community resources and parent support groups
    d. Postoperative care
        1) Monitor client for respiratory distress during postoperative period; monitor lung sounds, encourage deep breathing without placing stress on suture line
        2) No oral temperatures
        3) A logan bar may be used with lip repair to prevent tension on suture line; although short periods of crying will serve to clear respiratory tract, extended crying will place tension on lip's suture line
        4) No straws, pacifiers, spoons, or fingers in or around the mouth for 7 to 10 days
        5) For cleft lip, use of a rubber tipped asepto syringe prevents damage to the repair
        6) For cleft palate, liquids can be taken from a cup; no straws are allowed; soft foods can be taken off side of spoon but never introduced into the mouth as it may injure the suture line; child is not allowed to feed self to reduce risk of injury
        7) Clean lip from suture line out after feedings and PRN; palate area can be cleaned after a feeding by offering infant water to drink
        8) Apply antibacterial ointment as ordered
        9) Use elbow restraints to keep infant from putting fingers in mouth or touching surgical site
        10) No tooth brushing for one to two weeks
        11) Place infant in supine position to prevent damage to sutures through contact with bedding
        12) Monitor site for redness, swelling, excess bleeding, purulent drainage, or fever
        13) Assess pain using appropriate tools
        14) Provide comfort measures to decrease stress, such as crying, on suture line; encourage rocking, cuddling, and holding
        15) Provide analgesics and sedatives on a scheduled basis
        16) Provide age-appropriate activities for diversion
6. Client and family education
    a. Teach precautions to prevent aspiration of formula and provide emergency phone numbers in case of emergency

b. Provide instruction on CPR

c. Teach parents safety and care issues regarding the use of restraints

    1) Do not apply restraints too tightly

    2) Remove at least every two hours and play games to encourage flexion

    3) Remove only one restraint at a time

d. Stress importance of follow-up care and referral appointments

e. Make appropriate and early referrals for speech and language disabilities

f. Encourage early speech attempts and arrange for speech therapy

g. Encourage good dental hygiene and orthodontic follow-up

7. Evaluation: infant maintains a patent airway, completes a feeding within 30 minutes, and follows appropriate growth curve; parents verbalize and demonstrate an understanding of alternate feeding techniques, demonstrate bonding behaviors, and assume responsibility for infant's home care and follow-up care; surgical site heals without infection; pain control is achieved as evidenced by infant's engagement in age-appropriate activities, lack of irritability, and ability to sleep undisturbed

B. Pyloric stenosis

1. Description: pyloric stenosis results when circular areas of muscle surrounding pylorus hypertrophy and block gastric emptying; also called hypertrophic pyloric stenosis (HPS)

2. Etiology and pathophysiology

a. Exact cause remains unknown; however, heredity is thought to play an important role

b. Incidence is 1 in 500 live births; firstborn children and offspring of affected children are at highest risk; males are affected five times more often than females and full-term infants more than premature infants; there is also a higher incidence in white infants; commonly noted at 8 to 12 weeks of age

c. Pyloric canal narrows because of progressive hypertrophy and hyperplasia of circular pyloric muscle

d. Leads to obstruction of pyloric sphincter, with subsequent gastric distention, dilatation, and hypertrophy (see Figure 13-2)

e. Pyloromyotomy, creation of an incision along anterior pylorus to split the muscle, is commonly performed to relieve obstruction

---

Practice to Pass

What feeding techniques would you discuss with the parents of a newborn with cleft lip and cleft palate?

Figure 13-2

Pyloric stenosis

Source: London, Marcia L.; Ladewig, Patricia W.; Ball, Jane W.; Bindler, Ruth C.; Cowen, Kay J., *Maternal & child nursing care*, 3rd Ed., ©2011. Reprinted and Electronically reproduced by permission of Pearson Education, Inc. Upper Saddle River, NJ.

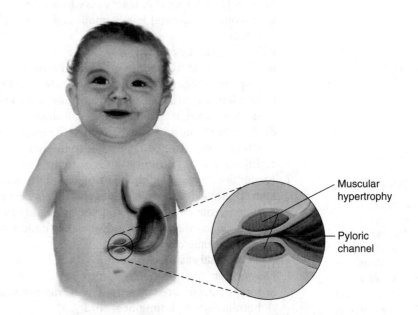

Muscular hypertrophy

Pyloric channel

3. Assessment

   a. Previously healthy infant with progressive, projectile, non-bilious vomiting
   b. Movable, palpable, firm, olive-shaped mass in right upper quadrant (RUQ)
   c. Visible, deep, peristaltic waves from left upper quadrant (LUQ) to RUQ immediately before vomiting
   d. Irritability, hunger, and crying
   e. Sunken fontanels, poor skin turgor, dry mucous membranes, and decreased urine output, constipation, jaundice, metabolic alkalosis
   f. Ultrasonography and upper GI series may reveal delayed gastric emptying and an elongated pyloric canal
   g. Laboratory findings may include an increased pH and bicarbonate level, indicating metabolic alkalosis; serum chloride, sodium, and potassium levels may be decreased; an increased hematocrit and hemoglobin may also be present, indicating hemoconcentration

4. Priority nursing diagnoses
   a. Risk for Aspiration
   b. Risk for Deficient Fluid Volume (hypotonic)
   c. Imbalanced Nutrition: Less Than Body Requirements
   d. Risk for Impaired Parenting

5. Planning and implementation
   a. Assess skin turgor, mucous membranes, and fontanels at least every shift; monitor urine specific gravity, weigh daily
   b. Maintain NPO status prior to surgery, monitor I&O hourly, administer IV fluids and electrolytes as ordered
   c. Maintain NG tube patency and monitor NG output
   d. Keep infant warm and quiet
   e. Initiate small frequent feedings of clear liquids as ordered within four to six hours after surgery; follow strict diet regimen of gradual advancement of feedings until normal formula feedings have been resumed
   f. Continue IV hydration until age- or weight-appropriate amounts of formula are tolerated
   g. Assess incision for redness, swelling, and drainage; immediately report signs of infection to physician
   h. Monitor vital signs at least every four hours
   i. Encourage parental involvement and rooming-in; support parents during feeding attempts

6. Client and family education
   a. Explain what pyloric stenosis is and how it is treated
   b. Explain all equipment such as NG tube and IV
   c. Discharge instructions for parents include to report any vomiting, abdominal tenderness, fever, incisional redness, or drainage to physician
   d. Provide verbal and written feeding instructions if client has not returned to full-strength formula feedings prior to discharge
   e. Inform parents of importance of follow-up care with physician

7. Evaluation: infant exhibits signs of adequate hydration, consumes age- and weight-appropriate amounts of formula and regains weight; incision is clean, dry, intact, and well-approximated; infant is free of signs and symptoms of infection; parents actively participate in infant's care and verbalize understanding of condition, surgical treatment, and home care

C. Omphalocele and gastroschisis

1. Description
   a. Omphaloceles are congenital malformations in which intra-abdominal contents herniate through umbilical cord

Practice to Pass

You have just admitted a child to the nursing unit. The child is scheduled for a pyloromyotomy. What information would you include in your preoperative teaching?

      b. Gastroschisis occurs when bowel herniates through a defect in abdominal wall, usually to right of umbilical cord, and through rectus muscle; there is no membrane covering exposed bowel

  2. Etiology and pathophysiology

      a. Omphalocele

         1) An omphalocele results from failure of abdominal contents to return to abdomen when abdominal wall begins to close by 10th week of gestation

         2) Viscera is outside of abdominal cavity but inside translucent sac covered with peritoneum and amniotic membrane

         3) Omphalocele is often associated with other congenital anomalies such as cardiac defects, genitourinary anomalies, chromosomal defects, craniofacial abnormalities, and diaphragmatic abnormalities

         4) Incidence is 1 in 3000 to 10,000 births

      b. Gastroschisis

         1) Controversy exists regarding etiology of gastroschisis; some suggest that at some point a tear occurs at base of umbilical cord, allowing intestine to herniate

         2) Viscera outside of abdominal cavity and not covered with peritoneal sac

         3) Gastroschisis is rarely associated with other major congenital anomalies, but jejunoileal atresia, ischemic enteritis, and malrotation may occur as a result of defect itself

         4) Gastroschisis occurs in about 1 to 3 in 10,000 births

  3. Assessment

      a. Obvious protrusion of abdominal contents present at time of delivery

      b. Size of omphalocele sac varies depending on extent of protrusion

      c. Rupture of sac or absence of sac results in injury to abdominal contents exposed to amniotic fluid over an extended period

      d. Defect may be noted on prenatal ultrasound

  4. Priority nursing diagnoses

      a. Risk for Infection

      b. Risk for Impaired Parental Attachment

      c. Risk for Impaired Gas Exchange

  5. Planning and implementation

      a. Assess body temperature continuously using skin probe; place infant in warmer immediately after birth

      b. Use sterile technique in dealing with defect

      c. Immediately cover with warm, moist, sterile gauze, and wrap with plastic to keep moisture in and preserve heat

      d. Minimize movement of infant and handling of intestines

      e. Assess respiratory status continuously during immediate newborn period by placing on cardiac and apnea monitor with pulse oximetry

      f. Monitor for circulatory compromise by monitoring temperature, pulses, capillary refill, skin color, and heart rate and respiratory rate

      g. Assess mucous membranes for moisture and skin for elastic turgor; monitor I&O, weigh daily, assess fontanels, monitor electrolytes, and maintain IV and administer fluids and TPN as ordered

      h. Maintain NG tube for decompression

      i. If amount of exposed intestinal material is large, abdomen will be too small for immediate replacement; a clear, plastic bag may be secured around bowel loops and suspended above abdomen to allow gravity to assist with return of bowel to abdomen; surgeon will decrease sac contents on a regular basis; watch infant closely for respiratory distress in immediate post-treatment period

      j. Monitor for signs of ileus by auscultating of bowel sounds, measuring abdominal girth, assessing bowel movements and maintaining an NPO status

        k. Assess parents' coping mechanisms

        l. Encourage parents to verbalize feelings of loss of "perfect" child and guilt that may accompany congenital anomaly

        m. Encourage parental participation in infant's care

    6. Client and family education

        a. Provide written and verbal information on growth and developmental needs

        b. Teach parents appropriate techniques for developmental stimulation

        c. Provide information regarding support groups and other community resources

        d. Teach parents signs of bowel obstruction

    7. Evaluation: infant maintains appropriate body temperature; infant is free from infection; infant maintains effective gas exchange as evidenced by absence of respiratory distress or circulatory compromise; infant maintains adequate hydration and nutrition status; parents verbalize feelings and actively participate in infant's care

D. Diaphragmatic hernia

    1. Description: congenital diaphragmatic hernia (CDH) results when abdominal contents protrude into thoracic cavity through an opening in diaphragm

    2. Etiology and pathophysiology

        a. CDH occurs when there is failure of transverse septum and pleuroperitoneal folds to completely develop and form diaphragm

        b. Intestines and other abdominal structures enter thoracic cavity

        c. Lung growth may cease; after birth, respiration becomes further compromised by pulmonary hypoplasia and compression of lung including airways and blood vessels

    3. Assessment

        a. Clinical findings depend on the severity of defect

        b. Fetal ultrasound shows abdominal organs in chest

        c. Postnatal diagnosis is confirmed by chest x-ray examination

        d. Diminished or absent breath sounds on affected side

        e. Bowel sounds may be heard over chest

        f. Cardiac sounds may be heard on right side of chest

        g. Dyspnea, cyanosis, nasal flaring, tachypnea, retractions

        h. Sunken abdomen, barrel-shaped chest

    4. Priority nursing diagnoses

        a. Impaired Gas Exchange

        b. Risk for Decreased Cardiac Output

        c. Risk for Impaired Parental Attachment

        d. Knowledge Deficit (parental) of disease process, medical interventions

    5. Planning and implementation

        a. Preoperative nursing care

            1) Assess vital signs frequently with ongoing respiratory assessment

            2) Elevate head of bed and position on affected side

            3) Maintain patency of NG tube to decompress the stomach

            4) Monitor IV fluids

            5) Maintain mechanical ventilation, extracorporeal membrane oxygenator (ECMO), chest tubes

            6) Provide minimal stimulation

        b. Postoperative care focuses on promoting lung function

            1) Monitor for signs of infection and respiratory distress

            2) Continue to support respirations by positioning in semi-Fowler's position on affected side; organize care to decrease exertion

            3) Promote nutrition when feedings resumed

            4) Support family through crisis

6. Client and family education
   a. Instruct parents on wound care, prevention of infection, and feeding techniques
   b. Provide written and verbal information on growth and developmental needs
   c. Provide information regarding long-term problems and necessity of regular follow-up visits
7. Evaluation: infant establishes effective breathing pattern, maintains adequate hydration status and is free from pain and infection; parents actively participate in infant's care and verbalize an understanding of condition, surgical treatment, and home care

E. Biliary atresia

1. Description: biliary atresia is a progressive inflammatory process that causes both intrahepatic and extrahepatic bile duct fibrosis
2. Etiology and pathophysiology
   a. Cause is unknown; because problem originates during prenatal period, viruses, toxins, and chemicals are believed to be a few of the suspected causes
   b. Obstruction of extrahepatic bile ducts causes obstruction of the normal flow of bile out of liver and into gallbladder and small intestine
   c. Bile plugs form and cause bile accumulation in liver
   d. Inflammation, edema, and irreversible hepatic injury occur
   e. Liver becomes fibrotic, and cirrhosis and portal hypertension develop, leading to liver failure
   f. Because of lack of bile in intestines, fat and fat-soluble vitamins cannot be absorbed; this leads to malnutrition, deficiencies of fat-soluble vitamins, and growth failure
   g. Without treatment this disease is fatal
   h. Treatment involves surgery (Kasai procedure), which may correct obstruction; liver transplantation may be required due to progressive cirrhosis
   i. Liver transplantation occurs in 66–75% of children with biliary atresia over time
   j. Without treatment, progressive cirrhosis will lead to death in most children by age 2 years
3. Assessment
   a. Healthy appearing infant at birth
   b. Jaundice occurs within two weeks to two months; usually diagnosed at less than 3 months of age
   c. **Acholic** stools: puttylike, clay-colored stools
   d. Increased direct bilirubin levels in infants older than 3 weeks of age
   e. Abdominal distention
   f. Hepatomegaly
   g. Increased bruising of the skin, prolonged bleeding time
   h. Intense itching
   i. Tea-colored urine
   j. Ultrasound shows atrophic or absent gallbladder; hepatobiliary iminodiacetic acid (HIDA) scan confirms no drainage or obstruction; liver biopsy is done at time of Kasai procedure and intraoperative cholangiography
4. Priority nursing diagnoses: Imbalanced Nutrition: Less Than Body Requirements; Anticipatory Grieving; Ineffective Family Processes
5. Planning and implementation
   a. Weigh daily
   b. Administer fat-soluble vitamins A, D, E, and K as ordered
   c. Monitor stool pattern
   d. Establish an open, caring relationship with family
   e. Refer parents to support groups

6. Client and family education
    a. Instruct parents in meticulous skin care
    b. Provide verbal and written information regarding nutritional needs
    c. Provide instructions on home medication regimen and allow time for return demonstration
     d. Inform parents of the signs and symptoms for which to call the physician, such as elevated temperature, clay-colored stools, abdominal distention, other concerns
     e. If a transplant is performed, post-transplant medications should be discussed in depth including their administration and side effects
7. Evaluation: infant's weight is maintained; skin remains intact; parents understand treatment plan and discharge instructions; if a liver transplant has been performed, parents identify signs of rejection

F. Hirschsprung's disease

1. Description: a congenital anomaly resulting from an absence of ganglion cells in colon; also known as congenital aganglionic megacolon
2. Etiology and pathophysiology
    a. Is believed to be a familial, congenital defect
    b. Rate of occurrence is about 1 in 500 live births and is about four times more common in males than in females; there is a higher incidence in children with Down syndrome and genitourinary abnormalities
    c. Rectosigmoid region is most commonly affected
    d. Absence of autonomic parasympathetic ganglion cells in one portion of colon results in lack of innervation in that portion
    e. Peristalsis cannot occur without proper innervation; lack of peristalsis causes accumulation of intestinal contents and distention of bowel proximal to defect, essentially creating a mechanical obstruction
3. Assessment
    a. Clinical manifestations vary according to client's age at time of diagnosis
        1) Newborns
            a) Failure to pass meconium stools
            b) Reluctance to feed
            c) Abdominal distention
            d) Bilious vomiting
        2) Infants
            a) Failure to thrive
            b) Constipation
            c) Abdominal distention
            d) Vomiting
            e) Episodic diarrhea
        3) Toddlers and older children
            a) Chronic constipation
            b) Foul-smelling stools
            c) Abdominal distention
            d) Visible peristalsis
            e) Palpable fecal mass
            f) Malnourishment
            g) Signs of anemia and hypoproteinemia
    b. Rectal examination typically reveals an absence of stool
    c. Laboratory studies and diagnostic tests commonly reveal an enlarged portion of colon and a rectal biopsy confirms absence of ganglion cells

4. Priority nursing diagnoses
   a. Constipation
   b. Risk for Deficient Fluid Volume
   c. Imbalanced Nutrition: Less Than Body Requirements
   d. Disturbed Body Image
5. Planning and implementation
   a. Medical treatment involves removing aganglionic bowel; a temporary colostomy is created soon after diagnosis or around 6 months, which is closed with bowel reanastomosis at a later time, usually around age 2 years; older children and some infants will have just one surgery, which is a pull-through at time of diagnosis

   b. Preoperatively, assess bowel function and characteristics of stool; measure abdominal circumference; monitor client for vomiting and respiratory distress
   c. Monitor urine specific gravity; monitor electrolytes; assess hydration status
   d. Prepare client and parents for surgery and temporary placement of colostomy
   e. Administer antibiotics as ordered
   f. Monitor vital signs; measure abdominal girth; assess surgical site for redness, swelling, drainage after surgery
   g. Assess stoma for color, bleeding, breakdown of surrounding skin
   h. Assess anal area after pull-through for patency of appliance, presence of stool, redness, drainage
   i. Provide meticulous skin care, use appropriately sized stoma supplies
   j. Notify physician of any fever, unusual drainage, redness, or odor
   k. Keep client NPO until bowel sounds return or flatus is passed, maintain NG tube, administer IV fluids as ordered, obtain daily weights, and begin intake when ordered with clear liquids and progress as tolerated
   l. Assess pain using age-appropriate scales, provide comfort measures and involve parents, provide pain medications on regular basis as ordered, notify physician if pain is not managed
   m. Avoid rectal temperatures to protect fragile rectal mucosa
   n. Involve client in quiet age-appropriate activities for diversion
   o. Assess parents' level of understanding of condition, home care, and treatment; encourage parents to share feelings, anxieties, and concerns about rectal irrigations and ostomy care; explain surgical repair and recovery process
   p. Refer to support groups and make appropriate referrals
6. Client and family education
   a. Encourage preschool and early school-age children to draw pictures, use dolls, and play to express concerns about bodily appearance, irrigations, and colostomy
   b. Provide parents with instructions about how to complete rectal irrigations and allow time for return demonstration

   c. Teach ostomy care during immediate postoperative period and encourage parents to participate and learn while in hospital, encourage client to assume care as soon as appropriate
   d. Teach parents how to assess for distention and obstruction, and importance of reporting these findings to physician
7. Evaluation: client has no fluid and electrolyte imbalances, breakdown of skin surrounding the colostomy, or signs or symptoms of infection; demonstrates adequate nutrition for age and age-appropriate hydration status; states pain is controlled and resumes age-appropriate play; client and parents verbalize and demonstrate an understanding of condition, rectal irrigations, colostomy care, and routine postoperative home care; client and parents verbalize feelings about condition and altered body image and use effective coping mechanisms

Practice to Pass

What information would you consider when planning your preoperative teaching with the parents of a child with Hirschsprung's disease?

IV. ACQUIRED GASTROINTESTINAL HEALTH PROBLEMS

A. Gastroesophageal reflux

1. Description
   a. Gastroesophageal reflux (GER) is regurgitation of gastric contents into the esophagus; is a result of relaxation or incompetence of lower esophageal sphincter (LES)
   b. Gastroesophageal reflux disease (GERD) is a more extensive disease involving esophageal damage secondary to the reflux of gastric acids into the esophagus.

2. Etiology and pathophysiology
   a. Exact cause is unknown, but is believed to result from delayed maturation of lower esophageal neuromuscular function or impaired local hormonal control mechanisms
   b. Repeated **reflux** (backward flow) of gastric contents can damage delicate esophageal mucosa
   c. GER is typically self-limiting, usually resolving by 1 year of age; in more severe cases child may require surgery, such as Nissen fundoplication, in which gastric fundus is wrapped around distal esophagus
   d. There is a higher rate of occurrence in children with neurologic impairments like cerebral palsy, Down syndrome, and head injuries
   e. GER is most common esophageal problem in infancy; some reflux may normally occur in infants, children, and even adults; however, GER is pathologic when it is severe or when complications arise
   f. Pathologic GER occurs in approximately 3% of all newborns, with a higher incidence in premature infants; boys are affected three times as often as girls, and almost all infants with GER are symptomatic by 6 weeks of age

3. Assessment

   a. Frequent vomiting, possibly with **hematemesis** (bloody vomitus), hiccupping
   b. Weight loss, failure to thrive
   c. Aspiration and recurrent respiratory infections, recurrent otitis media
   d. Near-miss sudden infant death syndrome and cyanotic episodes
   e. Esophagitis and bleeding caused by repeated irritation of esophageal lining with gastric acid

   f. Heartburn, abdominal pain, irritability, melena
   g. Laboratory studies and diagnostic findings indicate absence of gastric or duodenal obstruction on barium swallow and upper GI radiograph
   h. Low resting LES pressure on esophageal manometry
   i. Endoscopy and pH probe studies
   j. Anemia secondary to blood loss

4. Priority nursing diagnoses
   a. Risk for Aspiration
   b. Deficient Fluid Volume
   c. Imbalanced Nutrition: Less Than Body Requirements
   d. Knowledge Deficit (parental) of feeding techniques to reduce reflux

5. Planning and implementation
   a. Medical treatment depends on severity of condition

   1) Mild: change feeding habits; keep child upright during feedings and for one hour after feedings; rice cereal may be added to formula to thicken feedings; fatty foods and citrus juices are avoided; decrease amount of feeding
   2) Severe: surgical treatment may be required (Nissen fundoplication); a gastrostomy tube may be utilized for six weeks after surgery

       b. Assess breath sounds and respiratory status particularly before and after feedings

       c. Position infant upright to reduce respiratory complications, place on cardiac and respiratory monitor, keep suctioning equipment at bedside; best postfeeding position is prone with head elevated; parents are taught to avoid placing infant in an infant seat as this increases intra-abdominal pressure

       d. Administer GER medications as ordered, which may include drugs that promote gastric emptying or pyloric sphincter relaxation, or antacids to neutralize the acidity of refluxed contents (Table 13-1)

       e. Assess hydration status, monitor I&O, administer IV fluids as ordered, weigh daily

       f. Assess the amount, frequency, and characteristics of emesis, assess the relation of vomiting to the time of feedings and the infant's activity level

       g. Provide frequent, small feedings

       h. If taking solids, offer solids first and then liquids, improve nutritional status through feeding techniques such as thickening formula with cereal, enlarging nipple openings, and burping the infant frequently

       i. Assess for dumping syndrome 30 minutes after feeding if postoperative for Nissen fundoplication

       j. Assess parents' ability to provide home care

       k. Assess parents' coping mechanisms

       l. Encourage parental participation in client's care and offer positive reinforcement

    6. Medications: see Table 13-1 for drugs commonly used to treat gastroesophageal reflux

    7. Client and family education

       a. Explain proper feeding techniques, such as thickening the formula, cross-cutting the nipples and upright positioning of infant

       b. Provide information about medication administration

       c. Inform parents of problems that may arise and when to notify the physician

    8. Evaluation: infant tolerates diet, gains weight, maintains balanced fluid and electrolyte status, exhibits clear breath sounds, and is free from respiratory distress; parents verbalize and demonstrate proper feeding techniques, and comply with follow-up care

B. Appendicitis

    1. Description: inflammation and infection of vermiform appendix, a small lymphoid, tubular blind sac at end of cecum

    2. Etiology and pathophysiology

       a. Exact cause is poorly understood, but results from obstruction of lumen of appendix by hardened fecal material (**fecalith**), foreign bodies, microorganisms, or parasites

       b. Obstruction of lumen causes an accumulation of normal mucous secretions causing the appendix to become distended; this distention causes capillary and venous engorgement and increased intraluminal pressure

Table 13-1	Medications Used to Treat Gastroesophageal Reflux
Drug	**Action**
Histamine blockers Ranitidine (Rantac) Famotidine (Pepcid)	Decrease gastric acid secretion by inhibiting H_2 histamine receptors on gastric parietal cells; alleviates symptoms.
Proton pump inhibitors Lansoprazole (Prevacid) Omeprazole (Prilosec)	Blocks final common pathway of acid production by inhibiting activated proton pumps in canaliculi of gastric parietal cells; alleviates symptoms and helps heal esophagitis.

Source: Adapted from London, M., Ladewig, P., Ball, J., Bindler, R., & Cowen, K. (2011). *Maternal & child nursing care.* (3rd ed.). Upper Saddle River, NJ: Pearson Education, p. 1529.

    c. Process of ischemia can lead to necrosis and perforation of intestinal wall; if this occurs bacteria from bowel contaminates peritoneum and may lead to peritonitis and sepsis

    d. Is the most common reason for abdominal surgery in childhood; frequency increases with age with the peak incidence between ages 15 and 30 years old

    e. Appendicitis occurs equally in males and females

3. Assessment

    a. Generalized abdominal pain progressively worsening and localizing in right lower quadrant at **McBurney's point** (Figure 13-3)

    b. Nausea and vomiting, fever, and chills

    c. Anorexia, diarrhea, or acute constipation

    d. Elevated WBC count: 15,000 to 20,000 cells/mm^3

    e. Ultrasound indicating an enlarged incompressible appendix

4. Priority nursing diagnoses

    a. Acute Pain

    b. Risk for Infection related to potential rupture

    c. Risk for Deficient Fluid Volume

    d. Imbalanced Nutrition: Less Than Body Requirements

5. Planning and implementation

    a. Surgical removal (appendectomy) is done as soon as diagnosis made

    b. Preoperative nursing care

        1) Prepare client for an appendectomy; explain procedure and postoperative care to client and family

        2) Keep client NPO before surgery and prevent dehydration by administering IV fluids as ordered

Figure 13-3

McBurney's point in appendicitis

Source: London, M., Ladewig, P., Ball, J., Bindler, R., & Cowen, K. (2011). *Maternal & child nursing care* (3rd ed.). Upper Saddle River, NJ: Prentice Hall, p. 1537.

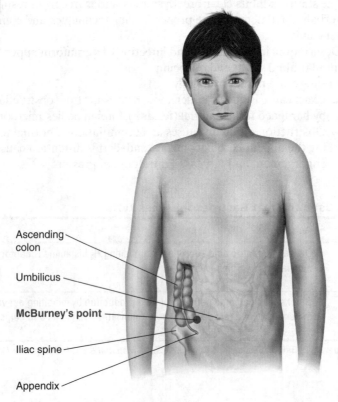

Ascending colon

Umbilicus

McBurney's point

Iliac spine

Appendix

        3) Place client in semi-Fowler's or right-side lying position to help localize and prevent spread of any infection; this position is used both preoperatively and postoperatively

        4) Assess bowel activity by evaluating for abdominal distention, auscultating bowel sounds, and observing elimination patterns

        5) Do nothing to stimulate peristalsis, which would hasten perforation; avoid laxatives, enemas, or heat applications

        6) Sudden relief of pain usually indicates a ruptured appendix

    c. Postoperative nursing care

        1) Monitor vital signs, assess for abdominal distention, and inspect surgical wound for signs of infection

        2) Encourage ambulation within six to eight hours after surgery, if not contraindicated

        3) Encourage client to turn, cough, and breathe deeply

        4) Monitor intake and output and ensure that spontaneous voiding occurs

        5) Assess for pain and administer analgesics as ordered

        6) If appendix ruptures, postoperative recovery is slowed; client will probably have NG tube to decompress stomach and a Penrose drain; antibiotics will be administered

6. Client and family education

    a. Explain to client and family diagnostic procedures, cause of appendicitis, surgical treatment, and anticipated postoperative care

    b. Provide instruction on assessing surgical incision for signs and symptoms of infection

    c. Provide information on other problems to report to physician, such as, fever, increased discomfort, and incision **dehiscence** (separation)

    d. Instruct parents to have client avoid lifting, stretching, and strenuous activities until all follow-up care is completed

    e. Provide information on fluids and nutrition during the recovery process and advancement of diet; include signs and symptoms to notify the physician for, including vomiting, abdominal distention, and increased pain

7. Evaluation: client expresses, through verbal and nonverbal behaviors, that pain is being controlled; client is free from fever and infection, remains hydrated, and demonstrates early ambulation; family and client verbalize feelings and understanding of condition and treatment

C. Umbilical hernia

1. Description

    a. A hernia is a protrusion of bowel through an abnormal opening in muscle wall

    b. An umbilical hernia is a soft, skin-covered protrusion of intestine and **omentum** (double fold of peritoneum) through a weakness in abdominal wall at umbilicus

2. Etiology and pathophysiology

    a. In an umbilical hernia, incomplete closure of umbilical ring results in protrusion of portion of omentum and intestine through opening

    b. The defect usually closes spontaneously by age 3 or 4 years; surgical correction is necessary if closure does not occur or if incarceration of herniated bowel occurs

    c. Is most common in low birth weight infants or black infants and commonly occurs in children with Down syndrome, hypothyroidism, and Hurler syndrome

3. Assessment

    a. Clinical manifestations of umbilical hernias typically include a soft swelling or protrusion around umbilicus, usually reducible with a finger; when the client cries, the amount of protrusion will increase

Practice to Pass

A 12-year-old just arrived at the emergency department. The admitting diagnosis is rule out appendicitis. What signs and symptoms would you anticipate this child has?

     b. An incarcerated hernia is one that cannot be reduced and increases risk of bowel ischemia; incarceration of umbilical hernias is rare, thus corrective surgery can safely be delayed to allow for spontaneous closure

     c. An incarcerated hernia produces such symptoms as irritability, tenderness at site, anorexia, abdominal distention, and difficult defecation and requires immediate intervention

4. Priority nursing diagnoses: Risk for Injury; Parental Anxiety

5. Planning and implementation

     a. Most umbilical hernias disappear spontaneously by 1 to 3 years of age

     b. No surgical repair is needed unless it causes symptoms, persists past 5 years of age, becomes strangulated, or continues to grow

     c. Binding is not effective in reducing or minimizing protrusion

     d. Monitor for changes in size of hernia

     e. Assess for increased bowel sounds and irreducible mass, which may indicate strangulation

     f. Postoperatively, assess for wound infection, maintain hydration, assess and manage pain, allow for self-expression

6. Client and family education

     a. Teach parents signs of strangulation, such as vomiting, pain, and an irreducible mass at umbilicus

     b. Instruct parents to avoid ineffective and potentially harmful home remedies such as "belly binders"

     c. Teach parents signs and symptoms of wound infection

     d. Inform parents of any precautions and restrictions, such as tub bathing or strenuous activity if surgery was performed

7. Evaluation: parents identify care of client with an umbilical hernia; parents avoid use of belly binders or coins as reduction devices; infant has an unremarkable postoperative period, including proper wound healing, effective pain management, and appropriate hydration status

D. Celiac disease

1. Description

     a. A genetic GI malabsorption condition also known as gluten-sensitive enteropathy, gluten induced enteropathy and celiac sprue

     b. Celiac disease is an immune mediated enteropathy of small intestine triggered by ingestion of gluten

     c. This disease results from inability to fully digest gliadin and glutenin or protein components of certain grains such as wheat, barley, rye, and oats

     d. This deficiency in digestion requires lifelong dietary modifications

2. Etiology and pathophysiology

     a. Exact cause is unknown, but there is likely an inherited predisposition with an influence by environmental factors and an immunologic abnormality

     b. Incidence of celiac disease ranges from 1 in 3000 to 5000 live births; is more common in white and European children and is rarely reported in Asians or blacks

     c. When exposed to gluten, changes occur in intestinal mucosa, which becomes damaged; villi will eventually atrophy, which reduces absorptive surface of small intestine and affects absorption of ingested nutrients; chronic diarrhea results

     d. Acute episodes that are characterized by a general flare-up of symptoms are precipitated by infections, prolonged fasting, ingestion of gluten, or exposure to anticholinergic drugs; these episodes are called celiac crises and can lead to electrolyte imbalance, rapid dehydration, and severe acidosis

3. Assessment
   a. Symptoms typically appear within three to six months after introduction of gluten (usually in form of grains) into client's diet
   b. Frequent bulky, greasy, malodorous stools with frothy appearance due to fat in stool (**steatorrhea**)
   c. Abdominal distention, vomiting, and anorexia
   d. Growth retardation with lack of fat deposits and muscle wasting
   e. Anemia, irritability, edema
   f. In a celiac crisis, severe diarrhea and dehydration ensue; electrolyte imbalances and metabolic acidosis can create life-threatening disease
   g. For unknown reasons, some children do not exhibit symptoms until after age 5, with growth retardation and delayed sexual maturation as predominant manifestations
   h. Laboratory studies and diagnostic tests
      1) Flat mucosal surface, absence or atrophy of villi, and deep crypts visible on biopsy of small intestine
      2) Steatorrhea on analysis of 72-hour quantitative fecal fat study
      3) Total IgA and tissue transglutaminase are gold standards for diagnosis; serum antigliadin antibody (AGA) and reticulin antibody levels are elevated but are not truly diagnostic
4. Priority nursing diagnoses
   a. Imbalanced Nutrition: Less Than Body Requirements
   b. Deficient Fluid Volume
   c. Impaired Growth and Development
   d. Deficient Knowledge (parental) of disease process and disease management
   e. Risk for Injury
5. Planning and implementation
   a. Nursing care focuses on supporting client and parents in maintaining a gluten-free diet (see Table 13-2)
   b. Assess client's growth and evaluate using a standard growth chart
   c. Administer fluids for hydration
   d. Monitor I&O, assess skin turgor, mucous membranes, and urine specific gravity
   e. Encourage participation in age-appropriate activities
   f. Inform parents of organizations such as American Celiac Society, Celiac Sprue Association/United States of America, and Gluten Intolerance Group
6. Client and family education
   a. Provide written and verbal instructions on gluten-free diet
   b. Instruct parents to read labels of processed foods, because most processed foods contain gluten as a filler

Table 13-2	Suggestions for a Gluten-Free Diet
Unrestricted Food Items	**Restricted Food Items**
Beef, pork, poultry, fish	Breaded items using wheat, oats, rye or barley
Eggs	Any food made from wheat, rye, oats, or barley (bread, rolls, cookies, cakes, crackers, cereal, spaghetti, macaroni)
Milk, cream, cheese	
Vegetables	Beer and ale, Ovaltine, instant tea mix, commercially prepared ice cream, malted milk, prepared puddings
Fruit	Canned baked beans, commercially seasoned vegetable mixes or vegetables with sauce
Rice, corn, gluten-free wheat flour, puffed rice, corn flakes, corn meal	Salad dressings and mayonnaise, ketchup, gravy

       c. Provide instructions about urgency of seeking medical care in event of celiac crisis

       d. Teach the importance of lifelong compliance with dietary modifications and follow-up medical care

7. Evaluation: client has soft, formed stools without diarrhea; client resumes normal growth pattern and participates in age-appropriate activities; parents verbalize an understanding of disease process, dietary modifications, and prevention of celiac crisis; parents contact one of suggested organizations for further information and support

E. Necrotizing enterocolitis

  1. Description

      a. Necrotizing enterocolitis (NEC) is an inflammatory disease of intestinal tract that occurs primarily in premature infants

      b. NEC is characterized by varying degrees of mucosal or transmural necrosis of intestine

      c. Usual onset is in first 2 weeks of life but can be later in very low birth weight infants

  2. Etiology and pathophysiology

      a. NEC can be caused by several factors, such as intestinal ischemia, bacterial or viral infection, and immaturity of gut; occurs most often in terminal ileum and colon

      b. Onset of pathology appears to begin when diminished blood flow to bowel leads to bowel wall ischemia; this ischemia allows bacteria to enter bowel wall and colonize

      c. Damage to bowel can lead to perforation, which leads to need for bowel resection

  3. Assessment

      a. History may include prematurity, small for gestational age, maternal hemorrhage, pre-eclampsia, cocaine exposure in utero, exchange transfusions, umbilical catheters, or asphyxia

      b. Typically, suspected NEC (stage I) consists of nonspecific clinical findings that simply represent physiologic instability and may resemble other common conditions in premature infants; these findings include the following:

        1) Temperature instability

        2) Lethargy

        3) Recurrent apnea and bradycardia

        4) Hypoglycemia

        5) Poor peripheral perfusion

        6) Increased pregavage gastric residuals

        7) Feeding intolerance, vomiting, abdominal distention

        8) Guaiac positive stools

      c. NEC (stage II) consists of nonspecific signs and symptoms plus the following:

        1) Severe abdominal distention

        2) Abdominal tenderness

        3) Grossly bloody stools

        4) Palpable bowel loops

        5) Edema of the abdominal wall

        6) Bowel sounds may be absent

      d. NEC (stage III) occurs when the infant becomes acutely ill; signs and symptoms include the following:

        1) Deterioration of vital signs

        2) Evidence of septic shock

        3) Edema and erythema of abdominal wall

        4) Right lower quadrant mass

        5) Acidosis (metabolic and/or respiratory)

        6) Disseminated intravascular coagulopathy

    e. Diagnostic testing includes an abdominal x-ray revealing free peritoneal gas, dilated bowel loops, bowel distention, and bowel thickening

  4. Priority nursing diagnoses

    a. Imbalanced Nutrition: Less Than Body Requirements

    b. Risk for Infection

    c. Risk for Injury

    d. Risk for Deficient Fluid Volume

    e. Ineffective Breathing Pattern

    f. Risk for Impaired Parenting

  5. Planning and implementation

    a. Nursing care focuses on early detection to minimize bowel necrosis

    b. Measure abdominal girth frequently

    c. Observe toleration of feedings

    d. Monitor cardiac and respiratory status

    e. Assess and maintain optimal hydration status

    f. Promote and maintain adequate body temperature

    g. Administer antibiotics as ordered

    h. Encourage family interaction and promote attachment process

    i. Provide developmentally appropriate activities

  6. Client and family education

    a. Encourage parents to state concerns about outcomes of surgery

    b. Instruct parents on signs of intestinal obstruction, strictures, poor tolerance of feedings, and impaired healing processes

    c. Instruct parents about care of ostomy and intravenous central line

  7. Evaluation: infant regains normal GI function; infant's growth improves as evidenced on growth chart; parents verbalize an understanding of home care and follow-up needs

F. Failure to thrive (FTT)

  1. Description

    a. A term used to describe a client whose weight falls below the 5th percentile on a standardized growth chart; growth measurements in addition to a persistent deviation from an established growth curve is generally a cause for concern

    b. There are two basic types of FTT: organic and nonorganic

  2. Etiology and pathophysiology: the type of FTT is determined by the causes involved

    a. Organic FTT is result of a physical cause; cystic fibrosis is leading cause of organic FTT; other physical causes include celiac disease, congenital heart defects, chronic renal failure, gastroesophageal reflux, malabsorption syndrome, or endocrine dysfunction

    b. Nonorganic FTT is caused by psychosocial factors and is suspected in the absence of history, physical, or laboratory findings of any organic disease; lack of bonding to primary caregiver is most common nonorganic cause; however, other factors that can play a role are poverty, health beliefs, inadequate nutritional knowledge, family stress, feeding resistance, or insufficient breast milk

  3. Assessment

    a. Physical findings

        1) Weight below the 5th percentile

        2) Sudden or rapid deceleration in growth curve

        3) Delay in developmental milestones

        4) Decreased muscle mass

        5) Abdominal distention

      6) Muscular hypotonia

      7) Generalized weakness and **cachexia** (malnutrition accompanied by wasting)

    b. Behavioral indicators

      1) Avoidance of eye contact or physical touch

      2) Intense watchfulness

      3) Sleep disturbances

      4) Disturbed manner, such as apathy, extreme irritability, extreme compliance

      5) Repetitive rocking, head banging, intense sucking, intense chewing of fingers or hands, or head rolling

    c. Diagnostic tests

      1) Developmental screening

      2) Tuberculin skin test

      3) Bone scan, chest x-ray, ECG, intravenous pyelogram, upper and lower GI series

      4) Urinalysis, complete blood count, sweat chloride test, stool tests, T4 test, celiac panel

      5) Bowel and muscle biopsies

  4. Priority nursing diagnoses

    a. Imbalanced Nutrition: Less Than Body Requirements

    b. Impaired Growth and Development

    c. Ineffective Family Processes

    d. Impaired Parenting

  5. Planning and implementation

    a. Document client's eating patterns, calorie count

    b. Document parent–child interaction

    c. Encourage parents to discuss positive and negative feelings of care, procedures, and interaction with child

    d. Feed on demand or increase intake as tolerated

    e. Offer high-protein, high-calorie snacks

    f. Offer frequent, small portions of a wide variety of foods

    g. Monitor I&O, daily weights

    h. Provide consistency in nursing care

  6. Client and family education

    a. Reinforce information about normal growth and development

    b. Provide written and verbal information on ways to make mealtimes less of a control issue

    c. Provide information on effective feeding practices

  7. Evaluation: infant gains weight and eats foods that are offered; parents participate in feeding infant, and demonstrate appropriate interactions with infant during meals

V. INFECTIOUS GASTROINTESTINAL HEALTH PROBLEMS

A. Hepatitis

  1. Description: an inflammation of liver; it ranges greatly in severity and can be caused by several different viruses, toxins, or disease states

  2. Etiology and pathophysiology

    a. Hepatitis viruses cause local necrosis of parenchymal cells of liver; an inflammatory response leads to swelling and blockage of liver's drainage system

    b. Hepatitis occurs in varying levels of severity from asymptomatic or mild cases, in which liver cells regenerate completely in two to three months, to more severe forms, in which hepatic necrosis and death may occur in one to two weeks

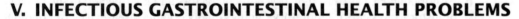

      c. There are five major hepatitis viruses

          1) Hepatitis A is transmitted via GI tract (oral–fecal route); hepatitis A is highly contagious and easily spread throughout households and day care centers

          2) Hepatitis B is bloodborne; hepatitis B is transmitted through exchange of blood or body fluids; hepatitis A and B are most common forms

          3) Hepatitis C, also called post-transfusion hepatitis, is spread by blood and body fluids; is most common cause of chronic hepatitis

          4) Hepatitis D, Delta-agent hepatitis, is transmitted by percutaneous route and occurs only in people infected with hepatitis B

          5) Hepatitis E is transmitted enterically

3. Assessment

    a. Children less than 5 years of age diagnosed with hepatitis A are usually asymptomatic or have mild, nonspecific symptoms

    b. Individuals with hepatitis B can be asymptomatic or have acute fulminating hepatitis, which can be fatal

    c. If symptomatic, symptoms usually occur in two stages: anicteric and icteric

        1) Anicteric (absence of jaundice), lasting five to seven days

           a) Anorexia, nausea, and vomiting

           b) Right upper quadrant (RUQ) abdominal or epigastric pain

           c) Fever, malaise, fatigue, depression, irritability

           d) Hepatosplenomegaly

        2) Icteric (presence of jaundice), lasting up to four weeks

           a) Jaundice, urticaria

           b) Dark urine and light-colored stools

           c) Client temporarily feels better as jaundice appears

    d. Acute fulminating hepatitis: bleeding problems, hepatic encephalopathy, ascites, acute liver failure, death; this complication is seen infrequently but quickly leads to liver decompensation that can lead to death within a week unless liver transplant is done

    e. Other assessment findings

        1) A positive history of exposure to jaundiced children

        2) A confirmed outbreak in day care center

        3) Percutaneous exposure to blood or body fluid

        4) Elevated liver function tests (AST and ALT), bilirubin levels, sedimentation rate

        5) Antigen identification markers (IgM anti-HAV and IgM anti-HBV)

        6) Positive liver biopsy

4. Priority nursing diagnoses

    a. Risk for Ineffective Health Maintenance

    b. Imbalanced Nutrition: Less Than Body Requirements

    c. Disturbed Body Image

    d. Activity Intolerance

5. Planning and implementation

    a. In uncomplicated cases, treatment is usually supportive; hospitalization is rarely indicated; in fulminating hepatitis, intensive care may be needed to provide homeostasis, nutritional, and hydration support, as well as neurologic assessment to increase chances of survival

    b. With cases of hepatitis A, controlling spread of infection is a major nursing focus; this is accomplished through disinfection of contaminated diaper-changing surfaces, use of standard precautions, and reporting to local public health department; exposed individuals should receive immune globulin as soon as possible

      c. With cases of hepatitis B, prevention is major health focus; hepatitis B vaccines are begun during neonatal period and are recommended for all infants as part of their well-child care

  6. Client and family education

      a. Teach parents how to maintain adequate nutrition

      b. Teach parents how to prevent spread of infection

      c. Advise parents to call for signs and symptoms of fulminant hepatitis

  7. Evaluation: client maintains a pre-illness weight, is free of vomiting and abdominal pain, and stools remain normal; family members remain free from infection; client does not experience fulminant hepatitis; family verbalizes an understanding of disease process, use of standard precautions, and complies with immunization recommendations

B. Vomiting and diarrhea

  1. Description

      a. Vomiting is forceful ejection of gastric contents through mouth

        1) Is common in children and is usually self-limiting

        2) Requires no specific treatment unless complications occur (including dehydration and electrolyte imbalances, malnutrition, and aspiration)

      b. Diarrhea is defined as frequent, watery, loose stools and is actually a symptom rather than a disease

        1) Accompanies many childhood disorders, including respiratory infections and GI disorders; can be an adverse effect of certain medical management modalities such as antibiotic therapy

        2) Can be acute or chronic, inflammatory or noninflammatory, or viral or bacterial in nature

        3) Can lead to a state of dehydration, electrolyte imbalance, hypovolemic shock, and even death in pediatric clients

  2. Etiology and pathophysiology

      a. Vomiting is a well-defined, complex, coordinated process that is under control of CNS; the act of vomiting involves both voluntary and involuntary muscles; a certain position is assumed, the glottis is closed, the diaphragm and abdominal muscles contract, and the lower esophageal sphincter relaxes while anti-peristaltic waves occur

      b. Can be an associated symptom of an acute infectious disease, increased intracranial pressure, toxic ingestion, food intolerance and allergy, mechanical obstruction of GI tract, metabolic disorder, or a psychogenic problem

      c. Client's age, pattern of vomiting, and duration of symptoms help to determine the etiology

      d. Color and consistency of emesis vary according to etiology

        1) Green bilious vomiting suggests bowel obstruction

        2) Curdled stomach contents, mucus, or fatty foods that are vomited several hours after ingestion suggest poor gastric emptying

        3) Vomitus having the appearance and consistency of coffee grounds (due to blood being mixed with stomach contents) is associated with GI bleeding disorders

      e. Associated symptoms also help to identify etiology

        1) Fever and diarrhea accompanying vomiting suggest an infection

        2) Constipation associated with vomiting suggests an obstruction

        3) Localized abdominal pain and vomiting often occur with appendicitis, pancreatitis, or peptic ulcer disease

        4) A change in level of consciousness or a headache associated with vomiting indicates a CNS or metabolic disorder

        5) Forceful vomiting (projectile) is associated with pyloric stenosis

      f. Diarrhea

         1) Increased intestinal motility and rapid emptying results in impaired absorption of nutrients and excessive excretion of water and electrolytes

         2) Electrolytes most affected are sodium and potassium; sodium is necessary for fluid and acid–base balance; potassium is a neurotransmitter necessary for muscle contractility

         3) Diarrhea can have many different causes (Table 13-3)

         4) Diarrhea is leading cause of death and a major cause of morbidity in children world-wide; children in daycare centers and those living in substandard housing environments lacking proper sanitation are at increased risk

      g. Fluid and electrolyte imbalance

         1) Body fluids are contained in extracellular and intracellular compartments and contain electrolytes, which perform varying functions, normal exchange of fluids between compartments occurs across the cell membrane; young children have more fluid outside the cell, interactions with environment can significantly compromise composition of that fluid

         2) The ratio of water and solute determines fluid and electrolyte balance; primary electrolytes are sodium, potassium, chloride, and calcium

         3) Extracellular sodium is responsible for degree of concentration of body fluids and whether cells swell or shrink; decreased sodium (hyponatremia) in children can occur with increased intake of water, dilute formula, or physiological causes

         4) Intracellular potassium is responsible for muscle function; imbalances cause flaccid skeletal muscles, GI cramping, and cardiac dysrhythmias (see Table 13-4)

      h. Acid–base imbalance

         1) Degree of acidity or alkalinity of body fluids determines how well cells of body function; body maintains proper balance by constantly producing acids and buffers, regulating concentrations via kidneys and respiratory system

         2) Acidosis is determined by number of hydrogen ions in fluid; increased hydrogen ions indicate acidosis; lungs attempt to compensate by increasing rate and depth of respirations to remove carbon dioxide; kidneys increase secretion of hydrogen ions, thereby raising serum pH

         3) Alkalosis refers to the buffer bicarbonate; increased levels of bicarbonate cause alkalosis, respiratory rate decreases and the kidneys conserve hydrogen ions and excrete bicarbonate

    3. Assessment

      a. Assessment of client's hydration status is highest priority (see Table 13-5)

      b. Assess amount, color, consistency, and time of stools and vomitus

Table 13-3	Common Causes of Diarrhea in Children
Causative Factor	**Effect on Bowel Function**
Colon disease	Trauma to intestinal wall
Stress	Increased motility
Food intolerance	Increased motility, increased mucus secretion in colon
Food sensitivity	Decreased digestion of food
Intestinal infection	Inflammation of mucosa, increased mucus secretion in colon
Medication	Irritation and superinfection
Surgical procedure	Reduced size of colon, decreased absorption surface

Table 13-4	Summary of Clinical Assessment of Electrolyte Imbalances	
Assessment Category	**Specific Assessments**	**Changes with Electrolyte Imbalances**
Skeletal muscle function	Muscle strength	Weakness, flaccid paralysis—hyperkalemia; hypokalemia
Neuromuscular excitability	Deep tendon reflexes	Depressed—hypercalcemia; hypermagnesemia
		Hyperactive—hypocalcemia; hypomagnesemia
	Chvostek's sign (not infants)	Positive—hypocalcemia; hypomagnesemia
	Trousseau's sign	Positive—hypocalcemia; hypomagnesemia
	Paresthesias	Digital or perioral—hypocalcemia
	Muscle cramping or twitching	Present—hypocalcemia; hypomagnesemia
Gastrointestinal tract function	Bowel sounds	Decreased or absent—hypokalemia
	Elimination pattern	Constipation—hypokalemia; hypercalcemia
		Diarrhea—hyperkalemia
Cardiac rhythm	Arrhythmia	Irregular—hyperkalemia; hypokalemia; hypercalcemia; hypocalcemia; hypermagnesemia; hypomagnesemia
	Electrocardiogram	Abnormal—hyperkalemia; hypokalemia; hypercalcemia; hypocalcemia; hypermagnesemia; hypomagnesemia
Cerebral function	Level of consciousness	Decreased—hyponatremia; hypernatremia

Source: Hogan, MaryAnn; Brancato, Vera; White, Judy; Falkenstein, Kathleen, *Prentice Hall Reviews & rationales: Child health nursing*, 2nd Ed., ©2007. Reprinted and Electronically reproduced by permission of Pearson Education, Inc. Upper Saddle River, NJ.

Table 13-5	Severity of Clinical Dehydration		
	Mild	**Moderate**	**Severe**
Percent of body weight lost	Up to 5%	6%–9%	10% or more
Level of consciousness	Alert, restless, thirsty	Restless or lethargic (infants and very young children); alert, thirsty, rest-less (older children and adolescents)	Lethargic to comatose (infants and young children); often consciously apprehensive (older children and adolescents)
Blood pressure	Normal	Normal or low; postural hypotension (older children and adolescents)	Low to undetectable
Pulse	Normal	Rapid	Rapid, weak to nonpalpable
Skin turgor	Normal	Poor	Very poor
Mucous membranes	Moist	Dry	Parched
Urine	May appear normal	Decreased output (<1 mL/kg/hr); dark color	Very decreased or absent output
Thirst	Slightly increased	Moderately increased	Greatly increased unless lethargic
Fontanel	Normal	Sunken	Sunken
Extremities	Warm; normal capillary refill	Delayed capillary refill (>2 sec)	Cool, discolored; delayed capillary refill (>3–4 sec)

Source: Hogan, MaryAnn; Brancato, Vera; White, Judy; Falkenstein, Kathleen, *Prentice Hall Reviews & rationales: Child health nursing*, 2nd Ed., ©2007. Reprinted and Electronically reproduced by permission of Pearson Education, Inc. Upper Saddle River, NJ.

       c. Assess daily weights; daily weights are best indication of fluid balance

       d. Assess I&O and client's activity level

       e. Assess for abdominal cramping, fever, and other related symptoms

       f. Laboratory and diagnostic tests

          1) Stool examination to rule out bacteria, ova, parasites, or rotaviruses if diarrhea is not self-limiting

          2) Stool examination for pH, leukocytes, glucose, and presence of blood

          3) Electrolytes, BUN, creatinine, and glucose

          4) X-rays, ultrasound, or endoscopy

    4. Priority nursing diagnoses

       a. Deficient Fluid Volume

       b. Impaired Skin Integrity

       c. Imbalanced Nutrition: Less Than Body Requirements

       d. Risk for Infection

    5. Planning and implementation

       a. Priority nursing interventions are focused on assessing signs and symptoms of dehydration

       b. Weigh client on admission and daily using same scale at same time of day

       c. Monitor and document I&O hourly, weigh each diaper after voiding and bowel movements, monitor urine specific gravity

       d. Monitor vital signs, avoiding rectal temperatures

       e. Client is usually NPO to allow bowel rest; administer IV fluids as ordered

       f. Begin oral rehydration with frequent, small feedings; oral rehydration fluids include commercial preparations such as Pedialyte; frequent small amounts of liquids should be offered—one to three teaspoons of fluid every 10 to 15 minutes; infants progress from clear liquids to a bland, milk-free diet; bananas, rice cereal, applesauce, and toast diets (BRAT) may still be prescribed for client recovering from diarrhea; as vomiting/diarrhea improves, client may resume regular diet

       g. Administer antidiarrheals, antibiotics, antiprotozoals as ordered

       h. Monitor lab tests (electrolytes, hematocrit, pH, serum albumin)

       i. Implement measures to reduce fever if needed

       j. Cleanse diaper area with mild soap and water after each stool, avoid the use of baby wipes

       k. Practice standard precautions

    6. Client and family education

       a. Provide information on causes of vomiting and diarrhea

       b. Provide instructions on oral rehydration therapy

       c. Demonstrate skin care to family

       d. Instruct parent about signs and symptoms that require medical attention

    7. Evaluation: client is well hydrated as evidenced by moist mucous membranes, elastic skin turgor, urine specific gravity of 1.005–1.020, 1–2 mL/kg/hr of urine output; client is free of frequent, loose stools as evidenced by soft, formed stools of less than four per 24-hour period; client is free from vomiting; client tolerates a regular diet; client maintains skin integrity

Practice to Pass

A mother brings her 4-month-old son to the pediatrician's office with a history of vomiting and diarrhea. What are your immediate assessments?

Case Study

A 4-year-old has been admitted for rule out appendicitis. She has just arrived in your nursing unit. The client is crying, stating her stomach hurts. No surgery has been scheduled, but close observation is warranted. The client and her parents are very anxious.

1. What questions will you ask her and/or her parents?

2. What general nursing orders do you expect for this client during her observation phase?

3. What can you do to help relieve this client's pain?

4. How can you decrease the parents' anxiety? The client's anxiety?

5. What postoperative nursing orders do you expect depending on whether there is rupture or no rupture?

For suggested responses, see pages 355–356.

POSTTEST

① A client who underwent cleft palate repair has just returned from surgery with elbow restraints in place. The parents question why their child must have the restraints. The nurse would give which of the following as the best explanation to the parents?

1. "This device is frequently used postoperatively to protect the IV site in small children."
2. "The restraints will help us maintain proper body alignment."
3. "Elbow restraints are used postoperatively to keep childrens' hands away from the surgical site."
4. "The restraints help maintain the child's NPO status."

② The nurse is caring for an infant vomiting secondary to pyloric stenosis. The mother questions why the vomitus of this child appears different from that of her other children when they have the flu. The nurse would explain that the emesis of an infant with pyloric stenosis does not contain bile because of which of the following?

1. The GI system is still immature in newborns and infants.
2. The obstruction is above the bile duct.
3. The emesis is from passive regurgitation.
4. The bile duct is obstructed.

③ The nurse is teaching the parents of a child with celiac disease about the dietary restrictions. The nurse would explain that the most appropriate diet for their child is a diet that is free of which of the following? Select all that apply.

1. Rice
2. Wheat
3. Oats
4. Barley
5. Corn

④ A high school experiences an outbreak of hepatitis B. In teaching the high school students about hepatitis B, the school nurse would explain which of the following?

1. Hepatitis B cannot exist in a carrier state.
2. Hepatitis B is primarily transmitted through the fecal–oral route.
3. Immunity to all types of hepatitis will occur after this current attack.
4. Hepatitis B can be prevented by receiving the HBV vaccine.

5 A 4-month-old infant is admitted to the nursing unit with moderate dehydration. Which of the following symptoms does the nurse recognize as consistent with this diagnosis? Select all that apply.

1. Elevated heart rate
2. Urine specific gravity of 1.038
3. Weight gain
4. Polyuria
5. Slow capillary refill

6 While performing a newborn assessment, the nurse notes the infant is having difficulty breathing, with nasal flaring, cyanosis, retractions, and an absence of breath sounds on the left side. The nurse auscultates the apical pulse on the right side of the chest. The nurse notifies the physician immediately, suspecting which of the following?

1. Diaphragmatic hernia
2. Pyloric stenosis
3. Cleft palate
4. Omphalocele

7 The nurse has taught dietary restrictions to a 7-year-old child who has celiac disease. After teaching, the child is allowed to choose a meal from the hospital menu. The nurse evaluates that teaching was effective when the child chooses which of the following?

1. Beef and barley soup, rice cakes, and celery
2. Ham and cheese sandwich with lettuce and tomato on rye toast
3. Beef patty on a hamburger bun and home fries
4. Baked chicken, green beans, and a slice of cornbread

8 An infant returns from initial surgery for Hirschsprung's disease. All of the following are routine postoperative nursing interventions. Because of the type of surgery this child had, the nurse would exclude which of them?

1. Maintaining the child NPO until bowel sounds return
2. Monitoring rectal temperature every four hours
3. Reuniting the parents with the child as soon as possible
4. Assessing the surgical site every two hours

9 A 3-month-old infant has gastroesophageal reflux (GER) but is thriving without other complications. The mother wants to know what she can do differently to decrease the reflux. Which intervention should the nurse suggest to minimize reflux?

1. Discontinue breastfeeding immediately.
2. Increase frequency of feedings and keep them small.
3. Place the baby in prone position with the head flat.
4. Place the infant in a car seat after feeding.

10 A 10-year-old boy has been admitted with a diagnosis of rule out appendicitis. While the nurse is conducting a routine assessment, the boy states, "It doesn't hurt anymore." The nurse suspects which of the following?

1. The boy is afraid of going to surgery.
2. The boy is having difficulty expressing his pain adequately.
3. The appendix has ruptured.
4. This is a method the boy uses to receive attention.

➤ *See pages 299–300 for Answers and Rationales.*

ANSWERS & RATIONALES

Pretest

1 **Answer: 3 Rationale:** During the immediate postoperative period, protecting the operative site is a priority in the nursing care of this child. Nothing is allowed in the mouth. The child might accidently stress the suture line with a toothbrush. The child should be using the tooth-

brush before this and thus it would not be frightening. Oral care will be performed according to the physician's orders but usually consists of cleansing the area with sterile water. At this age, the child should be close to having all deciduous teeth in place. Deciduous teeth are replaced by permanent (secondary) teeth around 6 years of age. The child will be on a full-liquid diet, although no straws are allowed. **Cognitive Level:** Applying **Client Need:** Reduction of Risk Potential **Integrated Process:** Teaching and Learning **Content Area:** Child Health **Strategy:** The core concepts for this question are cleft palate surgery and postoperative care. Since the stem states why use of toothbrush care is avoided, the learner must connect this to postoperative care. **Reference:** Ball, J., Bindler, R., & Cowen, K. (2010). *Child health nursing: Partnering with children & families* (2nd ed.). Upper Saddle River, NJ: Prentice Hall, p. 1136.

2 Answer: 3 Rationale: The goal after pyloromyotomy is to slowly increase the volume of feeding while preventing vomiting. Bubbling is essential after a feeding. Rocking is avoided as this might increase vomiting. Antiemetics are not helpful as the vomiting is not associated with nausea. **Cognitive Level:** Analyzing **Client Need:** Reduction of Risk Potential **Integrated Process:** Nursing Process: Evaluation **Content Area:** Child Health **Strategy:** Recognize the problem with pyloric stenosis is not related to vomiting but due to a tight pyloric muscle that will be incised. **Reference:** Perry, S., Hockenberry, M., Lowdermilk, D., & Wilson, D. (2010). *Maternal child nursing care* (4th ed.). St. Louis, MO: Mosby, p. 1419.

3 Answer: 4 Rationale: Omphaloceles are congenital malformations in which abdominal contents protrude through the umbilical cord. The protrusion is covered by a translucent sac; immediately after birth, the sac requires priority attention. The sac is covered with sterile gauze soaked in normal saline solution to prevent drying and injury. Weighing the infant is important but not the priority action. An orogastric tube may be inserted later but that is not the priority at the moment. Blood is not required for this infant. **Cognitive Level:** Analyzing **Client Need:** Physiological Adaptation **Integrated Process:** Nursing Process: Implementation **Content Area:** Child Health **Strategy:** The stem of the question is seeking the first action of the nurse. Ordering blood is not a nursing function. The nurse would not insert an orogastric tube without a medical order. Therefore, choose the most important action between the other two options. **Reference:** Ball, J., Bindler, R., & Cowen, K. (2010). *Child health nursing: Partnering with children & families* (2nd ed.). Upper Saddle River, NJ: Prentice Hall, p. 773.

4 Answer: 1, 3, 5 Rationale: Infants with Hirschsprung's disease usually display failure to thrive, poor weight gain, and delayed growth. Vomiting is usually bile stained. The child will demonstrate alternating constipation and diarrhea, but the stools are not bloody. Decreased urine output and intermittent sharp pain are nonspecific symptoms that can be associated with many different diseases and disorders. **Cognitive Level:** Applying **Client Need:** Physiological Adaptation **Integrated Process:** Nursing Process: Assessment **Content Area:** Child Health **Strategy:** Consider symptoms of Hirschsprung's disease without

looking at the options. Then review the options to determine which options match those symptoms. **Reference:** Perry, S., Hockenberry, M., Lowdermilk, D., & Wilson, D. (2010). *Maternal child nursing care* (4th ed.). St. Louis, MO: Mosby, p. 1392.

5 Answer: 4 Rationale: Small, frequent feedings followed by placing the infant at a 30- to 45-degree angle has been shown to be beneficial in treating gastroesophageal reflux. Diluting the formula would not be recommended because the infant needs the calories from the full-strength formula. It may be recommended to thicken the formula with rice cereal. It is recommended to burp frequently; to delay burping would only increase the occurrences of reflux. Gastroesophageal reflux is not related to milk intolerance, but rather to immaturity of the GI tract, so changing the formula would not help the child. **Cognitive Level:** Applying **Client Need:** Physiological Adaptation **Integrated Process:** Teaching and Learning **Content Area:** Child Health **Strategy:** Knowledge of the care of the infant with gastroesophageal reflux will aid in choosing the correct answer. Consider which activities will decrease vomiting. **Reference:** Perry, S., Hockenberry, M., Lowdermilk, D., & Wilson, D. (2010). *Maternal child nursing care* (4th ed.). St. Louis, MO: Mosby, p. 1395.

6 Answer: 1 Rationale: Omeprazole is a proton pump inhibitor to reduce acid secretions and alleviate symptoms. Amoxil is an antibiotic and is not indicated in this disorder. Simethicone is administered for gas issues. Donnatal is used to treat irritable bowel disorder, not GERD. **Cognitive Level:** Analyzing **Client Need:** Pharmacological and Parenteral Therapies **Integrated Process:** Nursing Process: Assessment **Content Area:** Child Health **Strategy:** Think of the problems associated with GERD to determine which drugs would be appropriate. **Reference:** Perry, S., Hockenberry, M., Lowdermilk, D., & Wilson, D. (2010). *Maternal child nursing care* (4th ed.). St. Louis, MO: Mosby, p. 1395.

7 Answer: 1 Rationale: Symptoms will return if dietary restrictions are not maintained. Anytime the child is exposed to gluten, irritation of the gastric mucosa will occur. Celiac disease is a lifelong disorder. The child does not outgrow celiac disease. Symptoms will return if dietary restrictions are not maintained. Celiac disease is a lifelong disorder. **Cognitive Level:** Analyzing **Client Need:** Health Promotion and Maintenance **Integrated Process:** Nursing Process: Evaluation **Content Area:** Child Health **Strategy:** Because celiac disease is a type of intolerance, the child will not outgrow the intolerance and must continue the diet throughout life. **Reference:** Ball, J., Bindler, R., & Cowen, K. (2010). *Child health nursing: Partnering with children & families* (2nd ed.). Upper Saddle River, NJ: Prentice Hall, p. 1179.

8 Answer: 4 Rationale: An early symptom of necrotizing enterocolitis is increasing abdominal girth. Measuring the abdominal girth frequently aids in early detection of necrotizing enterocolitis, which, in turn, minimizes loss of bowel. Assessment of gastric pH is not done. Frequent assessment of the neurologic status is not specific to this disease, as this is a gastrointestinal disorder. Rectal temperatures are contraindicated because of the increased risk of perforation. **Cognitive Level:** Applying **Client Need:** Physiological Adaptation **Integrated Process:** Nursing Process: Assessment **Content Area:** Child Health **Strategy:** Because the disease is a gastrointestinal disease, locate symptoms that relate to the GI system. **Reference:** Pillitteri, A. (2010). *Maternal & child health nursing: Care of the childbearing & childrearing family* (6th ed.). Philadelphia: Lippincott Williams & Wilkins, p. 1341.

9 **Answer: 2** **Rationale:** Hepatitis A is highly contagious and is transmitted primarily through the fecal–oral route. Washing hands will reduce the risk of transfer. Hepatitis A is spread by the fecal–oral route, not through simple contact. This disorder is not spread by a vector. The virus is transmitted by direct person-to-person contact or through ingestion of contaminated food or water, especially shellfish growing in contaminated water. The infectious organism does not live in carpets and upholstery. **Cognitive Level:** Applying **Client Need:** Safety and Infection Control **Integrated Process:** Teaching and Learning **Content Area:** Child Health **Strategy:** Consider how the virus spreads to determine the correct answer. Two options can be eliminated since they include a separate host. **Reference:** McKinney, E., James, S., Murray, S., & Ashwill, J. (2009). *Maternal-child nursing* (3rd ed.). St. Louis, MO: Saunders, p. 1133.

10 **Answer: 3** **Rationale:** Mucous membranes typically appear dry when moderate dehydration is observed. Other typical findings associated with moderate dehydration include restlessness with periods of irritability (especially infants and young children), rapid pulse, poor skin turgor, delayed capillary refill, and decreased urine output. Both anterior and posterior fontanels are closed on a preschool-age child. The skin is usually dry with decreased elasticity, not diaphoretic. Urine specific gravity increases with decreased urine output associated with dehydration. **Cognitive Level:** Applying **Client Need:** Physiological Adaptation **Integrated Process:** Nursing Process: Assessment **Content Area:** Child Health **Strategy:** Note there is only one symptom that is age related and is not associated with a toddler. Two options are not associated with dehydration, leaving only one response as correct. **Reference:** Perry, S., Hockenberry, M., Lowdermilk, D., & Wilson, D. (2010). *Maternal child nursing care* (4th ed.). St. Louis, MO: Mosby, p. 1382.

Posttest

1 **Answer: 3** **Rationale:** Elbow restraints are used to keep hands away from the mouth after cleft palate surgery. This precaution will be maintained at home until the palate is healed, usually four to six weeks. They are not used to protect the IV site, maintain NPO status, or maintain body alignment. **Cognitive Level:** Applying

Client Need: Physiological Adaptation **Integrated Process:** Nursing Process: Implementation **Content Area:** Child Health **Strategy:** Consider what movements elbow restraints will allow the child to determine the right answer. **Reference:** Perry, S., Hockenberry, M., Lowdermilk, D., & Wilson, D. (2010). *Maternal child nursing care* (4th ed.). St. Louis, MO: Mosby, p. 1414.

2 **Answer: 2** **Rationale:** In pyloric stenosis, bile is unable to enter the stomach from the duodenum because the pylorus muscle is hypertrophied, which causes the obstruction. **Cognitive Level:** Analyzing **Client Need:** Physiological Adaptation **Integrated Process:** Nursing Process: Implementation **Content Area:** Child Health **Strategy:** Consider the site of the pylorus to determine the correct answer. **Reference:** Ball, J., Bindler, R., & Cowen, K. (2010). *Child health nursing: Partnering with children & families* (2nd ed.). Upper Saddle River, NJ: Prentice Hall, p. 1140.

3 **Answer: 2, 3, 4** **Rationale:** Most children who remain on a gluten-free diet remain healthy and free of symptoms and complications. Gluten is a protein found in wheat, barley, rye, and oats. For this reason, appropriate foods need to be free of these grains. **Cognitive Level:** Applying **Client Need:** Physiological Adaptation **Integrated Process:** Teaching and Learning **Content Area:** Child Health **Strategy:** Children with celiac disease can eat corn and rice. All other grains need to be eliminated from the diet. **Reference:** Ball, J., Bindler, R., & Cowen, K. (2010). *Child health nursing: Partnering with children & families* (2nd ed.). Upper Saddle River, NJ: Prentice Hall, p. 1178.

4 **Answer: 4** **Rationale:** HBV vaccine provides active immunity, and current recommendations include immunizations for all newborns, as well as for several high-risk groups. Hepatitis B is spread by blood and body fluids, including sexual contact, not the fecal–oral route. The disease can exist in a carrier state. **Cognitive Level:** Applying **Client Need:** Safety and Infection Control **Integrated Process:** Teaching and Learning **Content Area:** Child Health **Strategy:** The student must know which forms of hepatitis are blood-borne and which are not. The only form of hepatitis for which there is a vaccine is HBV. **Reference:** McKinney, E., James, S., Murray, S., & Ashwill, J. (2009). *Maternal-child nursing* (3rd ed.). St. Louis, MO: Saunders, p. 1133.

5 **Answer: 1, 2, 5** **Rationale:** The nurse would expect an increased desire to drink fluids and a higher specific gravity caused by the concentration of urine. The heart rate would be elevated, and the fontanels sunken. The degree of dehydration is based on the percent of weight loss, so a weight gain would not be likely. Diminished urine output with elevated specific gravity is an expected normal finding in dehydration. Capillary refill is slowed, especially in children under 2 years of age. **Cognitive Level:** Applying **Client Need:** Physiological Adaptation **Integrated Process:** Nursing Process: Assessment **Content Area:** Child Health **Strategy:** Two of the options are age related and appropriate for the infant. Polyuria and weight gain would not be symptoms of dehydration. **Reference:** Perry, S., Hockenberry, M., Lowdermilk, D., & Wilson, D. (2010). *Maternal child nursing care* (4th ed.). St. Louis, MO: Mosby, pp. 1380–1382.

6 **Answer: 1** **Rationale:** Clinical findings will vary in infants born with congenital diaphragmatic hernias, but the first indications are of respiratory distress. Further assessment will reveal bowel sounds auscultated over the chest, cardiac sounds on the right of the chest, and a sunken abdomen with a barrel-shaped chest. Primary symptom of pyloric stenosis is vomiting. Cleft palate is the failure of the oral palate to close. Omphalocele is a herniation of intestinal contents outside the abdomen. It does not cause respiratory distress in the pre-treatment period. **Cognitive Level:** Analyzing **Client Need:** Physiological Adaptation **Integrated Process:** Nursing Process: Assessment **Content Area:** Child Health **Strategy:** Note that all findings indicate the absence of normal findings on the left side of the chest. **Reference:** Perry, S., Hockenberry, M., Lowdermilk, D., & Wilson, D. (2010). *Maternal child nursing care* (4th ed.). St. Louis, MO: Mosby, pp. 770–771.

7 **Answer: 4** **Rationale:** Celiac disease is characterized by intolerance for gluten. Gluten is found in wheat, barley, rye, and oats. This includes bread, cake, doughnuts, cookies, and crackers, as well as processed foods that contain gluten as filler. **Cognitive Level:** Analyzing **Client Need:** Physiological Adaptation **Integrated Process:** Nursing Process: Evaluation **Content Area:** Child Health **Strategy:** Determine which menu does not contain any rye, wheat, barley, or oats. Alternatively, select the menu that contains one or more items that are rice or corn. **Reference:** Ball, J. Bindler, R., and Cowen, K. (2010). *Child health nursing: Partnering with children & families* (2nd ed.). Upper Saddle River, NJ: Prentice Hall, pp. 1178–1180.

8 **Answer: 2** **Rationale:** Rectal temperature should be avoided since the rectal mucosa will be very fragile. Maintaining the child NPO until bowel sounds return is appropriate for the child postop for Hirschsprung's Disease. Reuniting the parents with the child as soon as

possible is appropriate for this client. Assessing the surgical site every two hours is an appropriate postop intervention. **Cognitive Level:** Applying **Client Need:** Reduction of Risk Potential **Integrated Process:** Nursing Process: Implementation **Content Area:** Child Health **Strategy:** The critical word in the question is *exclude*. With this in mind, choose the option that represents an incorrect or unacceptable nursing action. **Reference:** Ball, J., Bindler, R., & Cowen, K. (2010). *Child health nursing: Partnering with children & families* (2nd ed.). Upper Saddle River, NJ: Prentice Hall, p. 1151.

9 **Answer: 2** **Rationale:** Infants with GER should be given small, frequent feedings. After a feeding the infant should be placed in a prone position with the head of the bed elevated. A harness can be used to help maintain this position. Infant seats should be avoided because of the increased intrabdominal pressure this position creates. **Cognitive Level:** Applying **Client Need:** Physiological Adaptation **Integrated Process:** Teaching and Learning **Content Area:** Child Health **Strategy:** Consider which intervention decreases pressure on the abdomen. **Reference:** Ball, J., Bindler, R., & Cowen, K. (2010). *Child health nursing: Partnering with children & families* (2nd ed.). Upper Saddle River, NJ: Prentice Hall, p. 1144.

10 **Answer: 3** **Rationale:** Signs and symptoms of a ruptured appendix include fever; sudden relief from abdominal pain; guarding; abdominal distention; rapid, shallow breathing; pallor; chills; and irritability. **Cognitive Level:** Analyzing **Client Need:** Physiological Adaptation **Integrated Process:** Nursing Process: Assessment **Content Area:** Child Health **Strategy:** Read the question carefully and eliminate each of the incorrect options because there is no data in the stem of the question to support them. As an alternative, recall pain pattern in appendicitis before and after rupture to choose accurately. **Reference:** Ball, J., Bindler, R., & Cowen, K. (2010). *Child health nursing: Partnering with children & families* (2nd ed.). Upper Saddle River, NJ: Prentice Hall, p 1157.

References

Adams, M., Holland, L., & Urban, C. (2011). *Pharmacology for nurses: A pathophysiological approach* (3rd ed.). Upper Saddle River, NJ: Pearson Education.

Ball, J., Bindler, R., & Cowen, K. (2012). *Principles of pediatric nursing: Caring for children* (5th ed.). Upper Saddle River, NJ: Pearson Education.

Ball, J., Bindler, R., & Cowen, K. (2010). *Child health nursing: Partnering with children and families* (2nd ed.). Upper Saddle River, NJ: Pearson Education.

Hockenberry, M., & Wilson, D. (2011). *Wong's essentials of pediatric nursing* (8th ed.). St. Louis, MO: Elsevier.

Hockenberry, M., & Wilson, D. (2011). *Wong's nursing care of infants and children* (9th ed.). St. Louis, MO: Elsevier.

London, M., Ladewig, P., Ball, J., Bindler, R., & Cowen, K. (2011). *Maternal & child nursing care* (3rd ed.). Upper Saddle River, NJ: Pearson Education.

Perry, S., Hockenberry, M., Lowdermilk, D., & Wilson, D. (2010). *Maternal child nursing care* (4th ed.). St. Louis, MO: Elsevier.

Pillitteri, A. (2009). *Maternal and child health nursing: Care of the childbearing and childrearing family* (6th ed.). Philadelphia: Lippincott Williams & Wilkins.

Hematologic Health Problems

14

Chapter Outline

Overview of Anatomy and Physiology of Hematologic System

Diagnostic Tests of Hematologic System

Congenital Hematologic Health Problems

Acquired Hematologic Health Problems

Objectives

➤ Identify data essential to the assessment of the hematologic system in a child.

➤ Discuss the clinical manifestations and pathophysiology related to alterations in health of the hematologic system of a child.

➤ Discuss therapeutic management of a child with alterations in the health of the hematologic system.

➤ Describe nursing management of a child with alterations in health of the hematologic system.

NCLEX-RN® Test Prep

Use the accompanying online resource, NursingReviewsandRationales, to test yourself with hundreds of NCLEX®-style practice questions.

Review at a Glance

anemia a decrease in number of red blood cells, amount of hemoglobin, and volume of packed red cells to less-than-normal levels

ecchymosis initial black or blue mark resulting from release of blood into tissue; may occur because of injury or spontaneous leaking of blood from vessels

erythrocytes red blood cells

erythropoiesis red blood cell formation

hemarthrosis bleeding into joint spaces of bones

hematopoiesis production of blood cells

hemochromatosis presence of excessive iron stores in the body

hemoglobinopathy a group of disorders associated with abnormal forms of hemoglobin

hemolysis destruction of red blood cells

leukocytes white blood cells

petechiae pinpoint hemorrhages that cause tiny red or purple spots on skin or mucous membranes

thrombocytes platelets

x-linked recessive trait also called sex-linked recessive trait; a form of inheritance where mother passes defective gene to her sons; the defective gene is carried on the X chromosome; the mother does not have the disease but is a carrier of the disease; affected fathers do not pass the gene to their sons, but their daughters will be carriers of the disorder

PRETEST

1 The nurse has completed some child and family education for a child diagnosed with thalassemia. The medical plan of treatment includes blood transfusions when the anemia reaches a severe point. Which statement by the parents indicates a need for further education?

1. "Because of the anemia, my child will need extra rest periods."
2. "My child inherited this disorder from both of us."
3. "We should be alert to periods when our child seems paler than usual."
4. "My child needs an iron supplement."

2 The nursing assistant is setting up a hospital room preparing to admit a child with disseminated intravascular coagulopathy (DIC). Which item would the nurse remove from the set-up?

1. Rectal thermometer
2. Bedpan
3. Intravenous therapy start kit
4. Sphygmomanometer

3 At a hemophilia camp, several children with injuries arrive at the clinic at the same time. When prioritizing care for the children, the child who requires the most immediate care from the nurse is the child with which of the following symptoms?

1. A swollen knee
2. Abrasions on both arms
3. A slight head injury
4. A puncture wound in the foot

4 A 14-year-old boy with sickle cell anemia is admitted with severe pain in his abdomen and legs. He asks why the doctor ordered oxygen when he is not having any problems breathing. The nurse will be most accurate in stating that the main therapeutic benefit of oxygen is to do which of the following?

1. Prevent further sickling
2. Prevent respiratory complications
3. Increase the oxygen-carrying capacity of red blood cells (RBCs)
4. Decrease the potential for infection during the crisis

5 The nurse is administering a liquid iron preparation to a 3-year-old with iron deficiency anemia. It will be most appropriate to do which of the following?

1. Mix the medication in the child's milk and give it at lunch.
2. Give the medication after lunch with a sweet dessert to disguise the taste.
3. Give the medication in a small cup and allow the child to sip it through a straw.
4. Allow the child to decide whether to take the medicine with breakfast or dinner.

6 The nurse is admitting a child newly diagnosed with disseminated intravascular coagulopathy (DIC). Although the plan of care has been explained to the family, they continue to ask about each nursing activity, and seem unable to comprehend the answers. What is the best action by the nurse?

1. Notify the doctor because the family seems to have a comprehension problem.
2. Ask the doctor to write down the information for the family.
3. Recognize that the family is under stress and continue to answer their questions.
4. Assume they are a family with English as a second language (ESL).

7 The nurse is administering factor VIII to a child with hemophilia. The nurse should observe for which potential complication during the infusion?

1. Fluid overload
2. Transfusion reaction
3. Emboli formation
4. Contracting AIDS

8 The clinic nurse has organized a class for several parents of children newly diagnosed with sickle cell disease. The nurse explains that problems with the disease can include which of the following? Select all that apply.

1. Aplastic crisis
2. Sequestration of blood
3. Hemarthrosis
4. Polycythemia
5. Vaso-occlusive crisis

9 Which statement should the nurse include when teaching the parents of a 7-month-old infant about preventing anemia?

1. "Anemia is unusual in infancy as infants use fetal iron stores until 18 months of age."
2. "Cow's milk is an excellent source of iron, and infants should be changed from formula to milk as soon as possible after 6 months of age."
3. "Milk is a poor source of iron, and infants should be given solid foods high in iron such as cereals, vegetables, and meats."
4. "Anemia can easily occur during infancy, and all infants should receive iron supplements."

10 A child with an alteration in platelet function has been receiving intravenous fluids for two days. The nurse is discontinuing the peripheral IV. The nurse should do which of the following?

1. Restrict movement of the arm for 12 hours.
2. Obtain a culture of the tip of the IV catheter.
3. Place steri-strips over site and have child hold the arm above the level of the heart for 15 minutes.
4. Apply direct pressure to the site for at least 5 minutes.

➤ *See pages 320–322 for Answers and Rationales.*

I. OVERVIEW OF ANATOMY AND PHYSIOLOGY OF HEMATOLOGIC SYSTEM

A. Hematologic function

1. Hematologic system facilitates regulation of all other body systems directly or indirectly via blood and lymph circulating through every tissue and organ
2. Hematologic system supplies and transports oxygen to other cells of body
   a. It transports food, wastes, and hormonal messengers
   b. It functions as a part of immune system to protect against and fight infection
   c. It also helps prevent hemorrhage when there is injury

B. Hematologic system

1. Blood forming organs
   a. Early production of blood cells (**hematopoiesis**) in fetus begins in the yolk sac at two weeks' gestation then occurs in liver and spleen until five months' gestation; bone marrow then takes over function of hematopoiesis and this continues in extrauterine life
   b. At birth, hematopoiesis occurs in almost every bone; however only flat bones, such as hips, pelvic and shoulder girdles, ribs, sternum, and vertebrae maintain hematopoietic activity throughout life
   c. After birth, liver is primary site for production of most blood clotting factors and prothrombin
      1) Proper liver function requires vitamin K which is acquired from two sources—produced by bacteria in bowel and absorbed from digested food
      2) Vitamin K is essential to the development of clotting factors VII, IX, X, and prothrombin
      3) Clotting factors that are activated by vitamin K are lower in infants; many physicians recommend a preventative dose of vitamin K at time of birth
   d. Spleen helps balance red blood cell (RBC) production and destruction by destroying aged or imperfect RBCs and stores platelets

Table 14-1	Mean Values for Common Hematology Tests in Children
Test	**Mean Value**
Red blood cell (RBC)	$3.8–4.9 \times 10^{12}/L$
Hemoglobin (HB)	11.5–14.5 g/dl
Hematocrit (HCT)	35–43%
White blood cell (WBC)	$7.8–12.2 \times 10^{9}/L$
Platelets	$150–400 \times 10^{9}/L$

Source: Ball, J., Bindler, R., & Cowen, K. (2010). *Child health nursing: Partnering with children & families* (2nd ed.). Upper Saddle River, NJ: Pearson Education, p. 1028.

2. Blood is composed of cellular elements and plasma
   a. Cellular elements: see Table 14-1 for normal pediatric blood values
      1) RBCs or **erythrocytes** are formed through process of **erythropoiesis** and make up largest component of blood cells; normal lifespan of a RBC is 120 days
         a) Hemoglobin (Hgb) is a component of RBCs and transports oxygen from the lungs to the tissues as well as carrying carbon dioxide back to the lungs
         b) RBC count, hemoglobin (Hgb), and hematocrit (Hct) levels are high in infants
         c) These values will stabilize in childhood
         d) However, adolescent males demonstrate increased Hgb compared to the lowered value of adolescent females
      2) White blood cells (WBCs) or **leukocytes** are formed primarily in bone marrow; production also takes place in lymph tissue
         a) Leukocytes provide immunity and help protect against consequences of infection and injury
         b) Leukocytes are divided into five types, each having a specific purpose related to inflammation or immunity (Table 14-2)
         c) Alterations in levels of five different leukocytes can be seen in a differential blood count and may indicate a specific disease or condition
      3) Platelets (**thrombocytes**) are cell fragments that work to stop blood flow from an injury by adhering to walls of blood vessels and forming platelet plugs
         a) Platelets are produced in bone marrow and then are stored in spleen; from the spleen, they are released as needed by body
         b) On average, 20% of platelets are stored in spleen, and 80% are circulating; newborns will have lower levels of platelets

Table 14-2	White Blood Cells and Their Functions
Type	**Function**
Neutrophils	Phagocytosis
Eosinophils	Allergic reactions
Basophils	Inflammatory reactions
Monocytes (macrophages)	Phagocytosis, antigen processing
Lymphocytes	Humoral immunity (B cell), cellular immunity (T cell)

Source: London, M., Ladewig, P., Ball, J., Bindler, R., & Cowen, K. (2011). *Maternal & child nursing care (3rd ed.).* Upper Saddle River, NJ: Pearson Education, p. 1441.

       b. The liquid component of blood plasma contains three plasma proteins

         1) Albumin prevents plasma from leaking into tissue by increasing osmotic pressure of blood

         2) Fibrinogen molecules accumulate to form essential structures for blood clotting process

         3) Globulins are main components of antibodies and protect body against infection; globulins also transport other substances

       c. Lymphatic fluid is similar to blood plasma but contains less protein; it does not produce cells, but rather has a necessary role in regulating blood cells; it is the extra interstitial fluid that is returned to systemic circulation by components of auxiliary venous system known as lymph vessels or lymphatics; this balances the systemic circulation

II. DIAGNOSTIC TESTS OF HEMATOLOGIC SYSTEM

A. History

1. Assess for a history of easy or frequent bruising as well as frequent or heavy nosebleeds
2. Assess for history of recurrent or chronic infections
3. Assess for medication use that might impair hematologic function, including those that cause bone marrow suppression, **hemolysis** (destruction of blood cells), or those that disrupt platelet function
4. Remember to question family closely as to over-the-counter medications that client or family might not associate with impaired hematologic function
5. Assess for dietary patterns that might contribute to anemia or altered blood cell function
6. Assess for family housing, occupations, or hobbies that might indicate exposure to chemicals or agents that affect hematologic function
7. Assess for past medical history related to hematologic dysfunction: illnesses, surgeries, or injuries
8. Assess for family history of illnesses related to hematologic dysfunction

B. Physical assessment

1. Assess skin for presence of pallor or jaundice; assess mucous membranes and nail beds for pallor or cyanosis
2. Assess skin turgor and pruritus as dry skin and itching may be indicators of a hematologic dysfunction
3. Assess skin for **petechiae**, red or purple pinpoint hemorrhages; assess also for **ecchymosis** or bruising caused by release of blood into tissues
4. Assess for spontaneous bleeding or bruising; assess for bleeding or bruising disproportionate to causative trauma
5. Assess gums for active bleeding; as appropriate, also assess for excessive menstrual flow
6. If indicated, assess for bleeding from invasive medical interventions such as peripheral IV sites, central lines, nasogastric tubes, endotracheal tubes, or indwelling urinary catheters
7. Assess heart for increased rate or audible murmur
8. Assess for swollen or tender lymph nodes; assess for increased liver or spleen size at costal margins
9. Assess for level of activity, fatigue, needing more rest than usual, decreasing endurance during routine activities, or dyspnea upon exertion
10. Assess for frequent infections, fevers, or weight loss

C. Common diagnostic studies

1. Complete blood count (CBC) with differential
   a. Evaluates red blood cell counts, white blood cell counts, platelet counts, and hemoglobin and hematocrit; also evaluates shape of red blood cells
      1) The hemoglobin level is an evaluation of the amount of hemoglobin per 100 mL (dL) of blood
      2) The hematocrit is a comparison of the amount of RBCs in a volume of whole blood (percentage of solids to liquids); changes in amount of either solids or liquids will affect results; a low hematocrit can indicate a decreased number of RBCs or an increase in liquid volume of blood
   b. White blood cell (WBC) count indicates total number of circulating WBCs (body's primary defense against foreign organisms and other substances); work by phagocytosis and through antibody production
      1) There are five types of WBCs reported as WBC differential; results of each are reported as a percentage, so as one type increases, another type decreases
      2) The WBC differential gives health care provider information about cause of alteration in WBC count
      3) Neutrophils are most common type of WBC and can be further divided into segmented neutrophils or segs and immature cells called bands; neutrophils work by phagocytosis; an increase is often called a "shift to the left" and indicates bacterial infection
      4) Lymphocytes are second most common type of WBC and become T cells and B cells, which are responsible for cellular-type immune responses; elevations in lymphocytes often indicate a viral infection
      5) Eosinophils are elevated in allergic diseases and parasitic diseases
      6) Basophils are associated with chronic conditions
      7) Monoctyes are also associated with chronic infections
2. Direct and indirect Coombs' tests evaluate presence of antibodies associated with the RBCs
   a. Direct Coombs' test evaluates amount of antibodies coating red cells
   b. An indirect Coombs' test evaluates presence of unattached, circulating antibodies
3. Prothrombin time (PT) and partial thromboplastin time (PTT) evaluate clotting sequence, looking primarily at factor function
4. Bleeding time differentiates hemostasis disorders from coagulation defects
5. Platelet agglutination/aggregation evaluates platelet clumping ability
6. Hemoglobin electrophoresis differentiates types of hemoglobin present and notes abnormal forms of hemoglobins
7. Serum ferritin measures iron stores in body
8. Bone marrow aspiration and biopsy involves removal of a small amount of bone marrow to evaluate production of blood cells; iliac crest is site of choice for pediatric bone marrow aspirations

III. CONGENITAL HEMATOLOGIC HEALTH PROBLEMS

A. Hemophilia

1. Description
   a. A group of disorders characterized by a deficiency in a specific clotting factor
   b. A chronic inherited bleeding disorder
   c. Has no cure and is a lifelong condition
2. Etiology and pathophysiology
   a. There are three forms of hemophilia: the two most common types are inherited as an **X-linked recessive trait** expressed almost exclusively as carrier females and

affected males; when a female inherits the hemophilia trait from her father, she has a 50% chance of transmitting it to her son

    1) Hemophilia A (classic hemophilia) results from factor VIII deficiency (approximately 80% of hemophilia cases); hemophilia A affects approximately 1 in 5000 male births

    2) Hemophilia B (Christmas disease) results from a deficiency of factor IX (approximately 15% of hemophilia cases)

    3) A third inherited bleeding disorder is von Willebrand disease in which the affected individual has a deficiency of von Willebrand factor (vWF); is usually inherited as an autosomal dominant disease and thus affects both males and females

b. Approximately one third of cases of hemophilia occur because of a new mutation and have no ancestors affected

c. Bleeding tendencies may be mild, moderate, or severe; may first be recognized after a circumcision when client continues to ooze blood or may not be apparent until client becomes active and starts walking or crawling

d. Repeated bleeding into joint spaces (**hemarthrosis**) can lead to loss of joint mobility

e. Significant deep tissue and intramuscular hemorrhages may occur; airway obstruction may result from bleeding into tissues of mouth, neck, or chest; critical bleeding may be seen in retroperitoneal or intracranial areas

f. Extensive bleeding may be seen after circumcision, tooth extractions, lesser injuries, and minor surgical procedures

3. Assessment

  a. Diagnosed by history, presenting symptoms, and laboratory data

  b. Presenting laboratory data will include prolonged activated PTT and decreased factor VIII or IX levels; PT, thrombin time, fibrinogen, and platelet count are normal

  c. Genetic testing can be used to identify carriers; carriers and affected individuals can also be identified prior to birth via amniocentesis or chorionic villi sampling

  d. Obtain medical history, with close attention to episodes of bleeding as well as a history of familial bleeding disorders

  e. Assess for active bleeding, joint swelling, pain, or deformities

  f. Assess for hematuria or flank pain

  g. Complete a neurological assessment to rule out peripheral neuropathies secondary to intracranial bleeding

4. Priority nursing diagnoses

  a. Risk for Injury

  b. Pain

  c. Impaired Walking

  d. Deficient Knowledge (parental or client) of disease process and management of care

5. Planning and implementation

  a. Control localized bleeding through topical coagulants, providing rest of site, pressure, elevation, and ice

  b. Control bleeding for significant bleeds through administration of necessary replacement factor; monitor factor levels as ordered

    1) Factor VIII is now available in a freeze dried form and can be stored in home refrigerator for use as necessary

    2) Factor is a blood product (found only in fresh or frozen plasma) and carries risk of blood borne pathogens although safety of factor continues to improve with development of recombinant forms

        3) Many children now take replacement factor prophylactically; factor has a short half-life and should be administered in morning so factor levels are highest when client is most active

    c. Transfuse as ordered to help minimize disease complications

        1) Fresh whole blood would only be used for severe bleeds into critical areas; it would take a large volume of whole blood because the amount of factor per unit of whole blood is insignificant

        2) Platelets are not administered because client's platelet count is normal

    d. As indicated for mild hemophilia, administer desmopressin acetate (DDAVP) intravenously

    e. Take no rectal temperatures

    f. Manage pain utilizing analgesics as ordered

    g. If joint is involved in a bleed, joint damage can be reduced via immobilization, elevation, and ice packs

    h. Physical therapy is used to prevent flexion contractures and to strengthen muscles and joints

    i. Physical therapy is only initiated when bleeding is under control

    j. Provide opportunities for normal growth and development activities; as indicated, provide injury protection for activities

    k. Some children develop antibodies to replacement factor; these children will require higher doses of replacement factor to maintain a clot

6. Medications

    a. Factor VIII (8) and IX (9) are available

    b. Three forms of factor are available: intermediate, monoclonal, and recombinant; intermediate and monoclonal are extracted from plasma; recombinant forms are manufactured from human genes but do not include plasma

    c. DDAVP may be administered to children with mild Hemophilia A; it increases level of factor VIII and von Willebrand factor by releasing these factors from their storage sites

7. Client and family education

    a. Importance of wearing a MedicAlert bracelet

    b. Injury prevention appropriate for age

        1) Toddlers should wear clothes that contain extra padding to prevent injuries as they learn to walk

        2) Padding of furniture corners and providing a clean environment reduces falls and injuries by eliminating clutter

        3) Children and adolescents should avoid contact sports; however, noncontact athletics help maintain physical strength; swimming and golf are appropriate activities

    c. Signs and symptoms of internal bleeding and hemarthrosis

    d. Using a soft toothbrush and having regular dental checkups

    e. Importance of avoiding aspirin and aspirin-like medications that can affect platelet function; educate as to such over-the-counter products

    f. Medication administration techniques

        1) Replacement factor may be stored in refrigerator until needed

        2) Teach proper dilution of factor; diluent is provided with factor; swirl factor gently until completely mixed

        3) Teach IV administration; young clients may have a subcutaneous venous port placed to aid in home infusion

        4) Use a plastic syringe, not glass

        5) Once replacement factor is reconstituted, administer within three hours

8. Evaluation: client is free of pain and without joint deformities; client demonstrates an age-appropriate level of independence; family and client verbalize and demonstrate understanding of disease, management, and sequelae

B. **Sickle cell anemia**

1. Description: a hereditary **hemoglobinopathy** primarily affecting African Americans, but also may be seen in those of Mediterranean and Hispanic descent

2. Etiology and pathophysiology
   a. An autosomal recessive condition whereby normal hemoglobin is partially or completely replaced by the sickle-shaped, abnormal hemoglobin S (Hgb S)
   b. The sickle cell trait (carrying one gene for disease) presents in 1 out of 12 African Americans; the disease occurs in 1 out of 600 African-American infants
   c. When exposed to diminished levels of oxygen, hemoglobin S develops a sickle or crescent shape; these cells are rigid and obstruct capillary blood flow, leading to congestion and tissue hypoxia; cyclically, this hypoxia causes additional sickling and extensive infarctions
   d. Children with sickle cell disease have three types of problems
      1) Vaso-occlusive crisis where stasis of blood causes ischemia and infarction; seriousness of sequelae depends upon the site of the occlusive crisis; signs include fever, pain, and tissue engorgement
      2) Sequestration crisis is a potentially life-threatening crisis where blood pools in spleen; usually happens in younger children; signs include profound anemia, hypovolemia, and shock
      3) Aplastic crisis is **anemia** associated with increased destruction of fragile red blood cells; signs include profound anemia and pallor

   e. Hypoxia or low oxygen tension may trigger a crisis, as will any condition that increases body's need for oxygen or alters oxygen transport; sickling of RBCs can also be triggered by a fever or dehydration and emotional or physical stress

   f. Symptoms do not usually appear until 4 to 6 months of age as sickling of cells is prevented secondary to high levels of fetal hemoglobin
   g. Those with sickle cell trait (carriers of the disease) rarely experience crises or symptoms, unless under conditions where there is abnormally low oxygen

3. Assessment
   a. Newborns may be diagnosed via hemoglobin electrophoresis of cord blood

   b. The Sicklidex (sickle turbidity test) is a screening test used for children 6 years and older
   c. Hemoglobin electrophoresis verifies diagnosis
   d. Obtain a detailed history as to crises, precipitating events, medical management, and details of home management
   e. Obtain current and accurate height and weight to assess for failure to thrive
   f. Assess for any acute or chronic pain; if currently in crisis, also note any signs/symptoms of infection or inflammation

   g. An ill sickle cell client will necessitate a thorough multisystem assessment; fever must be considered an emergency and will require urgent treatment

4. Priority nursing diagnoses
   a. Impaired Tissue Perfusion
   b. Risk for Injury
   c. Risk for Infection
   d. Pain
   e. Deficient Knowledge of disease process, prevention of sickling, management of crisis

5. Planning and implementation

   a. Assist hydration through IV fluids and oral intake

Practice to Pass

You are teaching the family of a 1-year-old newly diagnosed with hemophilia. The mother states she will continue to use ibuprofen for injuries and fever as previously instructed by her pediatrician. What would your best response be?

      b. Increase tissue perfusion by administering oxygen and blood products as ordered; this helps prevent further sickling

      c. Promote and encourage rest; schedule activities of daily living (ADLs) and play to maximize rest and comfort

      d. Assist client and family to avoid emotional stress as much as possible

      e. Administer analgesics around the clock (ATC) when client is in crisis; utilize patient-controlled analgesia if appropriate; position for comfort and to decrease stress upon painful joints

      f. Assess for signs/symptoms of worsening anemia, shock, and altered neurological function

      g. Provide emotional support during crisis, as well as on an ongoing basis when client is well and in the home setting

  6. Client and family education

      a. Necessity of following plan of care as prescribed by health care team

      b. Signs and symptoms of impending crisis

      c. Signs and symptoms of infection

      d. Preventing hypoxia from physical and emotional stress

      e. Providing adequate rest as well as avoiding heat and cold stress

  7. Evaluation: client maintains adequate tissue perfusion as evidenced by oxygen saturation at level ordered by provider, experiences appropriate pain control and ability to resume age-appropriate activities, remains free of signs and symptoms of infection; family and client demonstrate an understanding of disease process and treatment regimen

C. Thalassemia

  1. Description

      a. Another of the group of hereditary blood disorders of hemoglobin synthesis, characterized by mild to severe anemia

      b. Most common type is β-thalassemia, also known as Cooley anemia; there are three types of β-thalassemia: thalassemia minor, thalassemia intermedia, and thalassemia major

        1) Thalassemia minor is also known as thalassemia trait and produces mild anemia

        2) Thalassemia intermedia produces moderate to severe anemia

        3) Thalassemia major produces anemia that requires transfusions; see Box 14-1 for transfusion procedures

  2. Etiology and pathophysiology

      a. Most commonly seen in those of Mediterranean descent; however, they may also be seen among the African, Asian, and Middle Eastern populations

      b. Is an autosomal-recessive condition; when both parents carry this gene, there is a 25% chance of passing disorder to child; if child only acquires one gene for this disorder, child will be a carrier

      c. Thalassemia causes synthesis of defective hemoglobin; RBCs are fragile and have a shortened life span; this leads to anemia and hypoxia

      d. Primary consequences of thalassemia result from chronic hypoxia and iron overload from multiple blood supplements, which are part of supportive treatment

      e. Body conserves iron from aged and broken down RBCs and from transfused cells, leading to high levels of iron in body or **hemochromatosis**, which causes cellular damage and resulting in long-term complications:

        1) Splenomegaly

        2) Cardiac complications

        3) Gallbladder disease

        4) Liver enlargement and cirrhosis

        5) Growth retardation and endocrine complications

Practice to Pass

Sickle cell anemia may not be diagnosed until after infancy. Explain the reason for this.

Box 14-1	
Pediatric Transfusions	• Always follow agency policy regarding transfusion of blood products. • Wear gloves when handling blood products. • Verify correct blood product and type, client name, identification number, and cross-matching before beginning to prevent potentially fatal error. Most agencies require identification of unit to be performed by two registered nurses. • Review physician's order in relation to premedications and rate of infusion. • Have intravenous site ready prior to blood arriving on unit. Start blood administration immediately upon its arrival on unit; do not store blood in the unit refrigerator. • Check blood products—products that appear purplish or are bubbling should not be used because of risk of bacterial contamination. • Obtain informed consent. • Assemble administration equipment with appropriate blood filter. A separate blood filter and tubing is used for each unit. A Y set is usually recommended with saline used to prime the entire line including both Y legs. • Start slowly. For the first 15 minutes, the blood is transfused slowly, and the client is monitored for transfusion reactions. • Monitor vital signs before, during, and after the infusion. Usually vital signs are taken every 15 minutes 4, then every 30 minutes throughout infusion, and 30 minutes after infusion is complete. Watch for other signs of reaction.

Source: Hogan, MaryAnn; Brancato, Vera; White, Judy; Falkenstein, Kathleen, *Prentice Hall Reviews & rationales: Child health nursing,* 2nd Ed., ©2007. Reprinted and Electronically reproduced by permission of Pearson Education, Inc. Upper Saddle River, NJ.

      6) Jaundice and bronze skin pigmentation
      7) Skeletal changes including enlarged head, thickened cranial bones, enlarged maxilla, and malocclusion of teeth due to activity of bone marrow
   f. If untreated, the child may die at a young age
3. Assessment
   a. Thalassemia can be diagnosed early in infancy when child presents with pallor, failure to thrive (FTT), hepatosplenomegaly, and severe anemia; see Box 14-2 for clinical manifestations of β-Thalassemia
   b. There may also be signs and symptoms of chronic hypoxia such as lethargy, headache, bone pain, exercise intolerance, and anorexia
   c. Diagnosis of thalassemia is made via hemoglobin electrophoresis, which shows a decreased production of one hemoglobin chain; erythrocyte changes may be detected as early as 6 weeks of age
   d. Lab data will reveal a decreased hemoglobin, hematocrit, and reticulocyte count; RBCs are described as microcytic, hypochromic and anisocytic
   e. A folic acid deficiency may be present
4. Priority nursing diagnoses
   a. Disturbed Body Image
   b. Risk for Activity Iintolerance
   c. Risk for Injury
   d. Pain
   e. Deficient Knowledge of disease process and management
5. Planning and implementation
   a. Administer blood products as ordered, observing for complications of multiple transfusions
   b. Assess for signs of iron overload (hemosiderosis) and hepatitis
   c. Observe for signs of infection and work to prevent infection through good handwashing, proper rest and nutrition, and avoiding those with infection
   d. Administer folic acid as ordered
   e. Work towards fracture prevention by encouraging and providing opportunities for physical activities that do not increase risk of fractures

Box 14-2 Clinical Manifestations of β-Thalassemia	

Anemia
Hypochromic and microcytic changes
Folic acid deficiency
Frequent epistaxis

Skeletal Changes
Osteoporosis
Delayed growth
Susceptibility to pathologic fractures
Facial deformities: enlarged head, prominent forehead due to frontal and parietal bossing, prominent cheek bones, broadened and depressed bridge of nose, enlarged maxilla with protruding front teeth, eyes with mongolian slant and epicanthal fold

Heart
Chronic congestive heart failure
Myocardial fibrosis
Murmurs

Liver/Gallbladder
Hepatomegaly
Hepatic insufficiency

Spleen
Splenomegaly

Endocrine System
Delayed sexual maturation
Fibrotic pancreas, resulting in diabetes mellitus

Skin
Darkening of skin

Source: Hogan, MaryAnn; Brancato, Vera; White, Judy; Falkenstein, Kathleen, *Prentice Hall Reviews & rationales: Child health nursing,* 2nd Ed., ©2007. Reprinted and Electronically reproduced by permission of Pearson Education, Inc. Upper Saddle River, NJ.

f. Implement iron chelation therapy as ordered; iron chelation aids in elimination of excessive iron

g. Provide support through opportunities for expression of feelings by client and family regarding the chronic life-threatening illness

h. Encourage client and family to allow child to live as normal a life as possible

i. Bone marrow transplantations may be offered to cure the disease

6. Client and family education

a. Nature of disease and its medical management

b. Possible complications including iron overload and signs of infection

c. Activity restrictions designed to reduce risk of fractures secondary to excessive iron stores

7. Evaluation: client is without pain, has no signs of infection, engages in age-appropriate activities and has as normal a lifestyle as possible, and demonstrates coping with body image changes; family and client describe disease process and medical plan of care

Practice to Pass

You are transfusing a client diagnosed with thalassemia major. You determine that a hemolytic reaction is occurring. What should be your first nursing action?

IV. ACQUIRED HEMATOLOGIC HEALTH PROBLEMS

A. Disseminated intravascular coagulopathy (DIC)

1. Description
   a. DIC occurs as a complication of another health problem; it is a secondary illness, not a primary one
   b. Is an acquired life-threatening pathological process involving abnormal simultaneous activation of body's thrombin (clotting) mechanism and fibrinolytic system
2. Etiology and pathophysiology
   a. A complex process involving simultaneous excessive bleeding and clotting
   b. Abnormal activation of clotting system leads to extensive clot formation in small blood vessels throughout body which can lead to organ damage
   c. Excess generation of thrombin occurs, leading to abnormal deposition of fibrin strands through body tissues; these thromboses interfere with blood flow; tissue hypoxia occurs, leading to tissue necrosis
   d. As fibrin fragments circulate, they begin to interfere with aspects of clotting mechanism including platelet aggregation; the resulting depletion of platelets leads to hemorrhage and anemia (see Figure 14-1)

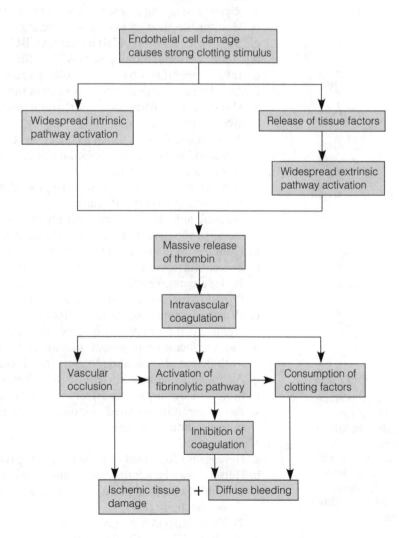

Figure 14-1

The process of disseminated intravascular coagulopathy (DIC)

   e. DIC may result from conditions causing cell or tissue damage; such damage can free up tissue thromboplastin, circulating endotoxins and immune complexes

   f. Primary conditions that can precipitate DIC include burns, cancer, hypoxia, liver disease, necrolyzing enterocolitis, sepsis, shock, trauma, and viruses

3. Assessment

   a. Onset of symptoms includes diffuse bleeding that may be seen as excessive bruising, hematuria, injection sites that do not stop oozing, and mild GI bleeding

   b. Assess progression that is indicated by petechiae, purpura, hypoxemia, renal failure, intracranial bleeding, ischemic pain, and progressive organ failure secondary to the ischemia

   c. Lab data will include low platelet count, deceased RBCs, prolonged prothrombin time (PT) and partial thromboplastin time (PTT), decreased fibrinogen levels, and increased levels of fibrin-fibrinogen split products

4. Priority nursing diagnoses

   a. Ineffective Tissue Perfusion

   b. Risk for Injury

   c. Anxiety

5. Planning and implementation

   a. Rigorous ongoing assessment of all body systems

   b. Monitor bleeding by assessing petechiae, ecchymoses, and oozing frequently

   c. Ongoing evaluation of lab including CBC, PT, and PTT

   d. Monitor arterial blood gases (ABGs) for indications of acidosis

   e. Take temperatures by oral or axillary route, not rectal

   f. Avoid trauma to delicate areas such as mucous membranes as much as possible

   g. Minimize administration of parenteral medications and invasive procedures as much as possible

   h. Areas of needle sticks such as injections or IV sites must be treated as an arterial stick and have pressure applied for at least 10 to 15 minutes; they must be observed every 15 minutes

   i. Observe regularly sites of invasive procedures such as nasogastric tubes, endotracheal tubes, or Foley catheters

   j. Measure any blood loss as precisely as possible; dependent areas are prone to blood pooling and must be assessed carefully

   k. Examine urine and stool for presence of blood

   l. Prevent further bleeding and injury by instituting bleeding control precautions

   m. Provide symptomatic treatment of primary condition

   n. Provide oxygen administration as necessary

   o. IV heparin administration is ordered to stop hemorrhage–thrombosis cycle; fluid replacement therapy may be given concomitantly

   p. Clotting factor replacement is achieved through transfusions of cryoprecipitate, fresh frozen plasma, and platelets (see Table 14-3)

   q. Assess anticoagulant and transfusion therapy and report any complications

   r. Monitor carefully for transfusion reactions (see Table 14-4)

   s. Assess for fluid overload as indicated by a slow bounding pulse and increasing central venous pressure

6. Medications

   a. Heparin is often used to reduce inappropriate utilization of clotting factors

   b. Heparin may be administered subcutaneously or intravenously (IV)

      1) Subcutaneous heparin is given slowly with sites rotated; injection site should not be massaged

      2) IV heparin may be given intermittently or continuously

   c. Monitor PTT and platelet count

Practice to Pass

The client with disseminated intravascular coagulopathy (DIC) is to receive multiple doses of heparin subcutaneously. Discuss the safety issues involved in administering this drug.

Table 14-3 **Administration of Blood Products**

Blood Product	Use	Comments
Whole blood	Used in trauma clients who have lost both cells and volume; occasionally used in other clients, although a blood component may be used in its place	Blood products must be kept refrigerated at a temperature between 0 and 10°C; normal refrigerators are inappropriate; prepare to administer product as soon as it arrives on unit and never store blood product in unit refrigerator; if length of administration exceeds blood bank's recommendations, blood bank can divide unit; transfuse through blood filter; one unit usually raises Hct by 3%, Hgb by 1 gram/dL; infuse only with 0.9% sodium chloride.
Packed red blood cells (PRBCs)	Often used in anemic clients who do not require volume expansion; PRBCs are developed by removing majority of plasma from a unit of whole blood	Transfusion completed within two to four hours to prevent bacterial growth; leukocyte-poor RBCs (filtered RBCs) may be used in clients with history of allergic reactions; these units have been exposed to extra processing which removes majority of WBCs; four-hour maximum infusion time; children with severe anemia are at risk for congestive heart failure if infused too rapidly.
Platelets	Used for clients with thrombocytopenia	May be pooled from several donor units or from one donor; a leukocyte-reduction filter for platelets may be used; pretransfusion medications may include antihistamines or acetaminophen.
Granulocytes	Usually only used for severely neutropenic client; sometimes used for neonates with sepsis	May be irradiated to reduce risk of graft versus host disease; risk of cytomegalovirus infection exists with granulocyte transfusion; pretransfusion medication with antihistamine or acetaminophen recommended.
Fresh frozen plasma (FFP)	Supplies clotting factors; may be used in severe liver disease or DIC	Half-life of plasma clotting factors short; must be fresh or fresh frozen to be of benefit; is transfused through a blood filter; may be given over 20 to 30 minutes.
Factor VIII or IX	Concentrated forms of specific factor; used for hemophilia type A and B; factor VIII may also be used for von Willebrand disease	Compatibility tests not required; quantity of factor varies for each vial; available in lyophilized concentrations, which can be kept in home refrigerator until needed; reconstituted with diluent provided; various forms refer to level of purity; recombinant forms available.

Table 14-4 **Transfusion Reactions**

Reactions and Cause	Signs and Symptoms	Treatment
Hemolytic reaction—ABO incompatibility	Fever, pain at insertion site, hypotension, renal failure, tachycardia, oliguria, shock; positive Coombs' test	Stop blood transfusion, maintain IV line; notify physician; send remaining blood and tubing to lab; lab samples will be obtained from client
Febrile nonhemolytic reaction—antigen-antibody reaction to something in donor blood	Fever, chills	Antipyretics; premedicate in future; use leukocyte-depleted products
Allergic reaction—client allergic to protein in donor blood	Rash, hives, respiratory distress, anaphylaxis	Pretreat with antihistamine
Viral transmission	Delayed fever	Treat symptomatically
Fluid volume overload—most frequently seen in severely anemic child	Signs and symptoms of congestive heart failure	Prevent by limiting speed of transfusion for the severely anemic child
Graft-versus-host disease—seen in immunocompromised client	Fever, bone marrow suppression, and death	Prevention is key—provide irradiated RBCs

          d. Protamine is a heparin antidote and should be available for emergency use

          e. Client should avoid use of aspirin and nonsteroidal anti-inflammatory drugs (NSAIDs)

    7. Client and family education

          a. Teach client and family about condition, its cause, and treatment

          b. Explain to client and family activities to reduce bleeding—using a soft toothbrush or gauze over finger to "brush" teeth, maintaining an obstacle-free environment, handling skin gently

          c. Instruct client and family about symptoms to report to health care provider

    8. Evaluation: client maintains appropriate organ function; bleeding from trauma is minimized; family and client verbalize concerns as well as demonstrate effective coping mechanisms

  B. Idiopathic thrombocytopenic purpura (ITP)

    1. Description

          a. Also known as autoimmune thrombocytopenia purpura (ATP)

          b. An autoimmune hematologic condition distinguished by increased destruction of platelets, despite normal platelet production in bone marrow

          c. ITP is most common bleeding disorder in children

    2. Etiology and pathophysiology

          a. ITP occurs most often in children ages 2 to 5

          b. ITP usually develops one to three weeks after a viral infection such as chicken pox, measles, or rubella

          c. ITP can manifest itself as acute and self-limiting or chronic, requiring treatment; acute type accounts for approximately 80% of ITP cases

          d. As platelet destruction exceeds production, the total number of circulating platelets decreases

          e. Blood clotting is slowed, and uncontrolled bleeding may occur

    3. Assessment

          a. Petechiae and multiple ecchymoses are characteristic; mucous membranes and sclera are particularly affected with petechiae

          b. Other symptoms include

             1) Excessive bleeding, especially nosebleeds

             2) Hematuria and bloody or tarry stools

          c. History of recent medical events

          d. Lab data that shows decreased platelet count, as well as anti-platelet antibodies in peripheral blood

          e. Physical assessment must include thorough neurological assessment to rule out intracranial bleeds

          f. Bone marrow aspiration is used to look for platelet precursors and rule out an oncologic disorder

    4. Priority nursing diagnoses

          a. Risk for Injury

          b. Deficient Knowledge (parental) of disease process, prevention of hemorrhage

    5. Planning and implementation

          a. Assess frequently for bruising or active bleeding including mucous membranes, sclera, nosebleeds, hematuria, or bloody stools

          b. Assess neurological status every shift and PRN

          c. Closely monitor platelet counts

          d. Monitor children who have undergone any invasive procedure closely

e. Use soft bristled toothbrush or toothettes on children with platelet counts less than 20,000 cells/mm^3

f. Avoid using rectal thermometers and aspirin-like products

g. If medications are not successful, a splenectomy may be attempted in an older child with one year of thrombocytopenia

6. Medications

a. Steroids are ordered to reduce inflammatory process

b. IV immunoglobulins may also be used to reduce autoimmune problem

7. Client and family education

a. Parents are instructed to obtain a MedicAlert bracelet for child

b. Teach client and family ways to prevent bleeding episodes

c. Give instructions about means to control bleeding and when to seek emergency assistance

d. Teach client and family safe administration of medications and potential side effects

e. Provide information to client and parents about splenectomy and surgical care as appropriate

8. Evaluation: client remains free of injury from bleeding episodes; client and family identify safety precautions related to medication administration and demonstrate behaviors designed to reduce bruising/bleeding

C. Iron-deficiency anemia

1. Description

a. Results from an inadequate supply of iron

b. Most common type of childhood anemia

2. Etiology and pathophysiology

a. Inadequate iron supply leads to smaller RBCs, a reduction in number of RBCs and quantity of hemoglobin, and a decrease in oxygen-carrying capacity of blood

b. Body stores of iron decrease and severity of symptoms is directly related to amount and duration of iron deficiency

c. Iron-deficiency anemia occurs as a result of blood loss or poor nutritional intake, or because of rapid growth with increased internal demands for blood production

d. It is most common nutritional-deficiency anemia in children

e. Premature or multiple-birth infants are at risk because of inadequate iron storage in latter part of pregnancy

f. After age of 6 months, infants who do not take appropriate solid food and are taking breast milk or formula without iron are at risk because of depletion of neonatal iron stores

g. Chronic blood loss can be a cause of iron-deficiency anemia; clients at risk include neonates who have experienced bleeding, hemophiliacs, those who have parasitic GI problems, or females who have heavy menstrual bleeding (menorrhagia)

3. Assessment

a. Classic symptoms include pallor, fatigue, and irritability, but the exact clinical signs will depend upon severity of anemia

b. Poor muscle development and growth retardation may occur; children with anemia may be at greater risk of infection

c. Nail bed deformities, tachycardia, and systolic heart murmurs occur with prolonged anemia; growth retardation and/or developmental delay may also be seen

      d. Laboratory data including hemoglobin levels, mean corpuscular volume, and serum iron-binding capacity all indicate decreased iron content; microscopic analysis reveals microcytic (small) and hypochromic (pale) red blood cells

      e. Low iron stores are easiest identified by a decrease in serum ferritin

      f. Assess nutritional intake through a dietary history and analysis

  4. Priority nursing diagnoses

      a. Deficient Knowledge related to sources of iron

      b. Imbalanced Nutrition: Less Than Body Requirements

      c. Activity Intolerence

      d. Risk for Impaired Growth and Development

  5. Planning and implementation

      a. Correct bleeding if it is the cause of anemia

      b. Implement dietary modifications to provide a high-iron diet

      c. Promote rest, protect from infection; monitor cardiac functioning

      d. If packed RBCs are administered, administer slowly; rapid administration can overload an already-stressed heart leading to congestive heart failure

      e. Some infants drink large quantities of milk and refuse solid foods, limiting their iron intake; for these infants it is often necessary to restrict their milk intake; milk intake should be limited to a maximum of one quart per day

      f. Client will also need protein and vitamin C to produce new cells; folic acid will help to convert iron from ferritin to hemoglobin

  6. Medications: oral iron supplements may be ordered; ferrous sulfate is preferred form as it is better absorbed

      a. Iron is best absorbed on an empty stomach; it may be taken with a vitamin C source such as orange juice to promote iron absorption; milk and antacids may inhibit absorption

      b. Oral iron preparations may temporarily stain teeth; liquid iron preparations should be taken through a straw to reduce contact with teeth; client should brush his or her teeth after administration

      c. Stools may be tarry and constipation may occur

  7. Client and family education

      a. Teach appropriate oral iron supplement administration technique

      b. Instruct client and family on dietary sources of iron

        1) For infants, iron-fortified formula and iron-fortified infant cereal

        2) Good sources of iron include organ meats, dried legumes, nuts, green vegetables, and iron-enriched flours

      c. Teach family about side effects of iron, such as constipation; encourage high-fiber diet and fluid intake to minimize this risk

      d. Instruct family to store iron preparation where children cannot reach it; iron supplement overdose could be fatal

      e. Provide parents with information about conserving client's energy and preventing trauma to blood cells to reduce red cell damage

  8. Evaluation: client demonstrates resolution of anemia with a return to normal lab values; family verbalizes an understanding of cause and treatment of iron-deficiency anemia

---

Practice to Pass

You are teaching the family of a 5-month-old with iron-deficiency anemia. In advising the family on how to minimize the side effects of the iron supplement, what administration guidelines will you give the family?

Case Study

You are caring for an 11-month-old male who has been admitted through the emergency department in order to treat a hemarthrosis of the right elbow and confirm a diagnosis of hemophilia.

1. What are the most pertinent questions you will ask his parents in your admission history?

2. What will be your priority nursing actions in regards to the client's physical comfort?

3. What diagnostics and medical interventions would you anticipate to be ordered by the physician?

4. What information will you give to his parents in explaining hemophilia when his diagnosis is confirmed?

5. What information will you give to his parents upon discharge?

For suggested responses, see page 356.

POSTTEST

1 A 2-year-old with hemophilia is being discharged, and the nurse is completing discharge teaching with his parents. Which statement by the parents indicates they require further teaching regarding hemophilia?

1. "It is good to know that his sister will not get hemophilia also."
2. "If our son has a temperature, we will not give aspirin or ibuprofen, only acetaminophen."
3. "We will get a MedicAlert bracelet for our son as soon as we get home."
4. "We will be sure to watch our son very closely to make sure he does not have another episode of bleeding."

2 The parents of a child with sickle cell anemia are asking for information about future pregnancies. Neither parent has sickle cell anemia. The nurse states that any future pregnancies will have what chance of producing a child with sickle cell anemia?

1. One in four chance of producing a child with sickle cell trait
2. One in four chance of producing a child with sickle cell anemia
3. One in two chance of producing a child with neither sickle cell disease nor trait
4. One in two chance of producing a child with sickle cell anemia

3 The nurse is working with the family of an 8-month-old infant who has severe nutritional anemia. In providing dietary recommendations, the nurse should instruct the family to do which of the following?

1. Switch the baby to cow's milk.
2. Delay the introduction of table food in the diet.
3. Restrict the amount of milk or formula in the baby's diet to one quart per day.
4. Provide dietary iron sources such as peanuts and unsweetened chocolates.

4 A child is being admitted to the unit with thalassemia major. In preparing client assignments, the charge nurse wants to assign a nurse to this child who can do which of the following?

1. Teach dietary sources of iron.
2. Administer blood transfusions.
3. Work with a dying child.
4. Monitor the child for bleeding tendencies.

5 The nurse is caring for a child who is being treated for extensive bleeding in the emergency department. The source and extent of bleeding are being determined as the nurse is trying to control the bleeding. The nurse places highest priority on which of the following activities?

1. Obtain the client's history.
2. Talk with the family regarding the risk of HIV and hepatitis C with blood transfusions.
3. Replace blood volume.
4. Provide psychosocial support to the family.

6 The nurse is working with the family of a toddler who is being treated for iron deficiency anemia. In teaching dietary considerations, the nurse will instruct the family to add sources of iron and which additional supplements?

1. Vitamin D and thiamine
2. Calcium and riboflavin
3. Carbohydrates and vitamins
4. Folic acid and proteins

7 The elementary school nurse is assessing and giving initial care to a client with hemophilia who has significant pain in his knee. The nurse suspects hemarthrosis. As the nurse waits for his caregiver to arrive, the nurse would take which action?

1. Maintain joint mobility with passive range-of-motion exercises.
2. Elevate the leg above his heart.
3. Administer children's aspirin or ibuprofen for pain.
4. Apply warm soaks to reduce the swelling.

8 A child who has recently been diagnosed with hemophilia will be placed on a recombinant form of antihemophilic factor (AHF). The parents are concerned about the possibility of the child being exposed to the HIV virus. What reassurance can the nurse provide?

1. AHF is not a blood product so there is no risk of HIV exposure.
2. AHF is sterilized so there is no risk of HIV exposure.
3. The recombinant form of AHF is made in a laboratory and does not contain human blood.
4. Although factor is a blood product, it does not contain RBCs or platelets so cannot spread the HIV virus.

9 The 10-year-old client in the emergency department has complete blood count (CBC) results that include hemoglobin (Hgb) of 8 grams/dL and hematocrit (Hct) of 24%. The nurse determines that, based on laboratory results, which nursing action has the highest priority?

1. Assessing and promoting skin integrity
2. Promoting hydration
3. Promoting nutrition
4. Reducing energy expenditure

10 The nurse is caring for a child diagnosed with thalassemia major who is receiving her first chelation therapy. The nurse reinforces teaching about chelation therapy with the parents by stating that it is done for which purpose?

1. To decrease the risk of hypoxia
2. To decrease the risk of bleeding
3. To eliminate excess iron
4. To prevent further sickling of red blood cells (RBCs)

➤ *See pages 322–323 for Answers and Rationales.*

ANSWERS & RATIONALES

Pretest

1 **Answer: 4** **Rationale:** A child diagnosed with thalassemia who will receive multiple transfusions throughout life will need chelation therapy for excessive iron stores. An iron supplement would be inappropriate in this child.

Cognitive Level: Analyzing **Client Need:** Physiological Adaptation **Integrated Process:** Nursing Process: Evaluation **Content Area:** Child Health **Strategy:** Consider which statements are appropriate for a child with thalassemia and eliminate those. That will leave only the response that indicates the need for more education. **Reference:** Perry, S., Hockenberry,

M., Lowdermilk, D., & Wilson, D. (2010). *Maternal child nursing care* (4th ed.). St. Louis, MO: Mosby, p. 1501.

2 **Answer: 1** **Rationale:** Rectal temperatures can traumatize the fragile rectal mucosa, leading to bleeding, and should be avoided. The vital signs will need to be measured on a regular basis. An intravenous start kit is appropriate as the child will need plasma and blood products. A bedpan will be needed if the child is on bedrest. Urinary catheters are avoided if possible. **Cognitive Level:** Analyzing **Client Need:** Safety and Infection Control **Integrated Process:** Nursing Process: Planning **Content Area:** Child Health **Strategy:** This child is at risk for bleeding. Consider equipment that might trigger a hemorrhage and eliminate that from the environment. **Reference:** Berman, A., & Snyder, S. (2012). *Kozier & Erb's fundamentals of nursing: Concepts, process, and practice* (9th ed.). Upper Saddle River, NJ: Prentice Hall, p. 539.

3 **Answer: 3** **Rationale:** All of the injuries require nursing care; however, the child with the head injury has a potentially life-threatening injury. The risk of permanent damage and death is greatest with head injury since the cranium does not expand easily, which results in increased pressure within the cranial vault. **Cognitive Level:** Analyzing **Client Need:** Management of Care **Integrated Process:** Nursing Process: Planning **Content Area:** Child Health **Strategy:** Consider which injury has the greatest opportunity for serious injury. Knowledge of the care of medical emergencies and prioritizing care of injuries will aid in choosing the correct answer. **Reference:** Perry, S., Hockenberry, M., Lowdermilk, D., & Wilson, D. (2010). *Maternal child nursing care* (4th ed.). St. Louis, MO: Mosby, p. 1503.

4 **Answer: 1** **Rationale:** RBCs sickle under conditions where low oxygen concentrations exist; therefore, administering oxygen will prevent additional sickling. The oxygen has no effect on the oxygen-carrying capacity of RBCs. It will not have an effect on development of respiratory complications. It will not decrease the potential for infection. **Cognitive Level:** Analyzing **Client Need:** Physiological Adaptation **Integrated Process:** Teaching and Learning **Content Area:** Child Health **Strategy:** Knowledge of the underlying rationale for the management of sickle cell disease will help to answer the question correctly. **Reference:** London, M., Ladewig, P., Ball, J., Bindler, R., & Cowen, K. (2011). *Maternal & child nursing care* (3rd ed.). Upper Saddle River, NJ: Prentice Hall, p. 1449.

5 **Answer: 3** **Rationale:** Iron preparations should be taken through a straw in order to prevent staining the teeth. While it is best to give toddlers choices in the hospital setting, the other options are not appropriate as iron is best absorbed on an empty stomach. **Cognitive Level:** Applying **Client Need:** Pharmacological and Parenteral Therapies **Integrated Process:** Nursing Process: Implementation **Content Area:** Child Health **Strategy:** Identify the side effects of iron preparations before reviewing the distracters. **Reference:** Kee, J., Hayes, E., & McCuistion, L. (2012). *Pharmacology: A nursing approach* (7th ed.). St. Louis, MO: Saunders, p. 227.

6 **Answer: 3** **Rationale:** In an acute care setting such as a hospital and with a potentially life-threatening disease such as DIC, the family may need help with coping with the stress they are feeling. This stress often interferes with communication. A patient response by the nurse with repetition of information will allow the family to absorb the information. The other options are not helpful. **Cognitive Level:** Analyzing **Client Need:** Psychosocial Integrity **Integrated Process:** Nursing Process: Implementation **Content Area:** Child Health **Strategy:** While one option might be true, the stem describes a difficult situation for the family. Choose the option that beset responds to this difficult situation. **Reference:** Chiocca, E. (2011). *Advanced pediatric assessment.* Philadelphia: Lippincott Williams & Wilkins, p. 51.

7 **Answer: 2** **Rationale:** Factor VIII concentrate is a blood product. Fluid volume overload is an unlikely concern, as the factor will be given in a comparatively small volume of fluid. There is no greater a chance of emboli formation with administration of factor than with any other IV preparation. Concern as to contracting AIDS from administration of a blood product is a long-term concern related to multiple administrations. It is not a concern during the actual administration of the factor. **Cognitive Level:** Applying **Client Need:** Pharmacological and Parenteral Therapies **Integrated Process:** Nursing Process: Implementation **Content Area:** Child Health **Strategy:** Since factor is a blood product, it carries many of the same potential complications as most other blood products. **Reference:** Kee, J., Hayes, E., & McCuistion, L. (2012). *Pharmacology: A nursing approach* (7th ed.). St. Louis, MO: Saunders, p. 685.

8 **Answer: 1, 2, 5** **Rationale:** There are three common problems seen in sickle cell anemia. First, there is the anemia crisis. This is a continuous problem for the sickle cell patient. Sequestration crisis occurs primarily in children under 6 and in older children and adults who have functioning spleens. The crisis is a pooling of the blood causing circulatory collapse. The third crisis is the vaso-occlusive crisis. **Cognitive Level:** Applying **Client Need:** Physiological Adaptation **Integrated Process:** Teaching and Learning **Content Area:** Child Health **Strategy:** Consider the definition of the terms. That will eliminate two choices, polycythemia and hemochromatosis. Knowledge of the etiology and pathophysiology of sickle cell disease will help to aid in the final selection. **Reference:** London, M., Ladewig, P., Ball, J., Bindler, R., and Cowen, K. (2011). *Maternal & child nursing care* (3rd ed.). Upper Saddle River, NJ: Prentice Hall, p. 1446.

9 **Answer: 3** **Rationale:** Anemia does occur easily in infancy, and infants have limited stores of iron. The first solid food offered to infants is often cereal, which is an excellent source of iron. All infants do not require iron supplements; it is preferable that the iron comes from dietary intake. **Cognitive Level:** Applying **Client Need:** Physiological Adaptation **Integrated Process:** Teaching and Learning **Content Area:** Foundational Sciences **Strategy:** Knowledge of infant iron needs and nutrition will help you to choose the correct answer. Note that two options are opposites, indicating one is more likely to be the correct answer. **Reference:** London, M., Ladewig, P., Ball, J., Bindler, R., & Cowen, K. (2011). *Maternal & child nursing care* (3rd ed.). Upper Saddle River, NJ: Prentice Hall, p. 913.

⑩ Answer: 4 Rationale: Alterations in platelet function necessitate treating a break in the skin's integrity as you would an arterial stick—apply pressure for 5 minutes or more. The goal of treatment is to apply pressure long enough that the defective clotting mechanism will have time to form a clot. Steri-strips would not close the wound adequately, and restricting arm movement will not assist in the initial formation of a clot. **Cognitive Level:** Applying **Client Need:** Pharmacological and Parenteral Therapies **Integrated Process:** Nursing Process: Implementation **Content Area:** Child Health **Strategy:** Platelet dysfunction refers to clotting problems. Two options refer to measures to prevent bleeding; one of these is the correct response. Knowledge of the care of the client with decreased platelets and IV care will help to make a final selection. **Reference:** Lewis, S., Dirksen, S., Heitkemper, M., Bucher, L., and Camera, I. (2011). *Medical-surgical nursing: Assessment and management of clinical problems* (8th ed.). St. Louis, MO: Mosby, p. 682.

Posttest

① Answer: 4 Rationale: It is not possible for parents of a hemophiliac to prevent a bleeding episode, no matter how careful they are. The nurse should reinforce this information along with methods for decreasing the chance of an injury that will lead to a bleeding episode. The other statements all indicate an appropriate understanding of hemophilia. **Cognitive Level:** Analyzing **Client Need:** Physiological Adaptation **Integrated Process:** Nursing Process: Evaluation **Content Area:** Child Health **Strategy:** Consider which statement would be inappropriate for a child with hemophilia. **Reference:** Ball, J., Bindler, R., & Cowen, K. (2010). *Child health nursing: Partnering with children & families* (2nd ed.). Upper Saddle River, NJ: Prentice Hall, p. 1055.

② Answer: 2 Rationale: Sickle cell anemia is an autosomal recessive condition. Therefore, if both parents have the trait, each pregnancy carries a 25% (one in four) risk that the child will have the disease. **Cognitive Level:** Applying **Client Need:** Health Promotion and Maintenance **Integrated Process:** Teaching and Learning **Content Area:** Child Health **Strategy:** Since neither parent has the disease, they are both carriers, meaning that they each have only one gene with the disorder. Affected children must have both genes affected. There are four combinations of the parents' genes. **Reference:** McKinney, E., James, S., Murray, S., & Ashwill, J. (2009). *Maternal-child nursing* (3rd ed.). St. Louis, MO: Saunders, p. 1282.

③ Answer: 3 Rationale: Many infants with nutritional anemia rely primarily on the milk/formula for dietary intake and refuse solid foods. When the milk/formula is limited, the child will be more willing to take solid foods. Cow's milk is a poor source of iron. Peanuts and unsweetened chocolates are sources of iron but are not appropriate for this child's diet. **Cognitive Level:** Applying **Client Need:** Health Promotion and Maintenance **Integrated Process:** Nursing Process: Implementation **Content Area:** Child Health **Strategy:** Recall that nutritional anemia means a diet with inadequate iron. Then recall that milk is a poor source of iron. **Reference:** Perry, S., Hockenberry, M., Lowdermilk, D., & Wilson, D. (2010). *Maternal child nursing care* (4th ed.). St. Louis, MO: Mosby, p. 1494.

④ Answer: 2 Rationale: Blood transfusions are utilized in order to maintain normal hemoglobin (HGB) levels. There is an excess of iron secondary to repeated transfusions, and, thus, iron supplements will not be necessary. The other therapies are inappropriate for the child with thalassemia major. **Cognitive Level:** Analyzing **Client Need:** Management of Care **Integrated Process:** Nursing Process: Implementation **Content Area:** Child Health **Strategy:** Because of fragile blood cells, the child will be anemic and require blood. Use this information to select the correct response. **Reference:** Pillitteri, A. (2010). *Maternal & child health nursing: Care of the childbearing & childrearing family* (6th ed.). Philadelphia: Lippincott Williams & Wilkins, p. 1310.

⑤ Answer: 3 Rationale: Appropriate oxygenation is not possible when there is significant loss of blood volume. Replacing the blood volume is critical to saving the child's life, and it is imperative that replacement occurs prior to any of the listed nursing actions. **Cognitive Level:** Analyzing **Client Need:** Physiological Adaptation **Integrated Process:** Nursing Process: Planning **Content Area:** Child Health **Strategy:** Use Maslow's hierarchy of needs to answer the question. The physiological intervention would be the first concern, as the child is actively bleeding. **Reference:** Berman, A., & Snyder, S. (2012). *Kozier & Erb's fundamentals of nursing: Concepts, process, and practice* (9th ed.). Upper Saddle River, NJ: Prentice Hall, p. 221.

⑥ Answer: 4 Rationale: Folic acid potentiates the removal of iron from ferritin, which makes it further available for heme production. The synthesis of albumin, blood proteins, fibrinogen, and hemoglobin is dependent upon the presence of proteins. None of the others are involved in building red blood cells (RBCs). **Cognitive Level:** Applying **Client Need:** Physiological Adaptation **Integrated Process:** Teaching and Learning **Content Area:** Child Health **Strategy:** Iron deficiency anemia refers to inadequate hemoglobin and RBCs. Look for nutritional additions that will help develop RBCs. **Reference:** Ball, J., Bindler, R., & Cowen, K. (2010). *Child health nursing: Partnering with children & families* (2nd ed.). Upper Saddle River, NJ: Prentice Hall, p. 1032.

7 **Answer: 2** **Rationale:** The nurse would elevate the leg above the level of the heart to reduce bleeding. Aspirin or aspirinlike products such as ibuprofen interfere with the clotting mechanisms. During active bleeds, the joint should be immobilized. Warm soaks would promote bleeding; ice packs should be used instead. **Cognitive Level:** Applying **Client Need:** Reduction of Risk Potential **Integrated Process:** Nursing Process: Implementation **Content Area:** Child Health **Strategy:** Since hemarthrosis is bleeding into the joints, look for strategies to reduce bleeding. **Reference:** Perry, S., Hockenberry, M., Lowdermilk, D., & Wilson, D. (2010). *Maternal child nursing care* (4th ed.). St. Louis, MO: Mosby, p. 1504.

8 **Answer: 3** **Rationale:** Recombinant factor is made in the laboratory and does not contain human blood. Therefore, it will not contain the HIV virus. All other responses have incorrect information in them. **Cognitive Level:** Applying **Client Need:** Pharmacological and Parenteral Therapies **Integrated Process:** Nursing Process: Implementation **Content Area:** Child Health **Strategy:** Think about the term recombinant and its definition **Reference:** Perry, S., Hockenberry, M., Lowdermilk, D., & Wilson, D. (2010). *Maternal child nursing care* (4th ed.). St. Louis, MO: Mosby, p. 1503.

9 **Answer: 4** **Rationale:** Such lab results indicate severe anemia. Fatigue results when the oxygen-carrying capacity of RBCs is impaired and cellular hypoxia is present. Fatigue can be diminished and oxygen depletion limited when the client's energy is conserved. The priority activity would be conserving energy and reducing cardiac stress. Skin integrity is not a high priority at this point. There is no indication of dehydration in this question. Additionally, increasing general hydration without transfusing RBCs will not positively affect the anemic state. Although improving nutrition is generally appropriate, the response would not be immediate and the cause of the anemia is uncertain. **Cognitive Level:** Analyzing **Client Need:** Reduction of Risk Potential **Integrated Process:** Nursing Process: Planning **Content Area:** Child Health **Strategy:** First recognize that these lab values are very low. Therefore, the child's oxygen-carrying ability is reduced. Select the option that relates to oxygenation. **Reference:** Pillitteri, A. (2010). *Maternal & child health nursing: Care of the childbearing & childrearing family* (6th ed.). Philadelphia: Lippincott Williams & Wilkins, p. 1300.

10 **Answer: 3** **Rationale:** Chelation therapy is to help the body remove excessive iron stores which have accumulated from the repeated blood transfusions needed to maintain adequate hemoglobin. Chelation therapy has no effect on hypoxia. Chelation therapy does not reduce the risk of bleeding. Sickling of RBCs does not occur with thalassemia. **Cognitive Level:** Applying **Client Need:** Physiological Adaptation **Integrated Process:** Teaching and Learning **Content Area:** Child Health **Strategy:** First determine the pathology of thalassemia as well as its treatment. Then determine which response relates to this knowledge. **Reference:** Perry, S., Hockenberry, M., Lowdermilk, D., & Wilson, D. (2010). *Maternal child nursing care* (4th ed.). St. Louis, MO: Mosby, p. 1501.

References

Ball, J., Bindler, R., & Cowen, K. (2010). *Child health nursing: Partnering with children & families* (2nd ed.). Upper Saddle River, NJ: Pearson Education.

Perry, S., Hockenberry, M., Lowdermilk, D., & Wilson, D. (2010). *Maternal child nursing care* (4th ed.). St. Louis, MO: Elsevier.

London, M., Ladewig, P., Ball, J., Bindler, R., & Cowen, K. (2011). *Maternal & child nursing care* (3rd ed.). Upper Saddle River, NJ: Pearson Education.

Pagana, K., & Pagana, T. (2009). *Mosby's diagnostic and laboratory test reference* (9th ed.). St. Louis, MO: Elsevier.

Van Leeuwen, A., & Poelhuis-Leth, D. (2009). *Davis's comprehensive handbook of laboratory and diagnostic tests with nursing implications* (3rd ed.). Philadelphia: F. A. Davis.

15 Special Considerations in Child Health

Chapter Outline

Congenital Health Problems
Acquired Health Problems

Accidents and Injuries Causing
Health Problems

NCLEX-RN® Test Prep

Use the accompanying online resource,
NursingReviewsandRationales, to test
yourself with hundreds of NCLEX®-style
practice questions.

Objectives

➤ Describe assessment findings and nursing management of a client
with attention deficit hyperactivity disorder, autism, or mental
retardation.
➤ Discuss the nursing management of the family experiencing the
loss of an infant to sudden infant death syndrome.
➤ Discuss assessment findings and nursing management of a client
who has sustained child abuse.
➤ Describe nursing management options for a client with the mental
health problems of substance abuse or suicide risk.
➤ Describe nursing management of a client who has experienced
accidental poisoning.

Review at a Glance

art therapy utilization of drawing as
a form of therapeutic strategy; drawing
exercises allow children of all ages an
opportunity to express feelings of fear,
anger, and pain

behavioral modification a method
utilized to alter inappropriate behaviors by
reinforcing desirable behaviors, usually by
stimulus or response conditioning (reward
system); often used by parents of children
with attention-deficit hyperactivity disorder
or mental retardation

child abuse infliction of physical,
psychological, or sexual harm on a child

physical abuse direct physical
injury to a child as a result of hitting,
striking, punching, kicking, shaking,
biting, or burning

play therapy a therapeutic strategy
that uses toys, dolls, art, or other creative
methods to allow child an opportunity to
reveal problems such as abuse; this
method is appropriate for preschool- to
school-age child

psychological abuse deliberate
failure of caregiver to provide emotional
nurturance, affection, and attention, significantly impairing child's self-esteem

sexual abuse sexual contact of a
child resulting from fondling, rape,
sodomy, intercourse, or exploitation
through pornography

suicide act of self-injury with intention
of the act to result in death

suicide attempt unsuccessful
effort to commit suicide

suicide ideation thoughts about
committing act of suicide

1 A 16-year-old has a history of writing a suicide note and then swallowing numerous anti-anxiety pills belonging to a friend. Which factor would indicate that the adolescent is at risk for a repeat attempt at suicide?

1. She stated that she wishes she hadn't made such a "stupid mistake."
2. Her grades dropped before her first suicide attempt.
3. Her father died recently.
4. She lives with her mother and stepfather.

2 The nurse is performing a health screening on an adolescent in the health clinic. The nurse determines the adolescent is at a higher risk of suicide than other adolescents of his age after the client makes which disclosure?

1. He sleeps late on the weekends.
2. He only has a small group of close friends.
3. He is gay/homosexual.
4. He often skips meals and does not worry about nutrition.

3 An 11-year-old female was discovered smoking cigarettes in the school bathroom. The school nurse implements which plan that has been shown to be most effective in the school-age child?

1. Assign the child to a peer-led program to teach the consequences of smoking.
2. Recommend that the child attend a community-based smoking prevention program.
3. Assign the child to view videos that demonstrate the effects of smoking.
4. Schedule the child to attend a session of health class that deals with smoking.

4 The nurse is providing care to a toddler who has ingested an unknown amount of his grandfather's medication, which is described as "a white pill." The physician has ordered the gastric lavage and administration of activated charcoal. What action should the nurse take?

1. Question the order because gastric lavage and activated charcoal are not to be used together.
2. Perform gastric lavage and then administer the activated charcoal.
3. Administer the activated charcoal, and then perform gastric lavage.
4. Perform gastric lavage, leaving the saline solution in the stomach, and then administer the activated charcoal.

5 A child is brought to the emergency department with excessive drooling, edema of lips and tongue, swollen mucous membranes, and is hypotensive and tachycardic. Based on this initial assessment, the nurse suspects that the child has ingested which agent?

1. A corrosive agent
2. Aspirin
3. A hydrocarbon
4. Acetaminophen

6 The nurse is teaching a class on child safety. During the discussion of ingestion of poisons, the nurse would teach the parents that safety measures include which of the following? Select all that apply.

1. Avoid placing leftover gasoline in a soda bottle.
2. Never encouraging a child to take medicine by telling the child it tastes like candy.
3. Keep syrup of ipecac available in case of an accidental poisoning.
4. Keep the poison control number by the phone.
5. Cover any lead-based paint in the house with a fresh layer of non-lead-based paint.

7 A 10-year-old child with mild mental retardation wants to join his younger brother's Cub Scout group. His parents are apprehensive about allowing him to join and ask the nurse for advice. Upon what information will the nurse formulate a response?

1. The child has the same need for socialization as children without mental retardation.
2. The child should not be encouraged to participate in clubs because of their developmental delay.
3. The child should participate in clubs especially created for children that are cognitively impaired.
4. The child does not have a need for socialization.

8 An 11-year-old child with attention deficit hyperactivity disorder (ADHD) being treated with methylphenidate (Ritalin) twice a day reports that he is having difficulty falling asleep at night. Upon questioning him, the nurse discovers he takes the morning dose before leaving for school and the evening dose after supper. Based on the information provided, the nurse would make which recommendation?

1. Continue taking the morning dose as previously, but take the evening dose earlier in the afternoon.
2. Stop taking the medication until he can be evaluated by his physician.
3. Take both doses of the medication in the morning before leaving for school.
4. Reduce the evening dose of medication to half the prescribed dose.

9 Parents who have just experienced the death of an infant from sudden infant death syndrome (SIDS) request time alone with the infant. The nurse should take which action?

1. Discourage the parents from seeing the infant because it will be too painful.
2. Allow the parents as much time alone with the infant as they need.
3. Allow the parents to view the infant, but remain in the room with them.
4. Deny the parents' request because they are emotionally distraught.

10 A 3-year-old child is brought to the emergency department with injuries the father stated occurred when the child fell off of his tricycle. Upon assessment, numerous bruised areas, old and fresh, are noted on the child's back, buttocks, and shoulders. Radiologic examination reveals fractured ribs and a healed fractured humerus. Based on these findings, what should be the nurse's next course of action?

1. Report the child as a victim of child abuse immediately.
2. Ask the father to provide further details of the incident, obtain a medical history of the child, and then interview the child separately.
3. Ask the father if he has been physically abusive to the child.
4. Ask the father if he believes the child's mother has been physically abusive to the child.

➤ *See pages 339–340 for Answers and Rationales.*

I. CONGENITAL HEALTH PROBLEMS

A. Attention-deficit hyperactivity disorder (ADHD)

1. Definition: ADHD is a persistence in hyperactivity, impulsiveness, or inattention that is observed more frequently than in other children at same developmental level
2. Etiology and pathophysiology
   a. Etiology is unknown; however, it is theorized that genetic and environmental factors can be attributed to ADHD; ADHD is associated with high blood lead level in childhood and prenatal exposure to alcohol
   b. Occurs more frequently in males, is diagnosed when symptoms appear, generally around ages 3 to 4
3. Assessment
   a. Easily distracted
   b. Difficulty waiting turns

      c. Excessive talking

      d. Leaves uncompleted task to begin another

      e. Does not appear to listen

      f. Constant squirming or fidgeting in chair

      g. Decreased attention span

      h. Impulsiveness

      i. Often loses things

4. Priority nursing diagnoses

      a. Impaired Verbal Communication

      b. Impaired Social Interaction

      c. Risk for Compromised Family Coping

      d. Risk for Caregiver Role Strain

      e. Risk for Injury

      f. Risk for Low Self-Esteem

5. Planning and implementation

      a. Assist with diagnostic procedures: MRI and psychological assessments

      b. Help establish plan for promotion of optimal growth and development

         1) Decrease excess stimulation (television, loud noises)

         2) Provide quiet environment for learning

         3) Promote self-esteem

         4) Establish reward programs for completion of tasks

         5) Provide parental support

      c. Refer parent(s) to Children and Adults with Attention-Deficit/Hyperactivity Disorder (CHADD) at www.chadd.org or 1-800-233-4050 and to the National Attention Deficit Disorder Association (ADDA) at www.add.org

! **6.** Medication therapy

      a. Methylphenidate (Ritalin, or Concerta as a longer-acting formulation) is a central nervous system stimulant

         1) In children with ADHD, it enhances catecholamine effects, which inhibit impulsiveness and hyperactivity; allows client to concentrate better and benefit more from school experience

         2) Should not be taken after 6 p.m. to allow client to sleep at night

      b. Dexmethylphenidate (Focalin), which is a stimulant and a schedule II controlled substance

      c. Amphetamine and dextroamphetamine (Adderall and Adderall XR), which is a schedule II controlled substance

      d. Atomoxetine (Strattera) is a selective norepinephrine reuptake inhibitor; as a nonstimulant, it is not a controlled substance; one side effect is that this drug may increase risk of suicide thoughts

7. Client and family education

      a. Teach safe medication administration of psychopharmacologic agents

      b. Educate parents and teachers to provide structure and decrease classroom stimuli to enhance school performance

      c. Educate client and family about disorder; provide family with strategies to deal with hyperactivity and inattentiveness

      d. Provide information to client and family about activities that serve to improve self-esteem

8. Evaluation: parents identify safe and effective drug administration; family identifies activities to decrease hyperactivity and promote learning; client exhibits symptoms of positive self-esteem

B. Autism (Autism Spectrum Disorders)

1. Description
    a. Autism is a developmental disorder of brain function characterized by deficits in behavior and often intelligence
    b. Involves abnormalities in behavior, interferes with ability for social interactions, and impairs verbal communication

2. Etiology and pathophysiology
    a. Autism Spectrum Disorders are diagnosed in about 6 children per 1000 and affects males more frequently than females
    b. Etiology is unknown but may be linked genetically, and to biochemical imbalances and brain dysfunction
    c. Most autistic children have cognitive impairment
    d. Severity ranges from the mildest (Asperger's disorder) to the most severe (autism)
    e. Symptoms usually become apparent by 3 years of age

3. Assessment
    a. Interview parent(s) regarding client's behavior
        1) Disinterested in being held or cuddled; stiffens when being held
        2) Avoids eye contact
        3) Poor language development
        4) Minimal facial responsiveness (does not smile)
        5) Appears not to hear when being spoken to
        6) Exhibits abnormal activities such as head banging
        7) Does not engage in social play with others

4. Priority nursing diagnoses
    a. Impaired Social Interaction
    b. Impaired Verbal Communication
    c. Delayed Growth and Development
    d. Compromised Family Coping
    e. Caregiver Role Strain
    f. Risk for Injury

5. Planning and implementation
    a. Decrease environmental stimuli (sounds and light)
    b. Maintain a safe environment, provide close supervision; self-abusive children need protective mechanisms in the least restrictive manner possible
    c. Promote parental coping
    d. Maintain hospitalized client's daily routine as much as possible to minimize stress
    e. Encourage activities and specialized educational programs to client's ability to promote optimal growth and development

6. Client and family education
    a. Teach family protective items that reduce child's risk of injury
    b. Educate parents about behavior modification methods
    c. Refer parent(s) to the Autism Society of America at www.autism-society.org or 1-800-3AUTISM

7. Evaluation: family identifies support systems within community; client demonstrates improved eye contact and ability to communicate, and remains free from self-injury

C. Mental retardation (sometimes referred to as cognitive impairment)

1. Description
    a. Mental retardation is defined as intelligence significantly below average, existing with limitation in adaptive skills

    b. IQ scores used to denote mental retardation are generally below the 70 to 75 range; IQ is a computation of an individual's mental age divided by his or her chronologic age times 100.

2. Etiology and pathophysiology

    a. Numerous causes are attributed to mental retardation including genetic factors (for example, Down syndrome), prenatal factors (such as fetal alcohol syndrome and maternal infections), and postnatal factors (such as trauma, errors of metabolism, and hypoxia)

    b. Mental retardation occurs more often in males than females

    c. Severity of mental retardation

        1) Mild retardation: an IQ between 50 and 70

        2) Moderate retardation: an IQ between 35 and 50

        3) Severe retardation: an IQ between 20 and 35

        4) Profound retardation: an IQ below 20

3. Assessment

    a. Prenatal and postnatal histories may provide clues to presence of mental retardation; family history of genetic disorders should be investigated

    b. Delays in motor and language developmental milestones; these delays are often first recognized by mother

    c. Associated seizure disorders and other injuries may indicate trauma

    d. Laboratory tests, including chromosomal analysis and blood levels for lead or enzymes, may be useful

    e. The Denver II developmental screening test provides information on developmental levels

    f. Neurologic exams may recognize soft neurologic signs such as a simian crease in the palms or abnormal hair swirls and low-set ears

4. Priority nursing diagnoses

    a. Delayed Growth and Development

    b. Self-Care Deficit: Toileting, Hygiene

    c. Impaired Verbal Communication

    d. Compromised Family Coping

5. Planning and implementation

    a. Early detection is beneficial; perform developmental screening to detect delays

    b. Support parent(s) in choosing educational programs; depending on severity, client may be "mainstreamed" into public school classrooms or attend special education classes

    c. Provide parental support and guidance, as they may experience shock and grief upon learning diagnosis

    d. When appropriate, perform a functional assessment to determine client's ability to provide self-care (toileting, feeding, dressing)

    e. Encourage socialization (may participate in scouting groups or other activities, depending on client's motor and developmental ability)

    f. May require occupational and/or speech therapy

    g. Promote optimal growth and development, encourage promotion of self-esteem and self-care

    h. Help parent(s) establish a behavior modification program if necessary

    i. Help parent(s) identify any potential complications (cardiac, pulmonary, gastrointestinal, motor) and seek medical assistance when necessary

    j. Educate parent(s) that client has same needs for exercise and play as other children, and this should be tailored to child's developmental age

6. Client and family education
   a. Teach safety precautions to prevent injuries caused by developmental delays
   b. Provide information that supports growth and development
   c. Teach parents to plan activities based on client's mental age rather than chronologic age
   d. Refer parent(s) to The National Parent Network on Disabilities (NPND) at www.npnd.org
7. Evaluation: parents make positive statements about their child; family provides stimulation appropriate to mental age of child; client displays evidence of a positive self-esteem

II. ACQUIRED HEALTH PROBLEMS

A. Sudden infant death syndrome (SIDS)

1. Definition: the sudden, unexplained death of an infant less than 1 year of age
2. Etiology and pathophysiology
   a. Death remains unexplained even after autopsy
   b. Most frequently occurs between ages 2 and 4 months
   c. Occurs more commonly in males
   d. Most often occurs in winter and spring
   e. Child is discovered in crib after period of sleep; a change of position may have occurred, and there may be frothy, blood-tinged secretions around mouth and nares
   f. The syndrome is usually considered unpreventable
3. Assessment
   a. Usually considered unpredictable; however, risk factors are known
      1) Prematurity
      2) Infections
      3) Brain stem defects
      4) Use of soft bedding (infant suffocates by rebreathing CO_2)
      5) Sleeping in prone or side-lying position
      6) Sleeping in room with decreased air movement
      7) Maternal smoking during pregnancy
      8) Sibling with SIDS
      9) Low birth weight
      10) Increased incidence in winter
      11) Increased incidence in lower socioeconomic groups
   b. Infant is brought to the emergency department and death is confirmed; an autopsy will be ordered to determine cause of death
4. Priority nursing diagnoses
   a. Compromised Coping related to death of child
   b. Fear
   c. Anxiety
   d. Grieving
   e. Risk for Sudden Infant Death Syndrome
5. Planning and implementation
   a. Nursing management of risk for SIDS includes educating parents about risk factors and activities that can reduce risk factors
      1) Children at high risk may be placed on an apnea monitor whenever client is asleep
      2) Parents need to be taught infant CPR
   b. Nursing management of family experiencing loss of child from SIDS

   1) Most often a nurse's first contact with suspected SIDS is in the emergency department after the infant is brought in for resuscitation
   2) Avoid questions that could imply parental negligence or involvement in the death
   3) Provide emotional support for grieving family; seek assistance from social services, clergy, and/or others that have experience in helping families deal with the death of a child

   4) Parent(s) may verbally express feelings of anger and guilt; assure parent(s) that there is nothing that they could have done to prevent infant's death
   5) Allow parent(s) an opportunity to hold child and say goodbye; infant should be presented cleaned and wrapped in a blanket
   6) An autopsy will likely be necessary to verify the cause of death; this should be explained to parent(s)
   7) Assess sibling response to death and intervene with counseling as necessary; a sibling may feel guilty or responsible for the infant's death
   8) Refer family to American SIDS Institute at www.sids.org or 1-239-431-5425

6. Client and family education

   a. Educate parent(s) that the American Academy of Pediatrics recommends placing infants on their backs, instead of prone, for sleep
   b. Encourage use of ceiling or free-standing fans in child's bedroom to increase air movement
   c. Educate parent(s) of high-risk infants on appropriate use of apnea monitors
   d. Provide information to parents of SIDS victims about what is known about syndrome

7. Evaluation: all parents place infants to sleep on their backs, not stomachs; parents of at-risk infants identify safety measures for using infant monitors and demonstrate infant CPR correctly; parents of SIDS victims state that child's death was unpreventable and participate in SIDS support groups

B. Child abuse

1. Description
   a. **Child abuse**, sometimes referred to as child maltreatment, is the infliction of physical, psychological, or sexual abuse on a child
   b. **Physical abuse** describes abuse that involves direct physical injury usually as a result of hitting, striking, punching, shaking, biting, or burning
   c. **Sexual abuse** describes abuse that involves sexual contact as a result of fondling, rape, sodomy, intercourse, or exploitation through pornography
   d. **Psychological abuse**, or emotional abuse, is characterized by deliberate failure of the caregiver to provide emotional nurturance, affection, and attention, significantly impairing child's self-esteem
   e. Child neglect is failure to provide basic needs such as physical, emotional, and educational needs
   f. Munchausen syndrome by proxy involves a distorted perception by parents that leads to situations of repeatedly seeking medical interventions for a healthy child; included in this syndrome can be deliberate injury to child by parent as a means of meeting own psychological need for attention

2. Etiology and pathophysiology; risk factors include the following:
   a. Prematurity
   b. Chronically ill child
   c. Child is viewed as difficult
   d. Unwanted child

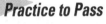

Practice to Pass

A 4-month-old infant is brought to the emergency department by the parents who found the infant dead in the crib when they woke up this morning. The initial cause of death is believed to be sudden infant death syndrome (SIDS). As the nurse who provided care to the infant and the family, what actions would you now take towards the parents?

      e. Adult abuser characteristically has low self-esteem and a low tolerance for frustration, lives in social isolation, and has an inadequate understanding of normal growth and development

      f. Incompatibility between a parent's (or parents') and child's temperament

      g. Parent abuses alcohol or drugs

3. Assessment

      a. Physical assessment includes a thorough examination of entire body; assess for burns, scalds, scars, bruising, fractures, dislocated joints, vaginal tears or bleeding, and other signs of abuse

      b. Height and weight to determine failure to thrive or other growth abnormalities

      c. Assess client and family interaction

      d. Assess for evidence of neglect (dirty, unkempt, withdraws from others)

      e. Assess for delays in psychosocial, psychomotor, and cognitive development

      f. Sexually abused client may exhibit bedwetting, frequent crying, excessive bathing, avoidance of family and peers

      g. Covert observation of the parent's interactions with the child will be a component of the assessment of this client

4. Priority nursing diagnoses

      a. Delayed Growth and Development

      b. Fear related to physical harm

      c. Risk for Injury

      d. Pain related to injuries

      e. Impaired Skin Integrity related to injury

      f. Ineffective Health Maintenance

5. Planning and implementation

      a. Maintain a nonjudgmental and nonthreatening attitude during interactions with client and parent(s)

      b. Document client and parent comments verbatim

      c. Be aware that incompatibility between the *history* and the *injury* is the number one criterion for suspecting child abuse

      d. Report all cases of suspected child abuse; health care professionals have a legal obligation to report suspected abuse

      e. Do not inform parent(s) that child abuse is suspected

      f. Child may be removed from home and placed in a safe environment to prevent further injury

      g. If child remains in custody of family, assist them in identifying support systems and resources such as Parents Anonymous

      h. Acknowledge client's fears during hospitalization and provide a consistent care-giver to encourage establishment of trust and security

      i. Refrain from stereotyping to decrease incidence of false-positive and false-negative accusations; there is no single predictor for who will commit child abuse

      j. Be aware of the types of therapeutic strategies utilized by therapists

         1) Play therapy utilizes toys, dolls, art, and other creative objects to allow client an opportunity to reveal problems such as abuse; this strategy is used mostly for the preschool- and school-age child

         2) Art therapy utilizes drawing exercises to allow expressions of feelings such as anger and pain; this strategy is appropriate for all ages

         3) Behavior modification applies methods to alter inappropriate behavior by reinforcing desirable behaviors, usually by stimulus or response conditioning; an example is the use of the "reward system"

   k. Refer family to the Parents Anonymous at www.parentsanonymous.org or 1-909-621-6184

6. Client and family education

   a. Teach child that he or she can report abuse without fear of repercussions

   b. All families need to know where to seek help when feeling overwhelmed

7. Evaluation: client is maintained in a safe environment; parents display appropriate parenting skills; client remains free of injury

C. Substance abuse

1. Definition: voluntary use of a substance to obtain a state of euphoria or a state of calmness

2. Etiology and pathophysiology

   a. Most commonly abused substances

     1) Tobacco (cigarettes, chewing tobacco)

     2) Alcohol

     3) Marijuana

     4) Volatile substances (inhaled) such as spray paint and plastic cement

     5) Cocaine, narcotics, heroin, ecstasy, CNS depressants, and CNS stimulants

   b. Risk factors for substance abuse

     1) Parent who engages in substance abuse

     2) Peer association (wants to "fit in")

     3) School drop-out

     4) Problems with conduct

     5) Biologic factors

     6) Depression (about 50% of adolescent drug abusers are depressed)

3. Assessment

   a. Physical, social, and psychological symptoms vary according to substance

     1) Cocaine produces euphoria, cardiovascular manifestations, and seizures

     2) CNS depressants have sedative effects such as drowsiness, decreased muscle tone and impaired speech

     3) CNS stimulants can lead to aggressive behavior, agitation, restlessness, paranoia, and boldness

     4) Narcotics use produces constricted pupils and respiratory depression

     5) Inhalants cause a feeling of euphoria or "high," loss of consciousness, respiratory arrest

   b. Assess for needle marks (tracks) on arms and legs

   c. Assess for behavioral changes

     1) Drop in school performance (grades, participation)

     2) Skipping school

     3) Socializing with a "new" group of friends

     4) No longer interested in activities previously enjoyed (sports activities, after-school functions)

     5) Engaging in risk-taking behavior

     6) Trouble resulting in intervention from law enforcement

4. Priority nursing diagnoses

   a. Risk for Injury

   b. Risk for Violence (other directed or self-directed)

   c. Impaired Social Interaction

   d. Chronic Low Self-Esteem

   e. Risk-Prone Health Behavior

5. Planning and implementation

   a. Encourage participation in educational programs that increase substance abuse awareness

b. Treatment for acute drug toxicity or withdrawal is specific to substance; gastric lavage or narcotic antagonists are most often utilized depending on route of substance involved

c. Acute management includes maintaining patent airway, adequate tissue perfusion, and fluid volume status

d. Treatment for chemical dependency/substance abuse often requires rehabilitation measures and involves a multidisciplinary approach

e. Encourage youth participation in prevention groups such as Students Against Driving Drunk (SADD)

f. Refer chemically dependent client to Alcoholics Anonymous or Ala-Teen at www.alcoholics-anonymous.org

6. Client and family education: educate parent(s) and teachers about signs and symptoms of substance abuse

7. Evaluation: client participates in substance abuse avoidance education program; parents and teachers identify symptoms of substance abuse; symptoms of acute substance abuse are recognized and emergency treatment is provided

D. Suicide

1. Description

   a. Suicide is defined as an act of self-injury, with intention that the act result in death; most common methods of suicide completion, in order, are using firearms, hanging, and overdose

   b. Suicide attempt is an intention to cause death that is unsuccessful

2. Etiology and pathophysiology

   a. Etiology of suicide is related to depression, poor self-concept, isolation, and family dysfunction

   b. For adolescents between 15 and 19 years of age, suicide is third-leading cause of death

   c. For children between 5 and 14 years of age, suicide is the sixth-leading cause of death

   d. Incidence of *completed* suicides is higher in males, but incidence of suicide attempts is higher in females

   e. Homosexual youths attempt suicide two to three times more often than heterosexual youths

   f. Risk factors for suicide

   1) Depression

   2) Previous attempts at suicide (suicide gesture)

   3) Family history of psychiatric disorders

   4) Family violence

   5) Substance abuse

   6) Homosexuality

   7) Chronic illness

   8) Overwhelming sense of guilt or shame

   9) Frequent risk-taking behaviors

   10) History of sexual abuse

3. Assessments of suicide risk

   a. Makes specific statements about suicide

   b. Gives away personal items

   c. Sudden calmness (suicide decision has been made)

   d. Any situation identified in risk factors (listed above)

   e. Suicide ideation: thoughts about the act of suicide

4. Priority nursing diagnoses

   a. Hopelessness related to fear and anxiety

   b. Ineffective Coping

   c. Ineffective Family Processes

Practice to Pass

A 16-year-old male is brought to the emergency department by a group of his friends who inform the nursing staff that "he took some drugs and now we can't get him to wake up." The adolescent is minimally responsive, pupils are constricted, and his respirations are 6 to 8 per minute. What immediate actions would you take?

        d. Risk for Injury

        e. Social Isolation

        f. Disturbed Personal Identity

        g. Risk for Suicide

    5. Planning and implementation

        a. Be supportive and nonjudgmental

        b. Use direct and clear approach; be physically available to decrease client's sense of isolation

        c. During hospitalization, take suicide precaution measures

        d. Help client develop coping strategies

        e. Help family develop coping strategies

        f. Refer to mental health professional

        g. Be aware that despair and hopelessness is not a normal part of adolescence

        h. Assess the degree of suicidality; take all suicidal remarks seriously and further investigate them; use acronym SLAP:

            1) S, Specificity: specific plan for suicide

            2) L, Lethality: intended method of suicide

            3) A, Accessibility: intended means of suicide is available

            4) P, Proximity: predetermined time to commit suicide

        i. Encourage "suicide contracts" with at-risk youths or those who have indicated a desire to commit suicide; client signs an agreement to not attempt suicide for a specified period of time; these contracts are usually renewed daily

        j. Community education: teach parents, teachers, health care providers, and children warning signs of suicidal ideation; emphasize that most people attempting or completing suicide have revealed their thoughts about depression and/or suicide to someone—*the key is to listen and intervene*

        k. Instruct parents to remove all firearms from household, especially in presence of high-risk youths; firearms are most commonly used method of suicide

        l. Provide anticipatory guidance to parents and adolescents to help them obtain an understanding of normal adolescent growth and development

        m. Refer parent(s) to the American Academy of Pediatrics: The Injury Prevention Program at www.aap.org or 1-847-434-4000

    6. Client and family education: educate parent(s) and client about pharmacotherapeutic agents (antidepressants or antipsychotic medications) prescribed for client

    7. Evaluation: client remains free of suicide attempts; client and/or family identifies coping strategies

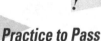

Practice to Pass

A 15-year-old female has been hospitalized numerous times for suicide attempts by swallowing various over-the-counter medications. You have provided care to her on several previous hospitalizations and are concerned because of the repeated attempts at suicide. What actions could you take to help this adolescent?

III. ACCIDENTS AND INJURIES CAUSING HEALTH PROBLEMS

  A Accidental poisoning

    1. Definition: accidental ingestion of poison or caustic substance

    2. Etiology and pathophysiology

        a. Most deaths from poisoning for young children occur during ages 1 to 4

        b. Most deaths from poisoning for adolescents occur during ages 15 to 19

        c. Risk factors for accidental poisoning

             1) Curiosity related to developmental age

            2) Lack of understanding of danger

            3) Lack of parental or caregiver supervision

        d. Most common agents of accidental poisoning

             1) Acetaminophen (Tylenol)

            2) Ibuprofen

3) Household plants

4) Cleaning solutions such as bleach

5) Cosmetic products (perfumes)

3. Assessments

  a. Acetaminophen: assess for nausea, vomiting, diaphoresis; later signs involve the hepatic system, with jaundice, coagulation abnormalities, and pain in right upper quadrant

  b. Aspirin: assess for nausea, vomiting, diaphoresis, tinnitus, seizures, oliguria, dehydration, coma

  c. Corrosive agents: assess for drooling or inability to clear secretions, swollen mucous membranes, edema of tongue, lips, burning in mouth, throat, and stomach, and signs of shock

  d. Hydrocarbons: assess for nausea, vomiting, weakness, pulmonary complications such as tachypnea and cyanosis, and alterations in sensorium

4. Priority nursing diagnoses

  a. Risk for Injury

  b. Risk for Ineffective Airway Clearance

  c. Risk for Impaired Gas Exchange

  d. Risk for Impaired Oral Mucous Membranes

  e. Risk for Decreased Cardiac Output

  f. Risk for Aspiration

  g. Risk for Poisoning

5. Planning and implementation

  a. Management is *specific to agent*

  b. Treat *client* first, not the poison

  c. Maintain adequate respiratory and circulatory function

  d. Be aware that condition may deteriorate rapidly

  e. Keep client warm

  f. Contact Poison Control Center for specific treatment of poisonings

  g. Refer to Table 15-1 for methods of treatment for poisonings

  h. Refer parent(s) to the American Academy of Pediatrics: The Injury Prevention Program at www.aap.org or 1-800-433-9016

6. Client and family education

  a. Teach families safety measures related to poisoning prevention

    1) Safe storage of household chemicals

    2) Use of child-proof medication bottles and keeping medications away from young children; remind family that toddlers can get access to medications in mother's purse

  b. Encourage all families to keep poison control center's phone number handy, such as taped on phone

7. Evaluation: parents identify interventions appropriate in an accidental poisoning; parents childproof child's environment; child remains free of accidental poisoning; accidental poisoning victim recovers without sequelae

Practice to Pass

A 3-year-old male is brought to the emergency department after eating acetaminophen (Tylenol). The client is treated and has no complications. Upon review, you discover that the client was treated four months ago for a similar situation involving vitamins. What actions should you take?

Table 15-1	**Management of Poisonings in the Pediatric Population**
Method of Treatment	**Indications and Usage**
Activated Charcoal The administration of a tasteless, odorless, black substance given to reduce systemic absorption of toxic agents	Given to reduce systemic absorption of toxic agents; may be mixed with sorbitol, water, or a saline cathartic. The client may drink the mixture through a straw, or it may be administered via nasogastric tube. If taken orally, administer in opaque container with lid to prevent visualization of black liquid. Not administered for ingestion of caustic substances or hydrocarbons.
Antidotes The administration of an antidote specific to the agent of poisoning	Acetaminophen poisoning:N-acetylcysteine (Mucomyst) Carbon monoxide poisoning: oxygen Digoxin poisoning/toxicity: digoxin immune fab (Digibind) Benzodiazepine overdose: flumazenil (Romazicon) Opioid overdose: naloxone (Narcan)*Note:* Gastric decontamination, if indicated, is still required when administering antidotes.
Cathartics The administration of cathartics is done to promote stimulation and evacuation of the bowel in order to decrease systemic absorption. Also administered to promote evacuation of activated charcoal.	Sorbitol Magnesium sulfate Magnesium citrate These solutions are administered orally, or via a nasogastric tube.
Gastric Lavage The insertion of a nasogastric tube and subsequent irrigation and removal of gastric contents	Insert largest bore nasogastric tube possible; lavage with prescribed solution. Contraindicated in corrosive poisonings.

Case Study

A 5-year-old female who is a victim of sexual abuse committed by her uncle is being admitted to your hospital unit for treatment of a urinary tract infection and labia lacerations.

1. As you admit the child to the unit, what will be your initial approach with her?

2. What measures can you take to promote a sense of security for the child?

3. The child tells you that she is "bad" because she told on her uncle. How would you respond?

4. The parents are arguing loudly in the child's hospital room. What actions would you take?

5. The child is exhibiting anger by throwing her breakfast tray and refusing to allow the nursing staff to assess her. What strategies could be initiated to support the child's well-being?

For suggested responses, see pages 356–357.

POSTTEST

1. A 17-year-old male has informed his friends and family that he plans to commit suicide. The school nurse's next action is determined after drawing which conclusion?

1. Most adolescents threaten to commit suicide.
2. Threats of suicide should not be ignored.
3. If he does not have a specific plan, then he is not serious.
4. No intervention is required because he has made these threats in the past.

2. The nurse overhears a group of student nurses in the break room discussing the role of the health care professional in suspected child abuse. The nurse concludes that the student who most accurately understands the role is one who makes which statement?

1. "Nurses should only report child abuse if they are certain."
2. "Nurses should tell the child's doctor if child abuse is suspected."
3. "Only the physician can report child abuse."
4. "Nurses are required to report any case of suspected child abuse to child protective services."

3. The nurse has spoken to the parents of a 2-year-old child about precautionary measures to be taken at home to help prevent accidental poisonings. The nurse determines that the parents require further instructions when the father makes which statement?

1. "I will have the Poison Control Center phone number available at every phone."
2. "I will lock up all medications, household cleaners, and other potentially poisonous substances."
3. "I will check for poisonous houseplants and remove them from the home or place them out of my child's reach."
4. "I will have syrup of ipecac available at home and administer it to my child if he swallows any type of poison."

4. The nurse has an order to administer activated charcoal to a child who has consumed numerous unidentified pills. Because the child has a decreased level of consciousness, the nurse should take which of the following most appropriate actions to administer the charcoal?

1. Administer the charcoal orally as long as the child has a gag reflex.
2. Do not administer the charcoal because the child has a decreased level of consciousness.
3. Insert a nasogastric tube and administer the activated charcoal as ordered.
4. Question the order for activated charcoal until the pills have been identified.

5. A 3-year-old child has been diagnosed with autism. The child has all of the following symptoms. Which symptoms are related to the diagnosis of autism? Select all that apply.

1. The child eats only a few preferred foods.
2. The child refuses to make eye contact.
3. The child's speech consists entirely of echolalia.
4. The child is a poor sleeper.
5. The child does not smile.

6. When performing a health screening on a 9-year-old boy with mental retardation, the nurse notes that his weight is in the 98th percentile. During follow-up assessment of the child's nutrition and exercise habits, the mother states that she does not allow her son to run and play because she is afraid he will be injured. The nurse then incorporates which information into a teaching plan for the child and mother?

1. This child requires a strict nutritional plan because he will not benefit from physical activities in the management of weight.
2. He is unable to engage in exercise or play activities because of the lack of coordination.
3. This child has the same need for exercise and play as other children, and it is beneficial to his health.
4. This child does not enjoy engaging in physical activities or participating in sports activities.

7 The parents of a 7-year-old child with attention deficit hyperactivity disorder (ADHD) have been taught to utilize a behavior modification plan to encourage completion of tasks such as homework. The nurse determines the parents understand appropriate behavior modification techniques when they do which of the following?

1. Punish him by taking away outside play privileges.
2. Utilize a reward system for accomplishments.
3. Allow him to choose what tasks he wants to complete.
4. Increase his medication when he does not complete his tasks.

8 When offering support to the family of a 5-month-old infant who died from sudden infant death syndrome (SIDS), the nurse anticipates that the infant's older sibling may experience which of the following?

1. Lack of concern about where the infant is
2. Acceptance of the infant's death
3. Guilt that he or she may have caused the infant's death
4. An understanding that the infant is dead

9 A mother brings her 6-year-old daughter to the health clinic with concerns about bedwetting and thumb-sucking. Her behavior in school has changed dramatically this year, and she also takes baths up to six times a day. She has also been treated for a urinary tract infection numerous times over the past few months. Based on this initial information, what should the nurse consider in order to determine next steps?

1. The child is experiencing school phobia.
2. The child is trying to gain her mother's attention.
3. The child needs psychological counseling.
4. The child may be a victim of sexual abuse.

10 In caring for an adolescent with suspected opioid (narcotic) abuse, the nurse would monitor the adolescent for which of the following? Select all that apply.

1. Constricted pupils
2. Euphoria
3. Hyperactivity
4. Aggressive behavior
5. Respiratory depression

➤ *See pages 341–342 for Answers and Rationales.*

POSTTEST

ANSWERS & RATIONALES

Pretest

1 **Answer: 3 Rationale:** Parental loss is a risk factor associated with suicide. A decline in grades is a symptom exhibited before her first suicide attempt, and without further investigation, there is no indication that there is a dysfunctional relationship between her and the mother or stepfather. Indicating remorse for the action is a positive step toward recovering. **Cognitive Level:** Applying **Client Need:** Psychosocial Integrity **Integrated Process:** Nursing Process: Assessment **Content Area:** Mental Health **Strategy:** Consider the option that would have the most longstanding effect on the adolescent. **Reference:** Pillitteri, A. (2010). *Maternal & child health nursing: Care of the childbearing & childrearing family* (6th ed.). Philadelphia: Lippincott Williams & Wilkins, p. 939.

2 **Answer: 3 Rationale:** Gay and lesbian adolescents are at a higher risk of suicide than other adolescents their age,

especially if the family does not offer support. Sleeping late on weekends and skipping meals without concern for nutrition is normal for adolescents, as is having a small group of close friends. **Cognitive Level:** Analyzing **Client Need:** Psychosocial Integrity **Integrated Process:** Nursing Process: Assessment **Content Area:** Mental Health **Strategy:** Eliminate findings that a large number of adolescents could report. **Reference:** Perry, S., Hockenberry, M., Lowdermilk, D., & Wilson, D. (2010). *Maternal child nursing care* (4th ed.). St. Louis, MO: Mosby, p. 1141.

3 **Answer: 1 Rationale:** All activities are appropriate to promote substance abuse prevention; however, peer-led programs have proven to be the most successful when teaching children about the hazards of substance and tobacco use and abuse. **Cognitive Level:** Applying **Client Need:** Health Promotion and Maintenance **Integrated Process:** Nursing Process: Planning **Content Area:** Child Health **Strategy:** This question requires the learner to

ANSWERS & RATIONALES

decide the most successful program for the school-age child. **Reference:** Perry, S., Hockenberry, M., Lowdermilk, D., & Wilson, D. (2010). *Maternal child nursing care* (4th ed.). St. Louis, MO: Mosby, pp. 113–117.

4 **Answer: 2** **Rationale:** Lavage is done first to remove as much of the poison as possible then the activated charcoal is given to reduce absorption if any chemical remains in the stomach. Both lavage and administration of activated charcoal may be used to prevent absorption of the poison. If lavage was performed second, it would remove the charcoal without allowing it to be effective. If the saline solution is left in the stomach then it is an instillation, not a lavage. The saline needs to be removed to rid the stomach of the poison. **Cognitive Level:** Applying **Client Need:** Reduction of Risk Potential **Integrated Process:** Nursing Process: Implementation **Content Area:** Child Health **Strategy:** Consider the purpose of the lavage and activated charcoal to determine the correct order of administration. **Reference:** Ball, J., Bindler, R., & Cowen, K. (2010). *Child health nursing: Partnering with children & families* (2nd ed.). Upper Saddle River, NJ: Prentice Hall, p. 600.

5 **Answer: 1** **Rationale:** Corrosive agents cause the signs and symptoms listed. Indications of aspirin overdose are nausea, vomiting, diaphoresis, and seizures. Hydrocarbons cause nausea, vomiting, cyanosis, and altered sensorium, and acetaminophen causes nausea, vomiting, diaphoresis, and later, jaundice. **Cognitive Level:** Analyzing **Client Need:** Physiological Adaptation **Integrated Process:** Nursing Process: Assessment **Content Area:** Child Health **Strategy:** The two medications can easily be eliminated as they would not cause the swelling of the mouth. It is then necessary to choose between the hydrocarbons and corrosive agent. **Reference:** Pillitteri, A. (2010). *Maternal & child health nursing: Care of the childbearing & childrearing family* (6th ed.). Philadelphia: Lippincott Williams & Wilkins, p. 1559.

6 **Answer: 1, 2, 4** **Rationale:** Syrup of ipecac is no longer recommended to be kept in the home of children. Covering lead-based paint with another layer of paint may not prevent exposure of the child. All other responses are correct. **Cognitive Level:** Applying **Client Need:** Reduction of Risk Potential **Integrated Process:** Teaching and Learning **Content Area:** Foundational Sciences **Strategy:** Consider nonfood substances that the child is likely to ingest and how to prevent ingestion. **Reference:** Perry, S., Hockenberry, M., Lowdermilk, D., & Wilson, D. (2010). *Maternal child nursing care* (4th ed.). St. Louis, MO: Mosby, pp. 1426–1430.

7 **Answer: 1** **Rationale:** Children with mental retardation have the same need for socialization as others and should be encouraged to participate in clubs and activities with children of the same developmental age. There is no need to encourage participation only in clubs exclusive to children with cognitive impairment; this would limit the child's social interaction. **Cognitive Level:** Applying

Client Need: Psychosocial Integrity **Integrated Process:** Nursing Process: Implementation **Content Area:** Foundational Sciences **Strategy:** Consider that two options are opposites. In some questions, there may be increased likelihood that one of these will be the correct response. **Reference:** Pillitteri, A. (2010). *Maternal & child health nursing: Care of the childbearing & childrearing family* (6th ed.). Philadelphia: Lippincott Williams & Wilkins, p. 1621.

8 **Answer: 1** **Rationale:** The purpose of Ritalin is to help the child concentrate in school so the second dose should be taken around noon. The nurse would not instruct a client to stop taking a medication unless it was an emergency situation. The doses should not be taken at the same time. If the physician had wanted that, the physician would have ordered the larger dose. Nurses do not change doses. **Cognitive Level:** Applying **Client Need:** Pharmacological and Parenteral Therapies **Integrated Process:** Nursing Process: Implementation **Content Area:** Child Health **Strategy:** The nurse would never tell a client to modify the dosage or to stop taking a medication. That leaves only the two choices related to timing of dosage. Consider that taking both doses at the same time would be inappropriate. **Reference:** Pillitteri, A. (2010). *Maternal & child health nursing: Care of the childbearing & childrearing family* (6th ed.). Philadelphia: Lippincott Williams & Wilkins, p. 1625.

9 **Answer: 2** **Rationale:** Parents need the opportunity to hold their infant and to say goodbye in private for as long as they wish. A peaceful, quiet, supportive environment should be provided. The other options are incorrect as they do not demonstrate compassionate care for parents who have just experienced the death of a child. **Cognitive Level:** Applying **Client Need:** Psychosocial Integrity **Integrated Process:** Nursing Process: Implementation **Content Area:** Mental Health **Strategy:** Knowledge of the supportive care for the family of an infant with SIDS will aid in choosing the correct answer. Consider which activity shows the most compassion for the family. **Reference:** McKinney, E., James, S., Murray, S., & Ashwill, J. (2009). *Maternal-child nursing* (3rd ed.). St. Louis, MO: Saunders, p. 1202.

10 **Answer: 2** **Rationale:** It is important to establish a thorough history and a detail of the incident before making assumptions of abuse. The child is safe from harm in the emergency department, allowing time to adequately assess the situation. The nurse should not make premature assumptions and, if abuse is suspected, the nurse should not inform the parent. **Cognitive Level:** Applying **Client Need:** Safety and Infection Control **Integrated Process:** Nursing Process: Assessment **Content Area:** Child Health **Strategy:** The nurse should always make a full assessment before proceeding with interventions. **Reference:** Perry, S., Hockenberry, M., Lowdermilk, D., & Wilson, D. (2010). *Maternal child nursing care* (4th ed.). St. Louis, MO: Mosby, p. 1069.

Posttest

1 **Answer: 2** **Rationale:** Threats of suicide should never be ignored. It is not normal for anyone to threaten to commit suicide, and the lack of a specific plan does not indicate the adolescent is not seriously contemplating suicide. **Cognitive Level:** Analyzing **Client Need:** Psychosocial Integrity **Integrated Process:** Nursing Process: Planning **Content Area:** Mental Health **Strategy:** Consider that further assessment is always required with suicide threats. **Reference:** Perry, S., Hockenberry, M., Lowdermilk, D., & Wilson, D. (2010). *Maternal child nursing care* (4th ed.). St. Louis, MO: Mosby, p. 1140.

2 **Answer: 4** **Rationale:** All health care professionals are required to report suspected child abuse to the appropriate authorities. Reporting the suspicions to the physician would not be sufficient. **Cognitive Level:** Applying **Client Need:** Management of Care **Integrated Process:** Nursing Process: Evaluation **Content Area:** Child Health **Strategy:** Recall the legal requirements about reporting child abuse to answer this question. **Reference:** London, M., Ladewig, P., Ball, J., Bindler, R., & Cowen, K. (2011). *Maternal & child nursing care* (3rd ed.). Upper Saddle River, NJ: Prentice Hall, p. 1178.

3 **Answer: 4** **Rationale:** Syrup of ipecac is no longer recommended for home administration. The other options all indicate correct statements. **Cognitive Level:** Analyzing **Client Need:** Safety and Infection Control **Integrated Process:** Nursing Process: Evaluation **Content Area:** Foundational Sciences **Strategy:** Note the critical words *require further instruction* in the stem of the question. Eliminate options that would be appropriate in providing a safe environment. **Reference:** Hockenberry, M., & Wilson, D. (2009). *Wong's essentials of pediatric nursing* (8th ed.). St Louis, Missouri: Mosby, p. 473.

4 **Answer: 3** **Rationale:** Activated charcoal is administered to decrease the systemic absorption of toxic agents and must be administered in a timely manner. Because of the risk for aspiration, oral solutions and medications should never be administered to those experiencing a decreased level of consciousness. Because the child has a decreased level of consciousness, inserting a nasogastric tube is the appropriate action to decrease the risk of vomiting and aspiration, which is a potential complication. **Cognitive Level:** Applying **Client Need:** Pharmacological and Parenteral Therapies **Integrated Process:** Nursing Process: Implementation **Content Area:** Pharmacology **Strategy:** Safety is the first issue. Recall that it is important that the activated charcoal not get into the lungs. **Reference:** Pillitteri, A. (2010). *Maternal & child health nursing: Care of the childbearing & childrearing family* (6th ed.). Philadelphia: Lippincott Williams & Wilkins, p. 1558.

5 **Answer: 2, 3, 5** **Rationale:** Typical symptoms of autism include echolalia, no eye contact, lack of response to social cues and repetitive behavior. Eating only preferred foods is common in 3-year-olds and being a poor sleeper is unrelated to autism. **Cognitive Level:** Applying **Client Need:** Psychosocial Integrity **Integrated Process:** Nursing Process: Assessment **Content Area:** Mental Health **Strategy:** Remember that autistic symptoms relate to difficulties relating to people and objects. **Reference:** Ball, J., Bindler, R., & Cowen, K. (2010). *Child health nursing: Partnering with children & families* (2nd ed.). Upper Saddle River, NJ: Pearson, p. 1399.

6 **Answer: 3** **Rationale:** Children with mental retardation need to exercise and play just as much as any other child does. Exercise and play are beneficial to the cardiovascular system, coordination, and weight control, as well as promotion of socialization. Emphasize that activities should be appropriate to the child's physical and developmental maturity. **Cognitive Level:** Applying **Client Need:** Health Promotion and Maintenance **Integrated Process:** Nursing Process: Planning **Content Area:** Foundational Sciences **Strategy:** Recall that the needs of all children are the same and that it is the implementation that varies. **Reference:** Perry, S., Hockenberry, M., Lowdermilk, D., & Wilson, D. (2010). *Maternal child nursing care* (4th ed.). St. Louis, MO: Mosby, p. 1180.

7 **Answer: 2** **Rationale:** Rewarding positive behavior is generally an effective means of encouraging the completion of tasks. Punishment is usually reserved for undesirable behaviors (negative reinforcement), and the child needs to participate in play and exercise activities. The child should be involved in some decision-making processes but should not be allowed to choose the tasks he desires to complete. No adjustment in medications should be made without the instructions from the primary care provider. **Cognitive Level:** Analyzing **Client Need:** Psychosocial Integrity **Integrated Process:** Nursing Process: Evaluation **Content Area:** Foundational Sciences **Strategy:** Recall that behavior modification techniques focus on positive shaping of behavior. **Reference:** Perry, S., Hockenberry, M., Lowdermilk, D., & Wilson, D. (2010). *Maternal child nursing care* (4th ed.). St. Louis, MO: Mosby, p. 814.

8 **Answer: 3** **Rationale:** It is not uncommon for older siblings to have bad thoughts or wishes toward a new sibling. They must be assured that their thoughts did not cause the infant's death. The understanding and acceptance of death depends on the child's developmental age. The children will express feelings of concern about where the infant is, the loss of the infant, and the expression of parental grief. **Cognitive Level:** Analyzing **Client Need:** Psychosocial Integrity **Integrated Process:** Nursing Process: Assessment **Content Area:** Foundational Sciences **Strategy:** No information is provided about the age of the older sibling; therefore, the response must be appropriate for most age groups. Recognize that everyone in the family will have some response to the death of the infant. **Reference:** Ball, J., Bindler, R., & Cowen, K. (2010). *Child health* *nursing: Partnering with children & families* (2nd ed.). Upper Saddle River, NJ: Prentice Hall, p. 733.

9 **Answer: 4** **Rationale:** Regressive behavior such as thumb-sucking and bedwetting, in addition to a sudden decline in school performance; excessive bathing, nightmares, and recurrent urinary tract infections are signs of sexual abuse and must be investigated immediately. There is no indication of school phobia, nor does she lack attention from her mother. The child may need psychological counseling, especially if sexual abuse is determined, but initially the abuse must be identified and appropriate interventions taken. **Cognitive Level:** Analyzing **Client Need:** Psychosocial Integrity **Integrated Process:** Nursing Process: Assessment **Content Area:** Mental Health **Strategy:** The core concepts of deterioration of behavior and repeated urinary tract infections should be clues to suspect sexual abuse. **Reference:** Ball, J., Bindler, R., & Cowen, K.

(2010). *Child health nursing: Partnering with children & families* (2nd ed.). Upper Saddle River, NJ: Prentice Hall, p. 593.

10 **Answer: 1, 2, 5** **Rationale:** Constricted pupils are a symptom of opioid use. Feelings of happiness are common with the use of opioids. If the amount of opioid taken is large, respiratory depression may be seen. Drowsiness is commonly seen in the individual using opioids. Aggressive behavior is not noted with opioid use. **Cognitive Level:** Applying **Client Need:** Physiological Adaptation **Integrated Process:** Nursing Process: Assessment **Content Area:** Pharmacology **Strategy:** The symptoms that the nurse will assess for are the same that would be seen in the client receiving a narcotic for a therapeutic purpose. **Reference:** McKinney, E., James, S., Murray, S., & Ashwill, J. (2009). *Maternal-child nursing* (3rd ed.). St. Louis, MO: Saunders, p. 1519.

References

Ball, J., Bindler, R., & Cowen, K. (2010). *Child health nursing: Partnering with children & families* (2nd ed.). Upper Saddle River, NJ: Pearson Education.

Deglin, J., Vallerand, A., & Sanoski, C. (2011). *Davis's drug guide for nurses* (12th ed.). Philadelphia: F.A. Davis.

Hockenberry, M., & Wilson, D. (2009). *Wong's essentials of pediatric nursing* (8th ed.). St Louis, MO: Elsevier.

London, M., Ladewig, P., Ball, J., Bindler, R., & Cowen, K. (2011). *Maternal & child nursing care* (3rd ed.). Upper Saddle River, NJ: Pearson Education.

Pillitteri, A. (2010). *Maternal & child health nursing: Care of the childbearing & childrearing family* (6th ed.). Philadelphia: Lippincott Williams & Wilkins.

Wilson, B., Shannon, M., & Stang, C. (2011). *Pearson nurse's drug guide 2011*. Upper Saddle River, NJ: Pearson Education.

Web sites

American Academy of Pediatrics: The Injury Prevention Program at www.aap.org

American Association on Intellectual and Developmental Disabilities at www.aamr.org

American SIDS Institute at www.sids.org

Autism Society of America at www.autism-society.org

Children and Adults with Attention-Deficit/Hyperactivity Disorder (CHADD) at www.chadd.org

National Attention Deficit Disorder at www.add.org

Parents Anonymous at www.parentsanonymous.org

Appendix

➤ Practice to Pass Suggested Answers

Chapter 1

Page 11: *Answer*—With normal motor development, a 10-month-old infant can do the following:

- Stand while holding onto furniture
- Sit down by falling down
- Cruise around furniture
- Crawl
- Use pincer grasp
- Say dada and mama
- Develop object permanence

Page 12: *Answer*—Safety precautions to be discussed will include the following:

- Continue proper use of car seat in automobile
- Supervision of indoor and outdoor play activities
- Risk for accidental poisonings: sources
- Avoid food such as cherries, hard candy, small pieces of hot dogs that can be aspirated by the young child
- Water safety
- Risks for burns, falls, and suffocation

Page 13: *Answer*—The child will need to have received the following:

- Diptheria, tetanus, and acellular pertussis (DtaP) #5
- Inactivated poliovirus vaccine (IPV) #4
- Measles, mumps, and rubella (MMR) #2
- Varicella #2
- Hepatitis A—in selected areas (4 to 18 years)
- Meningococcal vaccine (MCV4) to high risk groups

Page 15: *Answer*—The nurse will want to discuss with the parents these facts:

- Temper tantrums during toddlerhood are common. Children may display outbursts of negative behaviors such as screaming, yelling, and crying.
- Toddlers will have mood swings, fluctuating between pleasant temperament and displays of being difficult.

- Toddlers are striving to become more independent at this age, not as dependent on the parent(s). They seek autonomy within the environment.
- Common displays of negativism are observed in this age group.

Page 18: *Answer*—Activities to decrease anxiety include the following:

- Allow child to manipulate or play with equipment.
- Provide simple explanations: use visual aids such as dolls, pictures.
- Allow parent to be present with child.
- Use EMLA with IV starts and venipunctures.
- Avoid medical terminology.
- Use distraction during procedure.
- Use therapeutic play to facilitate expression of fear and feelings.
- Allow child choices that are realistic.
- Tell child it's OK to cry as long as he or she remains still.

Page 19: *Answer*—The nurse will be aware that a 15-year-old

- has a good understanding of illness related to death.
- views death as irreversible.
- perceives death as something that happens to old people, not "me."
- has common reactions: feelings of sadness, loneliness.

Chapter 2

Page 28: *Answer*—The nurse should have the environment at a comfortable temperature and free of distractions. Sitting at eye level with the informant will put the individual at ease. Demonstrate a nonjudgmental attitude. The nurse should explain simply and directly the reasons for needing particular information, directing questions to the child as appropriate based on age and developmental level.

Page 30: *Answer*—Some questions the nurse might ask include asking about the family's identification with a particular religious/ethnic group and what special religious or cultural traditions are practiced in the home—food choices and preparation for example. Other questions might include asking about languages spoken in the home or if there are any cultural or religious healers the family relies on at times of illness.

Page 36: *Answer*—To ensure an adequate examination of a toddler, the nurse should first allow the child to become familiar with the nurse's presence. In addition, allow the child to touch or hold equipment. The nurse should approach the child by first examining a doll or stuffed animal the child might have. Tell, rather than ask, the child what needs to be done and have the child participate if possible, lift arms for example. The child may sit on the parent's lap for much of the exam if that feels reassuring to the child.

Page 43: *Answer*—A 7-year-old who is otherwise healthy and has not had a recent hemoglobin or hematocrit level should be screened. If the child lives in a high-risk environment, a lead-level test would be appropriate. A family history of elevated cholesterol or triglycerides in a parent may indicate a desirability of checking those levels in a child to get baseline levels.

Page 43: *Answer*—The Denver II is used to assess a child's motor and social development. It is not a test of intelligence nor does it predict future academic ability. It is also not intended to diagnose specific developmental problems. The Denver II is part of a routine screening done on many children.

Chapter 3

Page 54: *Answer*—The child is no longer considered contagious after receiving antibiotic therapy for 24 hours. The nurse will need to emphasize that the child will continue the antibacterial eye drops or ointment as prescribed, usually 7 to 10 days.

Page 56: *Answer*—The nurse can perform the cover-uncover test and the corneal light reflex test as follows:

1. Cover-uncover test: Ask the client to fix his or her gaze straight ahead, focusing on a distant object. Cover one eye with an opaque card. As the eye is covered, observe the uncovered eye for movement. Remove the card while observing the eye just uncovered for movement. This is a screening test for deviation in eye alignment and eye muscle weakness. Eye muscle weakness is seen as movement of the "lazy eye" when it attempts to refocus during the cover test.
2. Corneal light reflex test (Hirschberg test): This test is done to assess parallel symmetry of the eyes. The examiner shines a penlight directly onto the corneas of both eyes, holding the penlight about 12 inches away from the client's nasal bridge while the client focuses on a distant object. The examiner should see the light reflected at the same spot in both eyes. An asymmetric light reflex indicates a deviation in the alignment of the client's eyes.

Page 59: *Answer*—After the health care provider has explained the procedure to the parents, the nurse should teach the parents about the following:

a. Admission procedures to the day-surgery area

b. Any necessary lab tests ordered prior to anesthesia
c. Preoperative medications for sedation (if prescribed)
d. What will happen in the period before transport to the operating room
e. What will happen when the child and family are reunited following the procedure in the postanesthesia care area

The child, if age and developmental level permit, should be taught similar developmentally-appropriate content to encourage cooperative behavior.

Postoperative teaching should include information about the following:

a. How to relieve pain (use of acetaminophen or other analgesic as prescribed)
b. How to administer medications prescribed (oral analgesics and ear drops are frequently prescribed)
c. How to prevent water from entering the child's ear during bathing or swimming activities; often ear plugs are recommended if the health care provider cautions against activity that might allow water to enter the ear and the tube

The child's caregivers should be taught to promptly report signs and symptoms of ear infection, such as fever and purulent ear drainage to the health care provider. They should be taught that tubes commonly extrude and fall out, and they should notify the physician if they note a tube visible in the ear canal. Information should be provided about how to resume the child's diet and activity, and when to see the health care provider for postoperative follow-up appointments.

Page 61: *Answer*—Because symptoms of pain and fever usually subside within 24 to 48 hours of antibiotic therapy, the child or family may have stopped the medication because the child experienced relief of symptoms. The nurse must research what antibiotic was prescribed to the child six days ago. If a 10-day course of antibiotic was prescribed, the antibiotic therapy is not finished, and the health care provider must be consulted because the infection is not eradicated until all of the prescribed medication is taken. If it is discovered that the antibiotics were not completed, it is important that the nurse reteach medication administration, including appropriate administration and side effects. The nurse should stress the need to complete the full course of antibiotics even though the child may feel better after a short period of time.

The nurse should assess the child's vital signs, including temperature, and assess the child's pharynx using a tongue blade and light source. The nurse could also assess the child's ears through otoscopic examination. The nurse should refer the child to the health care provider and supply all data collected in the nursing assessment.

Page 62: *Answer*—Humidify the air in the home, especially in the child's room during the night and during the winter. Discourage the child from picking at or forcefully blowing the nose. Encourage the child to blow the nose gently and release sneezes through the mouth. Encourage keeping the external nasal septum soft and moist by applying a layer of petroleum jelly twice per day.

Chapter 4

Page 72: *Answer*—A bronchoscopy is performed under general anesthesia. The child must be kept NPO until swallow and gag reflexes have returned. Reassure the mother that vital signs and respiratory effort are normal. Advise the mother that the child should be fully awake before being fed to guard against vomiting and aspiration. Encourage her to hold and cuddle the child. Listen to her concerns; encourage and answer all questions.

Page 76: *Answer*—The treatment of pulmonary infection in children with cystic fibrosis is a priority. Pathogens are unusually difficult to clear and the risk of chronic colonization with resistant organisms increases if antibiotic therapy is not aggressive. Although life expectancy for children with cystic fibrosis has increased, pulmonary infections continue to pose the greatest threat to survival. In this situation, the socialization needs of a child with a chronic illness are also important. The nurse could consider having the child attend the puppet show while his antibiotics are being administered via infusion pump. If there is sufficient time, perhaps the medication could be completed before the activity. The nurse could also ascertain the duration of the activity.

Page 79: *Answer*—BPD is a chronic pulmonary disease that primarily affects premature infants who received prolonged mechanical ventilation and oxygen therapy at birth. Full-term infants may be affected also. Respiratory distress or failure, requiring oxygen and ventilation for a minimum of three days, can contribute to development of BPD.

Page 82: *Answer*—Epiglottitis is a medical emergency. Laryngospasm, increased edema, and complete airway obstruction can occur rapidly if there is any manipulation or irritation of the mouth and throat. Airway obstruction can also occur as a result of anxiety and crying. For these reasons, a child with epiglottitis is kept as calm and quiet as possible. Parental presence reassures the child and decreases distress. The mother of this child should be encouraged to remain with her child and you can offer to telephone the husband. If there is a portable telephone available, it can be brought to the mother.

Page 86: *Answer*—Peanut butter is a common food to be aspirated by young children. The thick consistency easily occludes a child's airway and is difficult to remove. This dad needs safety information regarding appropriate snack foods and the danger of aspiration in a small child. Peanut butter, if offered, must be spread in a thin layer on a cracker and never fed from a spoon. Counsel this dad that aspiration is the leading cause of death in small children.

Chapter 5

Page 98: *Answer*—

1. The child should increase activity gradually.
2. Observe for signs of wound infection, fever, flu-like symptoms, an increased respiratory rate, and dyspnea.
3. The child may return to school in about three weeks.
4. The child should be monitored for signs of infective endocarditis (sudden onset of high fever and heart failure).

Page 100: *Answer*—

1. Following cardiac catheterization, it is important to limit activity for 24 hours to avoid disturbing the insertion site.
2. The child is instructed on intake of fluids. Maintaining hydration is important because the contrast medium used during the procedure has a diuretic affect.
3. The parents are instructed to monitor for temperature elevation, which is an early sign of infection.

Page 102: *Answer*—Transposition of great vessels is a condition whereby the two main arteries leaving the heart are reversed. The aorta, which is supposed to leave the left ventricle and take oxygenated blood to the body, actually leaves the right ventricle and directs blood back to the body without receiving oxygenation. The pulmonary artery, which is supposed to leave the right ventricle and take blood to the lungs, actually leaves the left ventricle and directs blood back to the lungs for reoxygenation. In effect, there are two closed systems. Families need to understand that the infant will need palliative surgery in order to survive. A medication called Prostaglandin E1 will be given to maintain an open ductus arteriosus that allows for mixing of the blood and provides a small amount of oxygen to the rest of the body.

Page 105: *Answer*—Rheumatic fever is an inflammation of collagen tissue. The cardiac muscle has much of this connective tissue within it. Increased activity can aggravate the inflammation and ultimately lead to damaged heart valves. If there is no evidence of cardiac involvement, activity can resume as normal; however, caution needs to be taken at the first sign of cardiac pathology.

Page 106: *Answer*—The child needs to be seen by a physician to identify the exact cause. Kawasaki's disease is one possibility. Kawasaki's is not communicated person to person, so isolation techniques are not needed. Laboratory data will help rule out a staphylococcal infection or other similar infections. Cardiac complications are serious complications of this condition, and hospitalization is usually required during the acute period.

Chapter 6

Page 120: *Answer*—One-third of children with cerebral palsy also have some degree of mental retardation and 50% have seizures. Many also have mobility challenges, feeding problems, and vision, hearing, and developmental delays. It is obvious that to address this requires a multidisciplinary team approach. The parent must be the core of this team since a high degree of coordination must take place. For optimal development to be fostered, all the therapy regimens must be maintained at home and supported by the family. Family-centered care recognizes the pivotal role the family plays in the health of children.

Page 123: *Answer*—There are clear differences in what a parent would be instructed to watch for as signs of shunt malfunction based on the physical development of the child. For an infant whose cranial suture lines have not fused and fontanels are still open, assess for increased head circumference, high-pitched cry, bulging fontanel, irritability when awake, and seizures. Toddlers and older children usually present with vomiting, irritability, and headache. As the condition persists, the child may exhibit setting-sun eyes, seizures, papilledema, decreased level of consciousness, and change in vital signs (increased blood pressure and widening pulse pressure). Older children may have difficulty with balance or coordination. All children can present with lethargy and Cheyne-Stokes respiratory pattern.

Page 125: *Answer*—Client education should focus on the following:

1. Parental understanding of what a seizure is and what triggers it for their child
2. The basic "first aid" or safety measures to take when their child has a seizure
3. The names of medications, a medication schedule, and potential side effect of the medications. Instructions specific to the administration of the medication should be included, such as Dilantin chewable tablets should not be swallowed whole
4. Whom to call with questions; referrals to support organizations allow the parents to talk to someone about their feelings and emotions
5. The need to inform people (teachers, day care workers, baby-sitters, etc.) who will have frequent contact with their child on the nature of the disease as well first aid measures

These are just a few of the possible approaches to ensure that the parents have a realistic understanding of the health problem, and the knowledge, skills, and adequate resources to cope to deal with seizures.

Page 132: *Answer*—The major cause of injuries in young children is falls—from changing tables, beds, sofas, etc. Initially a young infant lacks the ability to turn over. A caregiver who is not alert to the possibility of the child doing this places the child at risk for a fall. Young children are curious and want to explore their environment. If gates are not put up, they are at risk to fall down stairs. Child abuse or shaken baby syndrome is a possible cause of head injury in infants under one year of age. The brain is highly vascular and the dura is more likely to shear from shaking. Adolescents and older children often think of themselves as invincible and disregard both safety devices, such as use of seatbelts and bike helmets, and speed limits. Many head injuries result from motor vehicle accidents (MVAs) and bicycle, skateboard, snowboard, and skiing accidents, especially where the child did not wear a protective helmet. Teenagers may also be injured in alcohol- or drug-related MVAs and sports injuries.

Page 134: *Answer*—Glasgow scores are indicated in square brackets, [ ]. A child with a minor head injury might present with transient confusion [4] but no loss of consciousness,

spontaneous opening of the eyes [4], and will obey a command [6]. This child has a high score indicating good prognosis.

A child with a major head injury might present with loss of consciousness, some moaning but not oriented to time, person, and place [2], eyes open to pain [2], and the only motor response is to painful stimulation [4]. This child's score is much lower, reflecting the severity of symptoms. The prognosis would be less positive for this child.

Chapter 7

Page 142: *Answer*—

1. The renal system is responsible for the formation and excretion of urine. If this function were impaired, the client may present with decreased urinary output (oliguria) or absent urinary output (anuria).
2. The renal system regulates fluid and electrolyte balance within the body. If this function were impaired, the client may present with signs and symptoms of edema, dehydration, hyper-/hypokalemia, hyper-/hyponatremia, or hyper-/hypocalcemia. Elevated blood pressure may also be present.
3. The renal system regulates acid–base balance within the body. If this function were impaired, the client may present with signs and symptoms of metabolic acidosis or alkalosis.
4. The renal system regulates blood pressure. If this function were impaired, the client may present with hypertension or hypotension.
5. The renal system stimulates the production of red blood cells in bone marrow. If this function were impaired, the client may present with signs and symptoms of anemia.
6. The renal system regulates calcium metabolism in the body. If this function were impaired, the client may present with signs and symptoms of bone disorders.

Page 146: *Answer*—Infants: Clean-catch urine specimens are obtained with the application of a urine collection bag. The infant cannot voluntarily void and thus depends on a nurse or parent to apply and remove the collection device.

Toddlers: Clean-catch urine specimens are obtained with the application of a urine collection bag. The toddler cannot voluntarily void and depends on a nurse or parent to apply and remove the collection device.

School-age children: School-age children are able to void voluntarily. Instructions regarding correct specimen collection technique must be given to the parent if they are assisting in the collection process. The school-age child needs assistance with specimen collection.

Adolescents: Adolescents may collect their own specimens after instruction in correct specimen collection technique. Adolescents require privacy and may feel uncomfortable with this procedure.

Page 150: *Answer*—Discharge instructions should include demonstration and return demonstration of ostomy care and catheter care if applicable. Instructions should include monitoring for changes in urinary output, signs and symptoms of infection, and dehydration. If an appliance is present, instructions regarding skin care and odor management are necessary. Instructions are also provided in writing. A contact number for help should be provided. Community resources are also made available at the time of discharge.

Page 152: *Answer*—Nursing measures specific to caring for children with acute glomerulonephritis include prevention measures (prompt and thorough treatment of all group A beta-hemolytic streptococcal infections) and management of hypertension (medication administration, dietary salt restrictions, frequent blood pressure monitoring). Nursing measures specific to caring for children with nephrotic syndrome include parent education regarding signs and symptoms, treatment regimes, disease chronicity, and behavioral changes in the child that may manifest due to distorted body image secondary to massive edema and weight gain. How do they differ? Acute glomerulonephritis can be prevented; nephrotic syndrome cannot. Client education regarding treatment of strep infections can prevent acute glomerulonephritis; client education cannot prevent nephrotic syndrome. Distortions in body image do not usually occur with acute glomerulonephritis. Acute glomerulonephritis is not chronic in nature; coping skills and treatment regimes are necessary long-term for clients with nephrotic syndrome.

Page 156: *Answer*—The three types of renal replacement therapy are hemodialysis, peritoneal dialysis, and kidney transplantation.

- Hemodialysis: an advantage is better clearance of toxins from the bloodstream, while a disadvantage is disruption of family with travel to dialysis center three times a week or increased risk for infection related to needed vascular access.
- Peritoneal dialysis: an advantage is that it is continuous and easy to learn to do at home; a disadvantage is that the client is at risk for peritonitis or that clearance of toxins is not as effective as with hemodialysis.
- Renal transplantation: an advantage is that this regime provides for optimal return to homeostasis and provides for optimal growth and development of the child; a disadvantage is that organ procurement can be difficult or that immunosuppression can result from medications used to prevent organ rejection.

Chapter 8

Page 169: *Answer*—The nurse should explain that some of the signs and symptoms of congenital hypothyroidism will not be obvious at birth. If the screening is not done immediately, and the baby has the disease, he or she could suffer from irreversible brain damage. Other complications include lethargy, decreased peristalsis, scaly skin, poor feeding, thick tongue, and anorexia. The mother needs to be aware that state law mandates all infants be tested. If the mother continues to refuse the testing, the nurse should report the situation to the child's pediatrician or to the birth hospital for follow-up.

Page 170: *Answer*—Since adolescents like to possess control over their bodies and their life situations, it is imperative that the teenager is involved in this decision. As a school nurse, you could offer an opportunity for rest periods during study hall and recreational time at school. The nurse might want to seek a physician's release from physical education class. Other options might include a half-day school schedule or pursuing a GED diploma.

Page 172: *Answer*—Because children with PKU lack the pigment melanin, their skin is fair-colored and extremely sensitive. These children should actually avoid the sunlight, but when exposed, they should have a sunscreen with SPF 60 or higher for protection.

Page 180: *Answer*—By drawing up the regular (clear) insulin first, the likelihood of contamination of the regular insulin is reduced, resulting in less dose variance. That same regular insulin may be used alone at times for sudden high glucose levels. If it were contaminated with NPH, the rapid action of the regular insulin would be impaired.

Chapter 9

Page 198: *Answer*—The nursing care for the child with Legg-Calve-Perthes disease and for the adolescent with slipped capitol femoral epiphysis is very similar. Both clients should be on bedrest until the hip is surgically repaired or medical management is begun. With both clients, the nurse will assess neurovascular status of the lower extremities. Both clients will need pain assessments and appropriate pain management. Both clients will require age-appropriate diversional activities, as both will not feel ill and will have plenty of energy. The difference in care lies in client and family teaching, as the disease process is different and the treatment may be different. If a child with Legg-Calve-Perthes disease is treated medically with a containment device, the discharge teaching must include information about the care of and wearing of the device and reinforcing compliance with wearing the device for the long length of treatment. Discharge teaching for the child with either condition who had surgical containment or repair will include activity restrictions according to the surgeon, and need for follow-up care.

Page 200: *Answer*—

- Respiratory care is a priority for a postop client following a spinal fusion. Logrolling by two people must be done every two hours to mobilize respiratory secretions. This client must also engage in respiratory exercises such as deep-breathing, coughing, and incentive spirometry every two hours. The nurse carefully assesses respiratory status.
- A second priority for this postop client is pain management. Spinal surgery for scoliosis is very painful; pain assessments must be done frequently and pain medication is given frequently; PCA pain management is often

used. The client's pain must be under control in order to participate in the needed respiratory care.

- Other priorities of care include assessing neurological function of the lower extremities every hour for the first 24 hours postop and then every 4 hours; maintaining a nasogastric tube for decompression, along with NPO status and frequent assessments of bowel sounds; and maintaining antiembolism stockings to prevent venous stasis.

Page 201: *Answer*—By the time a male client with Duchenne's muscular dystrophy reaches 15 years of age, his muscles are usually quite weak. The client is usually confined to a wheelchair, as the child is unable to walk independently. The cough reflex becomes weak and ineffective by this time and pneumonia develops easily. The main priority of care is centered on his respiratory status with administration of intravenous antibiotics, aggressive turning, coughing, and respiratory exercises. To maintain his level of muscle strength and use, physical therapy should become quickly involved, as short periods of bedrest can lead to further muscle wasting and weakness.

Page 205: *Answer*—Bryant's traction is used to treat developmental dysplasia of the hip and fracture of the femur in children less than 3 years of age and weighing fewer than 35 pounds. Bryant's traction is skin traction that involves having the hips at 90-degree flexion, with both legs straight up in the air, and the buttocks just off the bed. The care of this child includes neurovascular checks of the extremities. The nurse ensures that the weights on the traction are the ordered weight and hang freely and safely. The bandages on the legs that hold the skin traction in place need to be checked to ensure they are not too loose or too tight. Good skin care must be maintained as well as assessments of elimination patterns. A normally energetic and busy toddler will not take to bedrest lightly, and appropriate diversional activities must be employed quickly and often.

Page 206: *Answer*—Immediately following cast application, the nurse must carefully assess neurovascular status of the involved extremity and compare it with the uninvolved extremity. Circulation to the affected extremity must be checked every 15 minutes for the first hour, hourly for 24 hours, and every 4 hours after that. Assess for color, warmth, presence of distal pulses, and sensations of numbness and tingling. Assess for pain. If the nurse's assessment revealed signs of impaired neurovascular function (pallor, pulselessness, severe pain in the casted part of the extremity, tingling sensation, severe swelling not relieved by elevation), the physician should be notified, as the constricting cast can lead to neurologic damage.

Chapter 10

Page 216: *Answer*—Some comfort measures the nurse could suggest include giving the child tepid baths followed by a gentle massage of nonaffected areas with nonperfumed lotion. Keeping the child in cotton garments with tags removed helps reduce itching. Put cotton mittens or socks on the child's hands to prevent scratching. Do not allow the child to get so warm that he or she begins to perspire.

Page 219: *Answer*—Lice and nits can survive on human hosts, so the environment must be deloused. All clothing the child has worn in the last week should be washed in hot water and dried in a hot dryer for at least 20 minutes. All bedding should be similarly washed and dried. Things that cannot be washed and dried (blankets or stuffed toys, for example) should be placed in plastic bags for about two weeks. Discard or soak all combs, brushes, and hair ornaments. Thoroughly vacuum all furniture, carpets, and floors. Check all members of the household for the presence of lice or nits.

Page 220: *Answer*—Scabies presents with intense pruritus, but impetigo is painless. Because scabies causes intense itching, the nurse can frequently see scratch marks that may almost obscure the small papules or vesicles at the end of a scabies mite burrow. Scabies is often found on particular body areas such as hands, feet, finger webs, or body creases. Impetigo typically presents on the face, arms, or legs.

Page 221: *Answer*—The nurse will ask about recent episodes of otitis media or sinusitis. It is also important to ask about any insect bites or scratches the child had in the recent past. The nurse will want to know when redness was first noticed and what treatment has been attempted at home. The nurse will get baseline vital signs. The site will be examined for the extent of redness, edema, and tenderness.

Page 223: *Answer*—A partial thickness burn has bright pink or red skin that may have blisters. It may also appear moist if blisters have ruptured. The skin will blanch on pressure. The child will experience intense pain at the site.

Chapter 11

Page 233: *Answer*—The body in response to any antigen produces a nonspecific immunity. It is the earliest response and is therefore not specific to any one antigen. This response includes protective barriers such as interferon, inflammation, and phagocytosis. Once the body has responded to an antigen in a nonspecific way, the body produces specific immunity in the form of an antibody. These antibodies match with the antigen in a key/lock manner. The antibody is specific to the antigen and will not attack other antigens.

Page 234: *Answer*—The patient and family need explanations of each of the tests. The patient needs to know that a bone marrow aspiration is painful and that analgesics will be given. WBC and differential involves a needle stick and blood aspiration. Allergy testing may involve blood aspiration and/or skin pricks with various allergens.

Page 234: *Answer*—Referring to the most recent Recommended Childhood Immunization Schedule, United States, from the American Academy of Pediatrics will ensure current knowledge of immunization schedules. These standards change periodically and nurses must ensure they are practicing by the most current standards.

Page 237: *Answer*—The child and family may need to evaluate the home setting for potential allergens. Carpets, bedding, and other upholstery may need to be taken up and changed. If it is impossible to change the entire house, the family should begin these changes in the child's bedroom. Because the child spends long hours at night sleeping in the bedroom, this room plays an important role in the child's allergic reaction. Laundry and cleaning procedures may need to be adapted to allow for more frequent cleaning. The family will be taught to store out-of-season clothes out of the child's room. All clothing should be stored in drawers or closets and these devices should be kept closed to decrease dust collection. The bedroom should be used as a room for sleeping, so toys should be removed from the room as much as possible in an attempt to reduce dust-collecting items. In addition, stuffed toys should be limited as they hold dust. Fresh flowers should not be kept in the home as they will hold dust and molds. Pets may need to find a new home, be kept outdoors, or restricted from the child's bedroom. If the pets are kept in the home, they need to be washed frequently to reduce dander. If the allergy is to foods, the family will learn to read ingredient lists before purchasing an item as it might contain the allergen.

Page 243: *Answer*—The first stage: The incubation period is the time period between exposure to the organism and the development of the first general symptoms. During this period, the organism is growing in numbers and in strength. It is not strong enough to cause disease symptoms at this time. Toward the end of this period, it may be communicable.

The second stage: The prodromal stage is when the organism has sufficient strength to cause generalized symptoms of illness. It is difficult to diagnose the organism but the patient is exhibiting symptoms. This is a communicable stage.

The third stage: This is the active stage. During this time, the specific symptoms of the disease are exhibited. It is possible to spread the disease through body fluids. The patient is communicable while there is an elevated temperature or secretion of body fluids.

The fourth stage: This is recovery stage. The infectious disease has abated and the body is rebuilding its stores. Immunity is diminished, and the patient is vulnerable to becoming ill if exposed.

Chapter 12

Page 255: *Answer*—This behavior would be very predictable given the life-threatening nature of this disease process. The family-centered goals would be that the parents will understand all tests and therapies and that they will be able to express their concerns freely. They would then continue to participate appropriately in the care of their child.

Page 257: *Answer*—This child is immunocompromised because of chemotherapy and is at risk for infection. His developmental tasks include increasing mental abilities and increasing independence. It would be appropriate to reason with this child and allow independence in the minimum of oral hygiene and perineal care.

Page 261: *Answer*—This tumor is intrarenal and is often accompanied by increased renin production with increasing blood pressure. The finding is expected.

Page 262: *Answer*—Encourage the parents to answer the child's questions honestly and simply. The parents should utilize their religious beliefs in the discussion with the child. The child will often have concerns about abandonment and separation. The parents should assure the child that he or she will not be alone. If the parents' religious beliefs involve an afterlife, the parents might refer to a relative who has gone before and is waiting for the child. Children of this age often view illness as a punishment and may feel that they have done something wrong. Assure the child that this is not the case. Preschool children still are preoperational and have magical thinking so they are less concerned with the scientific answer and are more concerned with feelings.

Page 263: *Answer*—It is not unusual for family members to be at different stages of bereavement. This puts tremendous strain on relationships. Parents need to understand there is no wrong way to grieve. As nurses, we must also recognize there is no schedule for grieving. Questions that the parents ask should be answered honestly and simply. When the father expresses anger at the nurses, it should not be taken personally but be recognized for what it is—a symptom of grief. A clergyperson can be offered, but the nurse should not abandon the parents to the clergy. Physical comfort can be offered by those who have developed a relationship with the parents, including medical personnel. Physical presence is important, and the nurse must be careful not to avoid contact because of personal discomfort. The nurse should listen attentively to the parents. Use the child's name when talking with the parents. Do not offer platitudes.

Chapter 13

Page 275: *Answer*—Your teaching includes feeding the infant in an upright position, feeding the infant slowly, and burping frequently. Also included in the discussion would be using an enlarged nipple, stimulating the suck by rubbing the nipple on the lower lip, and allowing the infant to rest after each swallow to allow for complete swallowing. You may also suggest using alternate feeding devices such as an elongated nipple or breast shield. Initial postoperative feeding instructions include refraining from the use of straws, pacifier, and spoons. No oral temperatures are taken in the immediate postoperative period.

Page 276: *Answer*—Ideally, you want to inform the client and family about preoperative and postoperative care. Therefore, you would inform the client and family that it is necessary to remain NPO prior to surgery and that feeding resumes within four to six hours postoperatively. Explain the purpose of intravenous therapy and strict I&O monitoring. Another important aspect of care to include is the necessity of the nasogastric tube to decompress the stomach. Briefly, you would discuss the pattern of resuming feeding with small frequent feedings of clear liquids, moving to full strength formula as tolerated.

Page 281: *Answer*—Routine pre- and postoperative care should be discussed, including remaining NPO, nasogastric tube placement, strict I&O and vital sign monitoring. However, the major topic for discussion is the placement of a temporary colostomy. Older children need to be emotionally prepared and educated, as will the caregiver of an infant. A colostomy represents a change in body image so misconceptions and concerns need to be addressed. Verbal explanation, drawings, and dolls can be effective methods for teaching this procedure.

Page 285: *Answer*—Signs and symptoms of appendicitis typically include generalized abdominal pain that gradually increases and localizes in the right lower quadrant at McBurney's point, nausea, vomiting, fever, chills, anorexia, diarrhea or acute constipation, and an elevated white blood cell (WBC) count.

Page 295: *Answer*—Evaluating the client's hydration status is the highest priority. You want to establish if there has been any weight loss, assess level of consciousness, blood pressure, pulse, skin turgor, mucous membranes, urine output, fontanels, skin color, and capillary refill. A complete and thorough history is also vital in determining the causative factor and will assist in the prescribed treatment plan.

Chapter 14

Page 309: *Answer*—Although the pediatrician previously recommended ibuprofen, it, like aspirin, can increase the risk of continued bleeding related to the effect on platelet function. Therefore, acetaminophen is now the OTC medication of choice for injuries and fever, unless otherwise indicated by the physician.

Page 310: *Answer*—Children affected with sickle cell anemia are usually asymptomatic until approximately 4–6 months of age because the sickling of red blood cells is inhibited by high levels of fetal hemoglobin. The level of fetal hemoglobin may mask the results of the hemoglobin electrophoresis test that is done on the infant's cord blood. After 6 months of age, the sickle-turbidity test (Sicledex) can be used for quick screening purposes. The results are then verified with hemoglobin electrophoresis.

Page 312: *Answer*—If you suspect a reaction of any type to a blood transfusion, no matter how mild, you should always first stop the transfusion. Keep the line open with normal saline and notify the physician.

Page 314: *Answer*—

- After verifying physician's orders and checking the medication, dose, and route, the nurse would also identify the patient.
- Subcutaneous heparin administration is an invasive procedure that can cause problems with bleeding.
- The subcutaneous sites should be rotated.
- The injection is given slowly and the site is not massaged after administration. Pressure is applied to the injection site for 10 to 15 minutes. The site is observed for at least 15 minutes after the injection.
- Protamine is an antidote for heparin and should be available.
- The nurse would monitor PTT and platelet count.

Page 318: *Answer*—The liquid iron preparations are to be given with a straw to minimize the possibility of staining the teeth. Giving the iron with a citrus juice can lessen the bad taste. Such juice will also help improve absorption. Constipation can be a problem with iron preparations. Instruct the family to encourage increased fluid intake and to have the child eat foods with a high fiber content such fruits and grains.

Chapter 15

Page 331: *Answer*—Maintaining a compassionate and caring attitude during this time of grief is essential. You should provide the parents with a quiet, supportive environment. The parents will be experiencing shock and overwhelming grief over the death of a child. The parents should be encouraged to hold the infant and to say goodbye. The infant should be cleaned and wrapped in a blanket. Support services should be available to offer grief counseling, and you should also be available to help the parents contact the family members, clergy or rabbi, and funeral home.

Page 333: *Answer*—Begin by asking the child nonthreatening questions. Avoid questions such as "Did someone burn you with a cigarette?" Ask the child to tell you what the areas on her legs are and how they got there. More information can be obtained by asking the child open-ended questions. If abuse is suspected or reported, you must notify authorities immediately to protect the child from further injury.

Page 334: *Answer*—The symptoms of constricted pupils, respiratory depression, and difficulty arousing suggest the ingestion of an opiate such as morphine. Initially, Narcan, an opiate antagonist, may be ordered to reverse the symptoms of respiratory depression. Support the airway since there is a strong potential for respiratory arrest, and monitor vital signs. Upon stabilization, the adolescent should be referred for counseling and further evaluated for substance abuse.

Page 335: *Answer*—The adolescent needs intense therapy and counseling to help her to develop problem-solving skills. She may require in-patient psychiatric treatment; therefore, you should request the adolescent be evaluated by a counselor, therapist, or psychologist to determine the best method of intervention for her. While she is hospitalized, it is important to maintain a nonjudgmental attitude. Establishing a strong nurse–client relationship, which includes trust, with the adolescent may provide you with the opportunity to help her develop problem-solving skills. During the hospitalization, maintain all precautionary measures for the suicidal adolescent.

Page 336: *Answer*—Obtain a full detailed history of the current incident and compare with the past incident for similarities. The family may need counseling on the developmental issues and safety measures for the 3-year-old child or there may be signs of parental neglect. It is recommended that social services make a home visit to evaluate the environment and safety measures being taken to prevent this type of incident from recurring.

➤ *Case Study Suggested Answers*

Chapter 1

1. The primary growth and development expectations for a 6-month-old include that the infant
   - doubles birth weight.
   - grows 1 in. (2.5 cm) monthly for first 6 months.
   - rolls from back to abdomen.
   - holds own bottle.
   - has taste preferences.
   - erupts lateral incisors.
   - begins to eat solid foods.
   - begins to fear strangers.
2. Common behaviors at this age include that
   - the child is able to discriminate between familiar and unfamiliar persons.
   - the child begins to fear strangers. Infants will show signs of fear and distress such as crying, clinging to the parent, pulling away from strangers.
3. Recommended immunizations at this age include the following:
   - Diptheria–tetanus–acellular pertussis (DTaP) #3
   - Haemophilus influenzae type B (Hib) #3
   - Inactivated poliovirus vaccine (IPV) #3 (6 to 18 months)
   - Heptavalent conjugant pneumococcal vaccine (PCV) #3
   - Hepatitis B #3 (6 to 18 months)
4. Appropriate toys would include the following:
   - Soft balls
   - Teething rings
   - Large blocks
   - Toys that child can manipulate
5. Anticipatory guidance would include the following points:
   - Developmental milestones for the first year
   - Safety: car seat facing the rear in the middle of the back seat of the car should be used for infants up to 20 lb (9 kg)
   - Infant becoming more mobile—never leave unattended on table, bed, bathtub, near stairs, balconies, or open windows
   - Avoid bottles at bedtime—can contribute to dental caries
   - Review injury prevention: sources of aspiration, poisonings, suffocation, falls, and accidental burns
   - Introduction of solids into the diet: cereals, vegetables, fruits, and meats

Chapter 2

1. Establishing the reason for the visit enables the nurse to focus questions in greater depth in specific parts of the review of systems, family history, and/or developmental areas. It also lets the client know that parts of the assessment might have to have greater depth of questioning.
2. The nurse should sit in a comfortable position on the same level as the parent. Keep the environment free of distractions and focus on the parent by listening attentively and asking questions that clarify data as needed. Explain what information is needed and why, as well as what will be done during the exam. Always ask if the parent has any questions or concerns as the history taking and the exam proceed.
3. The nurse should allow the child to "warm up" to the nurse. Direct questions and attention to the parent first. Ask questions of the child and display an interest in objects pertaining to the child. When proceeding with the examination, allow the child to help with undressing and to touch equipment first or to try it on the nurse. Explain to the child in understandable terms what will be done and what is expected. The nurse must not lie or deceive the child about anything that may be uncomfortable.
4. The nurse can ask the parent about what the child ate in the last 24 hours and if that was a typical day. The nurse can ask questions that ascertain how frequent representative foods from each section of the food pyramid are eaten as well as specific cultural or religious practices that determine the family's diet. The child's height and weight should be plotted on growth curves to see where they fall with respect to each other and to national percentiles. Assess the abdomen to see if it is gently rounded. Results from hemoglobin and hematocrit levels may indicate if the child is iron deficient.
5. It would be appropriate for the nurse to check hemoglobin and hematocrit if they have not been recently checked or if results are not available. Unless other familial or environmental risk factors or health problems are evident, further lab testing is not indicated.

Chapter 3

1. A complete health history should be taken because the child will likely be undergoing general anesthesia. Information about the child's primary problem (chief

complaint) should be obtained, as well as any concurrent illnesses. Information about current medications should be included. The history of the illness that preceded the need for surgery should be detailed. Past medical history, including allergies to medication, food, and environment should be elicited. The child's birth history and past medical and health history should be documented. A review of body systems should be completed. The nurse should inquire about familial and hereditary diseases and any difficulties with anesthesia (such as malignant hyperthermia) should be recorded. The health status of family members, including parents, siblings, and extended family should be explored during the health history interview.

2. One of the most important tests is evaluation of bleeding and clotting function. A complete blood count (CBC), which includes platelet count, may be ordered. Prothrombin time (PT) and partial thromboplastin time (PTT) are commonly ordered lab tests. The child's blood chemistry may also be analyzed prior to anesthesia and the tonsillectomy.

3. After the surgical procedure is explained by the health care provider, the nurse should reinforce the teaching about the procedure. The nurse should explain events related to the operation, such as admission procedures and preoperative lab procedures. Teaching should be provided about preoperative medications for sedation (if prescribed), what will happen in the period before transport to the operating room, and what will happen when the child and family are reunited following the procedure in the postanesthesia care area.

4. The child, if age and developmental level permit, should be taught similar, developmentally-appropriate content to encourage cooperative behavior. Special attention should be given to explaining the sight, sounds, smells, touches, and tastes that the child will experience in the operating room and when the child wakes up from anesthesia. A tour of the day surgery area, including operating room and postanesthesia care areas should be provided.

5. A complete physical assessment is indicated for the child undergoing surgery. The nurse should make certain the child shows no current symptoms of illness. A child of this age should have the oral cavity checked for any loose teeth.

Chapter 4

1. Peak expiratory flow is a pulmonary function test that measures the amount of air that can be exhaled forcibly. It monitors asthma and acts as a signal of an asthma episode. To use the peak flow meter, move the pointer to zero, take a deep breath and blow out hard and fast into the meter. Repeat three times and record the highest value. Peak flow should be done every day and values below a child's "personal best" indicate that an acute episode may be imminent.

2. Exercise is recommended for children with asthma to enhance self-esteem and encourage endurance. Physical education activities that do not require prolonged endurance are usually not a problem for children with asthma. Exercise-induced bronchospasm can be prevented by prophylactic treatment with inhaled cromolyn sodium before strenuous exertion.

3. Keep records of peak flow readings to establish a "personal best." A reading that is 50 to 80% below personal best is a caution. Other subtle signs may be increased nonproductive cough and episodes of shortness of breath.

4. A spacer deposits medication deeper into the airways and avoids large droplets of steroids on the oral mucosa, thereby minimizing the risk of oral yeast infections. A spacer is also useful for parents of infants and small children who are unable to manipulate the MDI. The spacer prevents the loss of medication.

5. The overall goal of asthma education is to prevent asthmatic episodes, improve respiratory capacity, and facilitate optimal psychologic and social development of the child and family.

Chapter 5

1. The nurse needs to assess parents' level of understanding of the condition. Second, the nurse needs to know how they cope in times of crisis and should help the parents to identify their coping strategies. Third, the family needs to have an emergency plan to respond to an acute cyanotic spell. The family needs to be knowledgeable about the medications that are ordered and be able to administer the medications effectively.

2. Assess for increasing cyanosis and note the activity that precipitated it, irritability (which may be a sign of hunger, pain, or air hunger) and fever, fatigue, and malaise (which can be signs of infective endocarditis).

3. Maintain venous access for infant receiving continuous infusion of prostaglandin E1. Have intubation and resuscitation equipment available. In the event of an acute cyanotic spell, place the child in knee-chest position and administer oxygen. Assess for postoperative bleeding. Assess cardiac performance.

4. The nurse should ensure that the parents are knowledgeable about the following:
   - Signs of infective endocarditis
   - Acute cyanotic spells
   - Promoting as normal activity and as possible
   - Administering medications
   - How to observe for abnormal delays in growth and development

5. Parents should be knowledgeable about cardiopulmonary resuscitation. They must be able to recognize and respond to an acute cyanotic spell (assist the child to the knee-chest position and administer oxygen). Emergency numbers need to be easily visible at the telephone,

including 911 and the number of the client's physician. Discuss that being prepared for an emergency is a good idea; however, they need to relax and enjoy their child in as normal a way as possible.

Chapter 6

1. The physical parameters the nurse should monitor include the following:
   - Vital signs, especially temperature for fever
   - Behaviors such as suck, cry, posture, muscle tone
   - Bulging fontanel and other indicators of increased intracranial pressure
   - Hydration status: mucous membranes, urine ≥ 1 mL/kg/hr, weight daily on same scale
2. Nursing interventions that would have priority during the first 48 hours include the following:
   - Monitoring respiratory status, heart rate, and blood pressure
   - Provide an environment that minimizes ICP elevation: head of bed should be at 30-degree angle, maintain head in neutral position, quiet environment
   - Administer antibiotic therapy as soon as prescribed
   - Maintain IV fluids as prescribed
   - Administer antipyretics as needed for temperature elevation
3. The usual medical treatment for meningitis is based on diagnosis from the results of a lumbar puncture. Cerebrospinal fluid is cultured to determine the causative organism and appropriate intravenous antibiotic therapy is initiated. Fluid status and serum sodium levels are closely monitored during the early period because clients with this diagnosis are at risk for developing syndrome of inappropriate antidiuretic hormone.
4. There are numerous developmental implications for this family. This infant is in a sensitive bonding period with her parents. Since she has an older sibling who also needs the attention of the parents, this poses the dilemma to the family of how to handle visitation. Parents will have some stress since they lack extended family in the geographical proximity; however, that does not rule out that they may have many friends and neighbors who can help out with babysitting when one of them cannot be home. The separation of family members because of the hospitalization could be more stressful for the preschooler than the hospitalized infant because of the preschooler's age-appropriate separation anxiety.
5. In planning for discharge, specific areas of support for or teaching with the family include the following:
   - When to return for follow-up visit
   - Resources in the community if indicated. Fifty percent of children with meningitis suffer some degree of neurological sequelae. This infant could develop deafness and then require referral to hearing and speech specialists.

Chapter 7

1. Dietary management for children with ESRD focuses on maximizing calories for growth while limiting demands on the kidney and minimizing fluid and electrolyte disturbances. Sodium-, potassium- and phosphate-restricted diets may be necessary. Daily fluid restrictions may also be necessary.
2. Renal transplantation is considered to be the optimal renal replacement choice for children. Transplantation provides for a normalization of physiology and the potential for normal growth and development.
3. Complications of hemodialysis are hypotension, rapid changes in fluid and electrolyte balance, and disequilibrium syndrome. Hemodialysis provides for more efficient clearance of toxins than peritoneal dialysis. Hemodialysis significantly lowers the BUN and creatinine levels in the bloodstream more quickly than does peritoneal dialysis.
4. Peritoneal dialysis is more widely used in the treatment of children with ESRD because it is a continuous process, can be done at home, and is an easier process for family or child to learn and implement. It is also less disruptive to the family social structure than hemodialysis.
5. Children with ESRD suffer body image disturbance related to small size and their perception of being and looking different than other children. Because their condition is chronic, they have altered health maintenance, which impacts their social and psychological growth. Psychosocial concerns for the child undergoing hemodialysis are care and maintenance of a vascular access site and travel to a hemodialysis center three times a week. Psychosocial concerns for the child undergoing peritoneal dialysis include caregiver role strain related to daily dialysis treatments and potential for frequent peritonitis resulting in hospitalization. Psychosocial concerns for renal transplantation include immunosuppressive therapy management and the potential for transplant rejection. Also, a living, related donor contributes to a higher kidney survival rate than does a cadaver kidney.

Chapter 8

1. It is necessary to obtain all necessary information regarding the teenager's present condition. Appropriate questions include the following:
   - How long has she been ill?
   - Is she able to keep fluids down?
   - What types and how much fluid has she taken?
   - Does she have fever?
   - What were her last four blood glucose results?
   - Is she urinating?
   - Are there any ketones in her urine?
   - Is she eating anything more than toast?
2. Continue to give insulin, but the teenager might need to use the sliding scale utilizing regular insulin only. Test blood

glucose every three to four hours and administer insulin as needed. Check urinary ketones also.

3. The teenager would benefit from calorie-free liquids to clear ketones in the urine, if necessary. Simple carbohydrates are allowed for nutrition, especially if the teenager has a poor appetite. Encourage frequent blood testing.

4. If ketones are present in the urine
   - encourage calorie-free fluid intake.
   - encourage rest.
   - discourage exercise at this time.

5. Notify the doctor or nurse practitioner for the following complications:
   - Moderate to high urinary ketones
   - Hyperglycemia
   - Acetone or fruity breath
   - Lethargy
   - Deep, rapid respirations

Chapter 9

1. The assessment findings in a newborn with developmental dysplasia of the hip (DDH) include a positive Ortolani or Barlow's sign. The nurse will also find limited abduction of the hips, asymmetry of the thigh and gluteal folds, and unequal knee and leg lengths. A wide perineum will be found in the infant with bilateral disease.

2. The exact cause of DDH is not known, though certain factors are known to increase the risk of it. Family history increases the risk tenfold. Prenatal conditions affecting the development of DDH, such as the frank breech position and maternal hormones of relaxin and estrogen, may cause laxity of the hip joint and capsule and lead to joint instability. Twinning or large infant size are additional conditions associated with DDH.

3. The priorities of care for this newborn include teaching the parents about the care of this infant, along with helping the parents deal with their feelings of their newborn having a deformity.

4. DDH is treated by keeping the hip in abduction by way of an abduction device. For infants less than three months, the most common treatment is use of a Pavlik harness, which is an adjustable chest halter that abducts the legs. Soft plastic stirrups hold the hips flexed, abducted, and externally rotated.

5. Teaching that should be completed with the parents of an infant who will be wearing a Pavlik harness includes proper application, the need for sponge bath, and assessing skin under the straps daily for irritation or redness. A t-shirt and knee socks should be worn under the brace to prevent skin irritation and the diaper should be placed under the straps and changed without taking the harness off. The harness is worn 23 hours a day, and the hips and buttocks should be supported carefully when not in the harness. The nurse should also discuss the necessary modification of the car seat and strollers, and modification of positioning for nursing

and eating. Parents need to ensure the child has adequate stimulation with toys and activities at appropriate eye level and should encourage activities that stimulate upper extremities.

6. Early detection and treatment enable the majority of children with DDH to attain normal hip function.

Chapter 10

1. The nurse saw a small area of papules and vesicles on skin that was otherwise clear. The child said they did not itch.

2. Impetigo is highly contagious, and the child could infect many of his classmates by holding hands or playing on the playground or sharing books.

3. The nurse will explain that the mother needs to seek medical attention for her child as this is a bacterial infection that requires antibiotics. The mother should gently wash the infected area with antibacterial soap and warm water and remove crusts. The antibiotic ointment that is prescribed should be applied to the site as directed for the full duration of therapy, a week to 10 days. The child's fingernails should be cut short and he should be reminded not to scratch or pick at the lesions. The child and all family members should wash hands frequently with antibacterial soap.

4. The primary goal is to prevent the spread of impetigo to other areas on the child and to other individuals.

5. The child should be able to return to school after using topical antibiotics for 48 hours.

Chapter 11

1. CBC with differential. Dependent on the differential results, the physician may begin treatment or may decide to do allergy testing. Frequently the physician will begin the allergy testing with the skin or scratch test. This test allows a quick evaluation of many possible allergens (antigens) with results within 30 minutes. There is a small risk of anaphylaxis from this type of testing. Based on the scratch tests results, the physician may order a RAST to further evaluate allergens. The RAST test is more specific and carries no risk of anaphylaxis.

2. The nurse will ask questions relative to recent exposures to communicable diseases. The nurse would want information about the risk of exposure, such as whether the child attends a preschool or kindergarten or if anyone else in the family has been sick. The nurse will question if the child has a history of allergies, including food allergies, skin allergies, and insect sting/bite allergies. The nurse would also be interested if there is a family history of allergies as the tendency towards allergies runs in families. Finally, the nurse will question the history of present illness looking for onset, prodromal symptoms as well as precipitating events.

3. Priority nursing diagnoses for this child would include the following:
   - Hyperthermia related to infectious disease process.
   - Risk for Fluid Volume Deficit related to increased insensible fluid loss and possible refusal to drink adequate liquids
   - Knowledge Deficit (parents) of infectious disease process (no etiology required for knowledge deficit diagnoses)
4. Nursing interventions appropriate for the child would include the following:
   - Monitoring the child's temperature and intervening as appropriate. If the child is hyperthermic, the nurse needs to reduce the temperature. Antipyretics would be administered as appropriate. The nurse would teach the parents to use acetaminophen (Tylenol) instead of aspirin. Studies have shown that in viral infections, the use of aspirin increases the risk of Reye syndrome. The nurse would also want to teach the use of a tepid bath, increased fluid intake, and minimal clothing to allow heat dissipation.
   - Blood and body fluid precautions. All patients should have the same precautions applied to their care. This is for the safety of the patients and the health care workers. If admitted to the hospital and while in the clinic, the child should be isolated from other children until the cause of the fever and potential rash is known.
   - The nurse would also provide information to the family about the potential rash. Antihistamines may be used if the child is itching. The child's nails should be kept short to decrease the risk of impaired skin integrity. Oatmeal (Aveeno) baths may make the child more comfortable.
5. Recovery will have occurred when
   - body temperature returns to normal parameters.
   - body fluid secretions decrease.
   - skin lesions decrease.

Chapter 12

1. It is essential to do a complete physical assessment as a comparison for changes that may occur during therapy. The child will have an increased risk for infection and injury subsequent to chemotherapy. The client will also need to be monitored for such side effects as nausea and vomiting, so baseline nutrition information and all other physical assessments are needed for accurate evaluation of response to interventions.
2. It would be important to look at the child's usual behaviors and coping abilities to evaluate response to treatment.
3. The priority of therapeutic medical management is to induce remission. Nursing management will focus on providing information so the family can learn about the disease and its treatment and providing emotional support to the child and family. Treatment for this illness lasts 2½ to 3 years, so goals need to be appropriate for this chronic, life-threatening cancer.
4. Initial information must include the reason for central venous line, while addressing the fear related to the unknown, pain, and threat to life. In addition, each test, treatment, and side effect must be discussed in a timely way. It is essential to allow time for questions. Families often need to have information repeated until they become more comfortable in the situation.
5. The planned vacation will have to be postponed. The parents may be using denial to cope or they may have a knowledge deficit about the length of treatment. It is very likely that this trip will be possible at another time in the treatment.

Chapter 13

1. It is imperative to complete a thorough pain assessment. Ask the client to point to the painful area and to describe the pain. Note the onset, location, and intensity of pain. Determine if there are precipitating factors or if any relief measures have been attempted. In addition to a thorough pain assessment, a complete history and head-to-toe assessment should be obtained. Vital signs and weight should be assessed for variances from the normal. Assessment of the abdomen includes observation, auscultation, and palpation; taking note of guarding, abdominal distention, rigidity, activity of bowel sounds, and rebound tenderness.
2. Orders should include frequent vital signs, keeping the client NPO, initiating IV therapy, intermittent antibiotics, strict I&O, apply cold packs as needed for comfort, and acetaminophen (Tylenol) every four hours as needed for fever.
3. Let the client assume a position of comfort, usually side-lying with knees bent. Administer analgesics if ordered and apply cold packs as needed to minimize discomfort. Demonstrate how to splint the abdomen for coughing and moving.
4. Many times this is the first hospitalization for a family, so anxiety and apprehension is to be expected. Providing emotional support is an important aspect of care that cannot be overlooked. Good preoperative teaching can reduce anxiety. Answering questions thoroughly and reviewing the plan of care is extremely beneficial. When interacting with children always remember the child's developmental level.
5. The postoperative care for a nonruptured appendix includes frequent vital signs, monitoring I&O, maintaining NPO status until bowel function returns, administering antibiotics if ordered, and maintaining IV fluids. Other orders include turning, coughing, deep-breathing, early ambulation, and management of pain. Monitoring the incision site and changing sterile dressings may be included. Postoperative care is short in duration; many times the client is discharged within 24 hours of surgery.

Postoperative care of the child with a ruptured appendix is more complex and longer in duration. The postoperative orders would include the same orders as for the nonruptured appendix with the addition of intermittent IV antibiotics for at least a 7-day regimen and maintaining a nasogastric tube to low intermittent wall suction until bowel function returns. The client who has experienced a perforated appendix may have a drain in place or large abdominal dressing, so care for these would also be included. The incision must be monitored, and temperature control measures will be ordered.

Chapter 14

1. In the complete medical history, including birth information, be sure to ask about any previous bleeding episodes, no matter how minor. Specifically, inquire as to any history of hemophilia or other bleeding conditions among other family members. Ask the parents as to any previous episodes of joint pain or swelling as well as a change in joint/extremity appearance. Check to see if there have been urinary problems such as hematuria or flank pain. Previously undiscovered cerebral bleeding may have caused peripheral neuropathies or neurologic impairment. Question the parents as to change in motor function/capabilities as well as cognitive abilities.

2. Pain and bleeding control with hemarthrosis will be managed through immobilization and elevation of the limb as well as ice pack. Oral or IV analgesics will also be administered per physician's preference. Analgesics that contain aspirin, aspirinlike substances, NSAIDs, or other medication that might affect platelet function are to be avoided.

3. Bleeding control is the first order of medical management. This will be accomplished through the administration of the missing factor. Laboratory tests including prothrombin time (PT), partial thromboplastin time (PTT), complete blood count (CBC), and fibrinogen levels will be monitored to assess the child's status. X-rays and/or a CT scan might be done to assess the degree of joint involvement or damage. Factor will be administered for a mild or major bleeding episode or if the child is in a life-threatening situation. If the child's situation were to include surface bleeding, a topical hemostatic agent might be applied to control capillary bleeding. Pain management will be handled as discussed above.

4. Hemophilia is a genetic disorder with an X-linked recessive trait. This means that it will result almost solely in carrier families and affected males. The disorder results from a deficiency in specific clotting factors. The missing factor will guide the treatment regimen. Classic hemophilia or hemophilia A is caused by a deficiency of factor VIII. Approximately 80% of hemophiliacs have hemophilia A. The occurrence rate is approximately 1 in 5000 male births. Hemophilia B, also known as Christmas disease, results from a deficiency in factor IX.

Approximately 15% of those with hemophilia have hemophilia B. Females with hemophilia trait do not often manifest the disease. However, they may experience prolonged bleeding time with dental work, surgery, or trauma. Males will have bleeding tendencies ranging from mild to severe. The presence of a child with hemophilia means there are implications for future childbearing, both for the parents as well as any of their children. Other family members may also be affected. Genetic testing and counseling are imperative.

5. Explain to the family that although the child may require hospitalization for diagnosis and management or with the first bleeding episode, most care can be managed in the home and outpatient clinic. Parents and child will need a good understanding of the origin of bleeding to understand the disease process and plan their lives accordingly. A medical identification bracelet is imperative for the child to wear at all times. The family must recognize that acetaminophen is to be used for fever and pain as opposed to aspirin or aspirin-like medications, including ibuprofen. The family needs to understand which situations and injuries can cause bleeding to occur. The family must learn how to identify internal bleeding and how to respond to all bleeding episodes, minor or not. It is particularly important for the family to recognize that abdominal pain, joint pain, and obvious bleeding are implications for an urgent infusion of factor. If the child is to receive factor in the home setting, the family will require instruction as to preparation and administration. If administration is to be on a regular basis, have the family verbalize the schedule and the principle that missing a scheduled infusion may lead to a bleeding episode. Assist the family to notify school officials and work with the appropriate personnel to handle any problems as they arise. Assist the family to plan for as normal a life as possible for the child at home and school. Overprotection should be avoided. However, the family should recognize that contact sports are not appropriate, but the child can engage in swimming. Certain other activities such as hiking, bicycling, roller blading, and so on can be done also with certain precautionary measures. Assist the family to schedule regular clinic visits and to coordinate with their regular pediatrician and dentist. If not already done, encourage the family to seek testing and genetic counseling for appropriate members. Lastly, place family in contact with appropriate support groups and social services.

Chapter 15

1. Begin by not having any physical contact with the child. She has been traumatized by someone she trusted, so establishing a nurse–client relationship will be more difficult. Maintain eye contact with the child by sitting in a chair or squatting down beside the child. Inform her of everything you are going to do. Ask her if she has any

questions and answer them truthfully. Remember that the abused child has the same developmental and physical needs as any other child.

2. Maintain consistent care providers and encourage a parent to stay with the child. Never attempt any type of invasive procedure or any other act that could be threatening to the child without fully explaining what is to be done, and always be truthful when answering questions. Encourage the child to participate in the routine playroom activities on the hospital unit.

3. The comment from the child is likely because the uncle told her she would be in trouble if she told anyone, a common ploy by sexual abusers of children. Assure the child that she did nothing wrong, and praise her for coming forward with the truth. It is important to allow the child to vent her feelings. The child will need counseling as a result of the abuse.

4. The parents should be asked to step into the hall or given a private area, if needed, until they can speak calmly in front of the child. When a child is the victim of sexual abuse, the parents feel guilt and anger, especially if the abuse is committed by a close friend or family member, as in this case. One parent may blame the other, and if interventions are not taken, the marriage could deteriorate from this incident. Consult social services, a counselor, or the available support services for parents of abused children to intervene and offer support through this traumatic event.

5. Therapeutic communication is essential during this crisis. Encourage the child to verbalize her feelings of anger, pain, and fear. Therapeutic strategies utilized by therapists such as art therapy and play therapy may be beneficial for the release of these feelings. Assure that the child is receiving appropriate counseling.

Index

Page numbers followed by b indicate box; those followed by f indicate figure; those followed by t indicate table.